CUCKOO CLUB

By Cairns Clery

'One million people commit suicide every year'
The World Health Organization

Published by:
Chipmunkapublishing
PO Box 6872
Brentwood
Essex
CM13 1ZT
United Kingdom

http://www.chipmunkapublishing.com

Dedication

For Colin Arnold. In memoriam.

PART ONE

That Was Then

Chapter   1.

Tow-rope loaded? Yes. Bottle of gin? Yes. Wooden kitchen chair to get up on and kick away? Yes.

Well. That's it, then. Or did she want a pen and paper for a last note? No, it would be quite obvious when they saw her dangling. There was no one she would want to write to anyway.

Shutting the front door with a purposeful finality, Rose McElvey stepped out to her car. Keys. Her car keys and house keys were on the same ring. Where were her keys? She looked through her bag and checked her coat pockets. No keys. What had she done with them? She went through her bag and her coat pockets again. Oh if that wasn't typical ! Just typical !

Except it wasn't actually. It wasn't typical of her at all. Usually she was a person who did everything with absolute regard for the finest detail. How *could* she have forgotten the keys? She must have left them inside. She bit her lip. The front door was self-locking. She couldn't get back in. Well, she'd just have to break back in then. It didn't matter now. Not any more. Go round the back and hope her neighbours remained invisible as ever.

She stepped past the dustbins to the rear of the house and picked up a brick from her long dead, overgrown vegetable garden. Its underside was covered in small black slugs. She had just had a bath, was nice and clean, so brushed them off with some distaste using a twig. Back in the spring she'd spent a whole weekend digging, raking and sowing her vegetable patch, measuring every line perfectly and ensuring the ratios between potential plant height and access to sunlight were properly balanced in terms of the shadows they would cast when they grew. But it was early November now, her radishes and runner beans had long since bolted and browned.

The brick was heavy. She took a couple of practice swings, the momentum of which almost sent her flying into the compost heap. She glanced down at her shiny, virtually unworn court shoes. They were still clean, not speckled with mud from the little puddle her efforts had just caused her to stand in. She had wanted to look her best for what would be her final act; she had put on her best silk frock and her most expensive shoes. It was somehow more appropriate to leave the world dressed in things that normally languished at the back of the cupboard. It showed you were carrying out your suicide efficiently, with due consideration and proper attention to detail; to the little things - the things which have to matter so much more when life has become meaningless. She had even put on the tarnished string of old pearls left to her by her mother.   All this dressiness wasn't belied by her beautiful old wine-red duffel coat with its original wooden toggles and its worn patches over the elbows and bum, because she loved her coat.

She went to the back door and threw the brick at its toughened glass panel, fearing that she knew what would happen even as she did it. Sure enough, it bounced back off the door onto the ground, hitting her shin painfully on the way. She hopped around for a moment wincing with the pain. Her leg was slightly grazed, her tights torn. Things were just not going well.

Still, at least that was consistent! She picked the brick up again, hating it, and tried once more. Again it bounced off the door, but this time she was ready and moved out of the way. She shook her head in frustration. She didn't have the strength for this, winced at the prospect of having to try a window. That would mean having to climb rather than walk back inside, which might be a bit awkward.

Oh well.

She used to be so proud of her windows, all of which had proper handmade lace curtains specially bought on lonely coach trips to places like Bruges, Amsterdam and Nottingham where it was still made in the traditional manner. Half an hour ago she had been arranging each one so that it hung perfectly and looked immaculate. Never mind, in a little while she would not have to be caring about anything like that anymore. All the same, if a window did have to be broken, she would prefer it to be one of the kitchen ones with blinds. She shook her head again. It was curious and mildly irritating that even now she still had some standards.

But she couldn't help closing her eyes this time as the brick sailed through her kitchen window in a perfect trajectory, shattering it with a resounding crash before landing plum in the middle of her pinewood table. She peered through the jagged gaping hole. Her half-drunk cup of coffee now lay on its side. It had knocked over the picture of her little boy which she had been looking at five minutes ago, and coffee was seeping through the broken glass into the frame. She thought of the cost of replacing the window, again felt a brief twinge of anger at her relentlessly trivia-conscious lack of focus. She glanced over at the houses of her neighbours on each side. Needlessly. No-one was interested. She reached in through the shards and gingerly undid the clasp. Then she knocked the remainder of the glass out. Clambering back in was an awkward ungainly struggle. She wasn't dressed for it and she wasn't young anymore. She was glad no-one could see her as she half-crawled, half-fell through the window onto the floor. She lay there for a moment, wallowing in ignominy, her heart pounding. If she'd been the type, she would have been crying by now.

She stood up, reached for a dish cloth and carefully brushed splinters and dust off her lovely old coat. It seemed to take ages before it looked pristine again. Through the broken window she could hear a neighbour's radio blaring and wondered how nobody could have heard the sound of shattering glass a few minutes ago. She looked at her watch.

Actually it wasn't a few minutes ago. Nearly half an hour had gone by.

Now that certainly *was* typical of her. She had been picking shards and tiny sparkling specks of glass off herself for a whole half hour! It made her feel angry. It was another reason why she just had to go. A life of being stuck in repetitive patterns of behaviour was just no life at all. She picked up the bigger bits of broken glass, thinking it would be so much easier to just take one, there and then, and slide it across the side of her neck. If only it wouldn't make such a mess. Shuddering at the thought, she wrapped the glass in some newspaper and deposited it in the bin. Then she got out the hoover out for the smaller bits, telling herself she would stop after five minutes no matter how much she felt the job hadn't been finished properly. She managed to switch it off and put it away again after six. Not bad. Very good in fact.

Her keys were by the front door. She unlocked it, made sure she put the keys safely into her purse and went upstairs to change her tights. Then she decided to have another cup of coffee before leaving.

The telephone rang. She ignored it with a childlike glee at being able to. For the last few years it had been so important to pick it up on the tenth ring – not before, not after – in memory of her son Luke who hadn't lived to see the age of eleven. Her ansaphone was programmed to answer on the eleventh, but the caller rang off as soon as the machine came on. She couldn't be bothered to find out who it was.

The coffee scalded her tongue.

I'm delaying things unnecessarily, she thought. Why? It's just scary that's all. Naturally. I've just got to get on with it. I wish, I wish, I wish I could do it here in my own home, but it wouldn't be right for anyone I know to find me here, and if no-one did actually find me for a few days the house would smell horribly which wouldn't be very fair on them, so I'm not having that. I've got to go away to do it. That's all there is to it.

As she drove down the motorway she was tempted at some points just to aim the car over the side, but feared it might not be successful. The airbag might cushion the impact, stop her from dying. She might endanger other people.

She drove too fast anyway, enjoying the rarely-felt sensation of staying on the very cusp of control. Tyres screeching, she took a slip road which curved interminably before joining an 'A' road which eventually passed through trees and woods. She pulled over into the first car parking area she came to.

It was 4.30, nearly dark. There was one other car present. Out of the woods a large man in boots and a hat was emerging with an equally large black dog. A labrador. He glared at her through her windscreen for a brief moment, before opening the back of his car to allow the dog in. Without another glance he got in himself and drove off.

She was alone.

She didn't like what she felt. Like a vagrant she took a swig from the bottle of gin on the seat beside her. She hadn't eaten anything since yesterday morning. The gin burned her throat on its way to her head. Suicide was stupid, selfish and hateful to the ones you love. She knew that. Not that she had anyone *to* love, absolutely nobody. So in her case it was just plain stupid. But in a curious and satisfying way, it did feel wonderful to be ending her life stupidly. She had always been so sensible. Everybody had always said so ever since she was a little girl.

Even so, not caring about the silliness of what she was doing would depend on getting herself seriously drunk now. She knew from past experience that getting pissed rendered her capable of anything, as long as it was driven by self-loathing. She took another swig.

Her head began ringing.

Tinitis. That was another thing she needed to get away from. Her head often rang when she drank, ever since she'd deliberately if inexplicably stood beneath a heavy pot she was dusting on a high shelf and knocked it down onto her head. There had been a lot of blood although it hadn't really hurt. Not as much as being patronised by the A and E nurse who sutured her, and who had blandly told her the bleeding obvious about having to be more careful because blood tends to gush more profusely from the head.

Well, hers wasn't going to ever again.

She put her hand on the tow rope holding her open bottle snug between its coils like a snake on the seat beside her. She had considered three different methods. All involved getting drunk first. She had decided against a hosepipe from the exhaust because it would be too easy to escape if she changed her mind. She had also decided against her preferred method – drowning herself by walking out into the sea. It was the wrong time of year and she didn't think she would be able to stand the cold as she waded out through the waves. And as for an overdose, well that was ridiculous. She had known so many people over the years who had done that only to find themselves in hospital a few hours later having failed to achieve their end.

She was going to take the torch and the rope and the chair, walk well into the woods and find a tree with a branch low and sturdy enough to take her weight, but high enough for her to hang from properly when she kicked the chair away.

Not wanting to wait around, she got out of the car. Where was the torch? Oh dear. It would be pitch dark out here soon and she'd forgotten the torch. How irritating! What *was* the matter with her? She had never known herself be as forgetful as she had been today. It just wasn't like her at all. Never mind, she would just have to make do without it. She would try and find the perfect tree in the dark and then maybe build herself a little fire beside it so that she could see what she was doing. She was only a quarter of the way through the gin and already she felt as if it would be difficult finding a path through the woods in the darkness, let alone finding a suitable branch and looping the rope around it properly. She put the gin bottle into her coat pocket, checked her purse again. In it were her birth certificate, driving licence, passport. Enough to identify her, spare someone who knew her from having to do so.

She wrestled the chair from out of the back of her little Peugeot and with the rope resting on it awkwardly, changed the habits of a lifetime by intentionally not locking the doors before setting off into the woods. She'd never left the car unlocked before. It simply wouldn't have occurred to her to do so, but she wouldn't be needing it again now. And if it was about anything, suicide had to be about breaking habits, all the habits of a lifetime. It felt good not to lock it.

She trudged off up the hill through the trees. It was a slow business, carrying the chair, the rope, and the bottle in her bag. With every other step her silly heels kept on sinking into the soft earth beneath the carpet of autumn leaves. But her eyes didn't take long to become accustomed to the dark and soon she felt she could see quite well even though it was a cloudy moonless night.

She peered left and right through the gloom looking for the right tree.

That one. It looked mature enough to provide the strength to carry her weight. At the same time its lower branches didn't look too big to get the rope around. She patted it. Her own special tree. Then leaned against it and looked back the way she had come. She couldn't see her car at all. Occasionally the yellow arc of passing headlights flickered by down below letting her know where the road was, but otherwise she was completely alone. She heard no night time noises – no owls or scuffling rats, thank goodness; just the gentle patter of falling leaves and the sound of her own breathing, punctuated by the occasional drone of passing traffic.

She uncapped the bottle again, rapidly swallowing a series of capfuls. Then she pushed the chair firmly into the moss, leaves and earth at the base of the tree, kicked off her shoes and gingerly climbed up on to it. It sunk unevenly a little further into the ground. She swayed to keep her balance, undid the rope and on her first attempt successfully managed to throw it over the branch immediately above. She knotted the rope together, stepped down off the chair, pulling on the rope as she did so to make sure it would be able to take her weight.

It did seem as if it would.

This is it then, a pathetic little end to a pointless little life!

She got back up on to the chair to make a noose of the other end of the rope. Satisfied it would do its work, she stepped down again, slipped back into her shoes and struggled to shift the chair, lift it back out of the ground and move it out of the way. For some reason, again perhaps because she wanted her last moments to be different, she didn't do the predictable thing by sitting down on the chair to gather her last thoughts. Instead she pulled her coat underneath her and sat down on the ground with her back to the tree, ignoring her poor old coat whimpering beneath her that she might be dirtying it beyond redemption. She felt stupid again. Like a child being made an example of in a school assembly or something. Yet here she was all alone. It was cold and she wasn't yet drunk enough to kill herself. Not by a long shot. I'm chicken, that's me. I've got all the way here and I'm just chicken.

She shivered, reached out and started sweeping leaves towards herself. Within a minute she had a whole mound built up in front of her. She felt pleased. Most of them weren't even slightly damp. It had been a dry autumn. She got up again and looked for dead wood or fallen twigs. She felt curiously excited as she did so. Much more interested than she had been a few moments ago attaching her tow-rope to the tree. Like a little girl who had never been a brownie, but had always wanted to be the one who gets to light the fire. Over the next ten minutes she lay sticks, twigs and small broken branches she found on the ground in a curving circle right around the top of the heap of leaves. Again like a little girl, she congratulated herself for the pattern she'd made. Like a circlet or a crown. When the leaves had burnt away, she thought, the wood would settle, fall inwards and the fire would last longer. Her sense of obsessional neatness felt right for a change, rather than neurotic.

If she wanted to have the perfect little bonfire to warm herself by before she went, so what? So damned what? As her husband used to say.

She reached into her bag again for her book of matches. She had put them there last weekend at the restaurant during her unsuccessful attempt at a romantic evening with the amorous, but uninteresting Alex. She lit one. It immediately went out. Did she really have nothing in the back of her car to help get it started? No, she was quite sure she didn't. She got her drivers licence out, opened it up and squeezed it roughly together into a taper. She lit the licence and placed it in a hole amongst the driest of the leaves. They took immediately. She fed more leaves and twigs into the flames until she felt satisfied it was going nicely. She clapped her hands with pride, like she had got to be a brownie after all, took another few swigs from the bottle which she had left leaning against the tree. Then she wiped her mouth with the back of her hand. She smiled with pride at that too. It was unheard of for her to be so uncontrolled and so uncouth. She looked up towards the crest of the hill. The glow of the fire lit up the canopy of leaves which were continuously dropping in twos and threes from the branches of the surrounding trees in a slow and silent dance.

'You better be careful or you'll burn your rope.'

She nearly jumped out of her skin.

'I don't mean to be rude or anything but your fire is right underneath it, you know.'

She turned round slowly, at once scared, relieved and angry. It was a young woman. She had a curiously bland sing-song voice, and a smallish fluffy dog which was now avidly sniffing at Rose's ankles. Annoyed, Rose pushed it away and stood up. In the light of the flames which were crackling now, she made out a small pale face, oval, shiny with make up, surrounded by soft curls of dark hair cut into a kind of a bob. Her eyes seemed to be gleaming, as shiny as her cheeks, or was that a trick of the firelight? Despite her pallor she wasn't obviously English. There was a Mediterranean, even slightly Asian look about her. Young, not yet out of her teens, she was slightly taller than Rose.

'I want to kill myself too', the girl said, looking up at the rope with a small, pensive frown as if assessing its effectiveness. Then she looked at Rose, smiled and said, 'Maybe I could be Jan first and then you could hang yourself afterwards!

'Jan?'

'Jeanne d'Arc! Joan of Arc. You know. She was burned at the stake. Died like a man, they said, never cried or anything. My dad's French,' she added inconsequentially. 'Well, Moroccan really, but he was born in France. So it made me interested in history. You know?'

What Rose knew was that she didn't like this and she didn't understand it either. It felt almost surreal. The girl was conversing with her in a polite tone as if they had been just introduced to one another at some social function.

'But I don't know what Milly would do,' she gabbled on. 'Perhaps she'd eat me if I was roasted,' she said with a silly laugh. 'And I really wouldn't like that very much'. The lilting upward emphasis she placed on every other syllable made her sound anodyne. No, just young, thought Rose, very young. And very unwelcome.

What on earth was going on? Why was this bloody girl here of all places? And now? And what was she talking about for heavens sake? Cannibalism?

Anyway, she was a distraction Rose could quite do without. She wanted to tell her to go away, leave her alone. But what she actually said was,

'Milly?'

'Yes.' The girl laughed at Rose's bemused, angry face and pointed at the dog.

'Milly. She eats anything. Anyway, I'm sorry to have disturbed you and of course I won't use your fire for such a purpose, but, well, I suppose you'll have to wait a little while anyway till it dies down, won't you?'

'It is my business what I will or won't have to do thank you very much. I would be very grateful if you and your dog just went on your way now please.'

The girl made no movement to go whatsoever. She just gave Rose a friendly smile and ignored her.

Maddening.

'What are you doing here?'

'Walking Milly. I come here most nights with her, after dark. It's quite safe. There's never anybody around. Not usually.'

Rose glared at her until she finally moved a few steps away from her as if she was frightened.

'You have to think of others, you know, when you want to do things that might upset them'. The girl was almost defensive, apologetic.

'*You've* upset me!' Rose barked.

'Oh. Well, I'm so sorry! But when I saw your rope and the flames I didn't know what to do. I wanted to run home and dial 999, but then I thought I couldn't do that if you were going to be hanging by the time I'd got back and spoken to the police.'

Rose's anger evaporated as quickly as it had boiled up. She would have come to the same decision herself if their positions had been reversed.

'Do you want to sit down?' Rose patted her chair. 'I'm so sorry I shouted at you. This is a difficult time for me. I won't do you any harm, I promise.' She moved her kitchen chair closer to the fire and sat herself down on the ground again with her back against the trunk of the tree. 'I know you meant well.' She paused, cleared her throat delicately. 'Thank you'.

'You're welcome'. She sounded like a supermarket checkout girl, warmly insincere yet coldly genuine. She looked down the wooded hill into the murk, made to go, but then seemed to change her mind and sat down on the chair.

'So why do *you* want to kill yourself?' Rose asked her as if they were waiting in a queue.

'Why do *you*?' the girl said back to her. 'You're the one who's actually trying to do it!'

'Fair enough, my dear, but I'm afraid I can't really answer it. It's so complicated, you see. I'm terribly sorry.'

The girl glared at her. It was clear she resented being taken for stupid.

'But I will try,' Rose continued, curiously mollified. 'Since you've been kind enough to ask. I am all alone. In some ways. No! In most ways. In far too many ways anyway,' she laughed. 'I feel dead already. There's nothing I like about myself. I don't care about anybody else. I'm fed up feeling this way. I can't remember when I didn't. My life has been a treadmill for years and I've had enough!' Rose heard the bitterness and the lack of shame as she laughed at the litany she'd made of her feelings. 'The list of reasons why is endless. I could go on and on, but all the things I would say to you would simply amount to that same thing. I've had enough. That's all.'

'Why didn't you get help?'

'I did. And it didn't.'

'I'm sorry.'

'How can you be? You don't know me,' Rose laughed. 'Actually, if you did you would probably say I was doing the right thing.'

'I wouldn't think that about anybody!' The girl protested. 'You make me feel worse about living than I do already, doing what you're doing'. Her bright, cheery way of speaking continued to jar with what she was actually saying. 'I hate anything upsetting, I really do,' she added chirpily. 'Especially violent things like suicide'. She finished with a silly, inappropriate little giggle.

She could have been talking about the weather.

Intrigued, Rose poured herself another capful of gin and saw the girl frown with disapproval. Grinning, she held it out towards her anyway. Her anger had now gone completely. She wanted to say, 'Cheers' and drink with her. The girl looked at her and shook her head. Alright young lady, thought Rose, intrigued into impulsivity, if you won't join me then I'll join you in your abstinence!

Somehow young people always seemed to sit on the moral high ground as if it were a natural right. She threw the booze away and then poured what was left of the bottle into the flames whose tongues flared, reaching up greedily for more.

'So?' Rose said.

'So what?'

'It's your turn. Why do you want to do yourself in?'

'My mum said never to talk to strangers.'

'I'm not really a stranger, am I? Not anymore. Not now. And anyway I already know you feel the same way about life as I do'. She paused, giving her a big sisterly smile. 'So in that sense we're not strangers at all, are we? I promise I won't do you any harm', she repeated. 'I suppose, if I think about it, you could actually be said to have saved my life.'

The girl pulled her long skirt further down over her knees and huddled up closer to the fire which had now begun to settle down. At the same time her expression was one of wanting to get away from Rose as soon as possible. It was clearly written on her face by the light of the flames.

14

'I mean it,' said Rose. 'You have stopped me doing what I was going to do. For now anyway! But don't be frightened. You don't have to tell me if you don't want to. Of course you don't. You and Milly can go whenever you want, can't you? Right now, in fact. I'm certainly not going to stop you! And please don't feel you have to stay in order to prevent me continuing with my plans because I can assure you I'm not going to. I've changed my mind. And it's all down to you, I think!'

She stared out into the dark listening to her own words and deciding they were true. When she turned back to look at the girl she saw that she was studying her face.

'To be honest, I don't feel the same way as you do about life at all,' said the girl. 'I was lying. But then I am a liar and I always have been. It's something I am good at and it was all I could think of to stop you'.

She flashed a bland, dazzling smile at her again and Rose noticed that her face in the yellow glare of the flames was actually quite pretty despite being overly made-up and doll-like. Her eyes looked dark and sad and bore no relation whatsoever to the smile on her lip-glossed mouth gleaming incongruously in the light of the flames. What was she doing looking like that in the dark in the middle of nowhere with no-one about?

'What's your name, dear?'

'I'm sorry, but I don't think it's any of your business actually'.

She saw Rose looking apologetic again and seemed to soften. 'My mum used to call me 'chick' but she's been calling me 'hen' these last few months', she said, 'and I like that! So I don't know. I don't see as much of her as I would like so I was thinking it's got to have something with an 'en' in it at the moment to remind me of her. At the moment I like Jenny, Helen or Karen,' she laughed, 'take your pick. Not that it's got anything to do with you! Jenny's nice, don't you think? You can always lengthen it, if you need to be a Jennifer. But it doesn't matter what my name is really.'

What was going on? Was she mentally ill? A multiple personality maybe?

'Look, your rope has gone all black underneath,' the girl said.

Rose glanced up at it, not really caring. When she looked back at the girl again she saw she was still staring at her, smiling vacuously; till she switched it off like a light and turned away.

'I don't think you were lying at all, er, Jenny', she said slowly, still and always the empathic intuitive therapist. 'Or Helen or Karen or whoever you are.' They both laughed for a few moments at their mutual silliness. 'My name is Rose.' She paused for a moment, made a face. 'Definitely,' she said, 'by no other name am I known.' This made the girl giggle like a younger child altogether. 'Why *are* you unhappy?' she asked softly, 'a pretty young girl like you.'

'Oh it's nothing serious,' the girl replied, 'just a teenage thing. You know.' She seemed to search for a story. 'A girlfriend is upset with me because I keep on borrowing her things. Only stuff she lets me borrow, mind you. I don't just take them. Things she doesn't fit anymore. She's put on a bit of weight. You know.'

She picked at her skirt.

'This is one of hers. I love it. Don't you think it's nice?'

She wasn't saying she was a thief, so what was she really saying? Rose lifted a cynical eyebrow at her obvious evasiveness. It was a trick she had learned when she herself was in her teens. Clearly not stupid, 'Jenny' nodded her head, added, 'and, you know, the usual teenage thing: I don't know who I am.'

She smiled almost apologetically at Rose then her eyes widened in alarm.

'You are safe aren't you? It's only your own self you would harm, isn't it? Not others? And – you promised – you're not going to do that anymore now, are you?'

Rose shook her head reassuringly. How on earth could she? Even if she did still want to? It was quite out of the question now. Her gin was gone.

'I get so scared,' the girl said. If you really want to know I was upset because till now I'd always thought – no, hoped – I might be a lesbian. I wanted to be! I really did. But I always knew I wasn't really, cos you can't help what you feel, can you? But the trouble is I've never ever *liked* boys. And it was always the boys who used to tease me and make me cry at school. But tonight I was feeling unhappy because I realised I had to stop running away from myself. I prefer girls and women as people. As friends. I really do, but I'm afraid I'm, you know, actually attracted to… men.'

She almost spat the last word out, looked directly at Rose and shrugged before giving her a tragic-comic smile. 'And I always do really sensible things like telling my most intimate personal problems to complete strangers who are trying to commit suicide!' She shook her head. 'Never mind.'

Rose liked her.

'We all have to come to terms with who we are, don't we? Please believe me when I say I really don't mean to be patronising, dear, but I remember feeling exactly the same as you do now when I was young.'

'Well look at you now then – you're trying to kill yourself!' Rose couldn't believe it, but the girl's intense, almost angry look berated her for not having been the slightest bit reassuring. Not as far as she was concerned. Yet the warm familiarity of such a glance was somehow intimate, as if they known each other for ages instead of having just met now. Ridiculous, but nice somehow too.

16

'I'm sorry,' the girl apologised. 'I didn't mean that horribly.' Her eyes sparkled and she seemed to have a revelation. 'But I can and I will say what I like cos of what you've just been trying to do! And because it's, like, just the two of us alone here and not knowing each other at all, and everything. Do you mind?'

Rose's intent look and slow shake of her head prompted the girl to visibly relax herself, then smile with the contentment of a kitten curling up in front of the fire.

'So, okay, you are right, actually,' she said, holding out the palms of her hands to the flames. 'I wasn't lying just now. I do feel like doing myself in a lot of the time, just like you do. But the difference is I've got Milly. Haven't I, Mills?'

She rubbed the dog's ears and then looked sideways at Rose. 'I didn't want anything to do with men, did I Milly? I just wanted to be a lesbian. That's all. But don't get me wrong, I'm not. I know I'm not.' She shuddered. 'It's as simple as that. I'm silly really, I know. It's nothing important. It's just – I don't know – I'm always finding that I'm not who I think I am. Or who I want to be, you know?'

Rose nodded though she didn't understand precisely what the child was talking about. Young people were so confusing nowadays. It had been a long time since she was young. As if she could see these thoughts written on Rose's face in the firelight, 'Jenny' sat upright in her chair. She gave Rose an unnecessary, defiant glance, let out another little laugh. Then she extended her arms with an almost too elegant shrug, gesturing towards her own body. She seemed to be both nodding and shaking her head at one and the same time.

'I'm not what I seem. Except that I am really,' she said. She bit her lower lip and straightened her back, clearly bracing herself again. 'I'm ashamed,' she went on, paused for a moment then stared at Rose and blurted out 'I'm transgendered. And I hate it. I just want to be normal, but I need to have a sex change for that.'

Rose frowned, failing to understand for a few moments. Then it dawned on her.

'I didn't realise. You're saying – I'm sorry, I don't mean to be rude – you're not really a girl?'

'Jenny' nodded and shook her head a few more times.

'Well! You certainly don't look or sound like a boy at all. Are you sure, dear? You're not having me on?' She laughed easily, despite feeling a little perturbed.

Jenny, or whoever she or he – really? – was called, looked simultaneously pleased and insulted.

'I'm – I'm never sure about anything. I'm all mixed up. All I know is who I am. And what I am not. I will *never* be a man. But I'm eighteen years old today. And if I don't get surgery to correct my body soon, it will be too late.

I've been on the pill – the contraceptive pill – for nearly five years now and I think it has helped stop any manliness developing, thank goodness. I would rather die than have that happen. You just can't be what you're not, can you? But without hormones and an operation, I can't be what I am either. So I'll never be me, just something hopeless and stupid in between. The pill is better than nothing, but it's not doing enough. I've got tits like a ten year old! It's so unnatural. At least my voice hasn't broken.'

Despite herself, perhaps because it was cold, Rose gave a little shudder of revulsion, but more out of empathy than disgust. It would indeed be awful to have a man's voice. Unless you were one, of course.

'I've always got on better with girls and women then with boys. Always. Because of my nature. Because I *am* a girl. As a person, you know? But I'm getting frightened if I don't have the op soon, I'll lose my nature and I'll lose myself.' She looked at Rose for acknowledgement, for confirmation; her gaze demanding it. Rose smiled, nodded her head automatically – the expert comforter. Goodness, how bizarre this was. As soon as she did so, 'Jenny' nodded too. 'So you do understand then. That's great!'

'Of course I do. But, if you don't mind my asking, how on earth did you manage to get on the pill?'

'Mum! They're Mum's. She gets them on prescription and gives them to me when I visit. She doesn't need them anymore.'

With pathetic defiance she added, 'My mum is wonderful. She's known who I really am all my life. And she's always thought I should have the operation too. She took me to see some doctors when I was younger and we asked them – begged them – to change me. They did some tests and wanted me to see a therapist, and I did, but he was a *man*! So he couldn't really understand. He said they couldn't do anything until I was grown up, but he still wanted me to come and see him for counselling. But I didn't bother. I mean, what was the point? I wished I had now though. I'm so scared. What will I do if my body turns? I won't be able to live.'

The hysteria in 'Jenny's' voice was almost palpable. Rose noticed her fascination was diverting from her own plight and found herself wanting to offer the child comfort and cuddles. She restrained herself, made a little sympathetic cooing noise instead. She thought she should be appalled, but she wasn't; although she would certainly have been ever so much more careful if she had met such a person professionally at work.

'I can't go private,' 'Jenny' said. 'I hardly earn enough money to live, let alone pay for all the pills and creams and surgery I need. I've been thinking I'll just have to go on the game. Earn money that way for my operation.'

'Surely that won't be necessary?' Rose said inadequately, even as she understood it probably might be.

'Girls like me have to – unless they've got a Sugar-Daddy, and I don't – to pay for what we need. I *need* to be myself. I'm completely fake at the moment. But you have to try, don't you? Do the best you can. Try or die! That's what I say. So when I saw what you were doing I thought, why not? Perhaps I'll join you. I'll die too. I've enough reason.'

What Rose now recognised as 'Jenny's' exaggeratedly feminine timbre lost its softness for a moment. Her eyes misted and she no longer sounded like an announcer in a supermarket when she whispered, 'I come out here to cut myself sometimes anyway. It's better than nothing.'

Taken completely out of herself by all this and now feeling utterly unafraid, Rose decided this definitely called for some motherly comfort from her. After all, she *wasn't* at work.

She got up off the ground. Her bottom was a bit damp and she needed to wee. She went over to the 'girl' called Jenny who sat still on the chair staring into her fate and despite all her reservations and all her professional training, she put her arms around her. 'Jenny' started shaking. Rose didn't let go.

'So that's why *I* want to kill myself! Sometimes,' she said the sing-song cheeriness back in her voice. 'On bad days. Like birthdays.' She reached down for her bag, took out a tissue, wiped a tear from her cheek carefully. 'I don't want to cry,' she said, 'and I'm not going to.' For some strange reason Rose was reminded of not wanting to ruin her net curtains an hour and a half ago.

'Thank you for saving my life, Jenny. For being there when I needed you, even though you didn't know me.'

Rose held her for a few moments, then gave her a squeeze and let go. This was ridiculous. Quite ridiculous. And quite possibly dangerous. At the same time she felt almost ecstatic that her own eyes were watering and wetness was freely flowing down her cheeks. She couldn't remember when she had last cried. Certainly not since the night her son died nearly five years ago. She always tried to think of him as little as possible because it always felt like yesterday. And always would.

'Are you going to take *your* turn now? You really haven't told me anything about why you've come out are here to kill yourself in – in my secret garden,' 'Jenny' sniffed. She wiped her nose, gave a timorous smile which Rose warmly returned. Then she felt her own pain again.

'You're lucky you've actually got your mum' said Rose. 'There is no one in this whole world who needs me'.

'I haven't got her! I can only sneak round and *see* her on Mondays when I've got the day off and if my dad is at work.'

' I shouldn't make assumptions, but you know what I mean. My mother and father are both dead. And – and so is Luke. My son.'

19

'Luke?' 'Jenny' repeated and then went silent, stared into the fire and looked away. Some minutes later and as if it were an afterthought she asked 'Is it alright to ask you how he died?'

'He drowned aged ten in the pus produced by his own lungs.' Rose didn't care how brutal she sounded. The facts *were* brutal. 'Cystic Fibrosis. They usually live into their teens. He was lucky I suppose, my golden boy.'

'You were wanting to join him just now, weren't you?' 'Jenny' looked up at the rope now swaying a bit in the slight breeze which had got up.

'No. I didn't think of it like that at all. But it is true I have always wanted to be with him again.'

'What about your – I mean Luke's dad?'

'Richard? He left me six months after Lukey died. We couldn't bear it. We were just hurting each other. There was no acrimony after he'd gone. We were both relieved, actually. We still meet for a chat sometimes. He's married again since. He's got three lovely step-children now. I send them a Christmas card each year.

'When did Luke die?'

'Five years ago. Just before Christmas. He'd have been fifteen next week. We have – I mean had – the same birthday. It's wonderful how life throws up coincidences like that.' Now she was the one putting on the tra-la-la voice.

'I don't know if you could call this a coincidence cos loads of people have the same name, don't they! But it's a bit spooky and I don't want to upset you or anything, but my name, I mean the name I was given when I was born was Luke. At work I make them call me Lucie, short for Lucille. It's French. My mum told me that they would have called me Lucille if I had been born with the right body. But I want to get away from that altogether now I think. I want to be Jenny from now on. Let the past go completely.'

Rose looked at her, saw no trace of Luke in her at all, but felt a sudden intense bodily connection with the child. In her belly, her breasts, eyes, lap – everywhere. For a brief blissful moment she felt just like a mother again.

'Oh, that is unbelievable! It truly *is* a coincidence. How wonderful! You're not lying again to stop me getting too maudlin, are you?'

'I don't know what that means. But I'm not lying. Why should I? And I don't mean to offend you – about your taste in names, I mean – but I've always hated that name. Lucille's alright I suppose, but 'Luke'?' She shuddered. 'Yuck.' Then she seemed to recollect herself, whispered, 'Sorry! I just meant it's not for me, because I'm a girl. You know.'

'I understand dear, I do understand,' Rose murmured, squeezing 'Jenny's' arm. Or should that be 'Lucille's'? Truly, it couldn't be 'Luke's'. This just wasn't a boy.

'Now you know all my names I suppose we should be formally introduced?' She grinned, stood up and held out an elegant little hand, her slim wrist adorned with masses of tiny Indian bangles. 'How do you do!' She said, moving hair out of her face with her other hand with the exaggerated grace of a princess.

'I'm very pleased to meet you,' Rose replied formally, laughing as she shook it.

'It's nice to meet you too, Rose,' said this girl who wasn't one.

Rose held onto her hand and carried on laughing with her for a moment. There was definitely as much intimacy between them now as if they were family and had known each other all their lives. It was utterly amazing how a little suicidality could bring two complete strangers together like this! Milly stood up on her hind legs and started whining and pawing at them, trying to separate them or join in.

Glowing orange fragments and the occasional whole leaf began to blow off the top of the fire into the trees. A breeze had come up.

'I think I better put the fire out,' said Rose disengaging, 'or it'll set the whole woods alight, the rate this wind is getting up.' She did feel a little bit anxious about it.

She began sweeping at the fire with the outside of her foot to remove the leaves on the outer edges of the heap which had not yet started burning. She didn't want to think about what this was doing to her shoes, told herself again to stop having such irrelevant thoughts. But the fact that she thought them at all told her that the idea of suicide had been a conceit. She just needed someone to care for. That was why she had the job she had, no doubt. She laughed with the exhilaration as she and 'Jenny' who was wearing boots with only slightly more sensible heels, jumped from smouldering leaf to smouldering leaf stamping out the embers.

Then suddenly it wasn't funny anymore. Everywhere she looked there seemed to be another little pocket of leaves with flames licking up around it. The fire itself was now flattened, but the sea of leaves around them was spotted with little orange and yellow tongues flickering up every now and then. Though by no means a gale, the wind nevertheless seemed to want to blow them down the hill, and no sooner had they put one fire out, than another seemed to pop up. The dog was barking with excitement, but was sensible enough to stay beyond the spread of the flames which despite the rapidity with which they arose, were not large. Nor were they putting the trees at risk. They were easily stamped out. The trouble was they seemed to just as easily spring up again.

'Jenny' joined her in stomping away at them vigorously, pointing to new ones as they popped up. They were laughing together as they stamped their feet, slightly hysterical, on an adrenalin high dealing with the danger.

'I always wanted to know what a fire fighter did,' 'Jenny' said, grinning before falling over backwards into brambles, having tripped herself up in her eagerness to put out the flames. She tried to get up again immediately, but was not able to.

'I think I've twisted my ankle or something,' she said, whimpering. 'I can't get up.' She tried again. 'Ouch.'

'Give me a moment, there's only a couple more to put out, then I'll help you,' Rose replied breathlessly. She continued stamping out what few little fires remained for another few minutes. She waited a while after the last one was out, but no more sprang up.

Satisfied, she trudged over to 'Jenny' with a smile and bent down holding out her arms to her to hoist her up. 'Jenny' was looking worried.

'Thank you ever so much for helping me. I'm not sure I would have managed without you. The whole forest would have caught fire! Is your foot very painful?'

'Only when I move.'

'You're biting your lip. You must be in a lot of pain, you poor thing.'

'I'm not. Really.' She took hold of Rose's hands who tried to pull her up. 'Not very much anyway. I'll be alright.'

Rose pulled her up without difficulty. She was as light as a feather.

But in fact she could hardly stand without support, let alone walk.

'I'll drive you home. No, I insist. Please let me. It was all my fault, after all.'

'No! I'm alright. I'll manage. Really. Thank you.' She disengaged from Rose and half-hopped, half-walked around the blackened ground trying to put her weight on to her foot. She couldn't do so without limping. The pain was obviously acute. Rose picked up her kitchen chair and placed it behind her. She sat back down on it with a sigh. 'That's better! Thanks! I'll be right as rain in a minute.'

'I don't think so, Jenny.'

'I have to be. I have to.'

'Why can't I take you?'

'Because, because you might meet Ron and I don't want you to. Thank you.'

'I won't come in if you don't want me to. Who is Ron?'

'He's Grainne's boyfriend, or meant to be. And my landlord. Well, it's Council really, the house I mean, but he takes my money.'

'And Grainne?'

'My best friend. But not for much longer if she finds out what Ron's been doing with me. She's the one who lent me this.' 'Jenny' patted her skirt, then pulling it up, she gingerly unzipped her boot and took it off to massage her ankle.

'What's Ron been doing to you, Jenny?'

'You wouldn't want to know, believe me.'

'Please tell me.'

'Jenny' hesitated, then shrugged. 'Grainne's a nurse and she works shifts and every time she works a late and after I come in from work at six thirty – I work in a hairdressing salon – he makes me, forces me to give him, you know, French. Before I take Milly out. He always waits till I've got out of my work clothes, and only does it when he knows I'm properly dressed as a girl and have done my face and hair and everything. He says he only likes women, that's why, and that he's doing me a favour letting me find out what it's really like for a woman. But afterwards he usually calls me a – well never mind what he calls me! He works as a welder all day and he smells disgusting, of metal and sweat and urine.' She shuddered. 'The first time he made me, I felt sick and tried to pull away, and wipe his – you know – off my face and clothes. But he hit me and said he'd do that to me every time unless I swallowed it. So now I just do what he tells me. And he says if I ever tell Grainne he'll cut both our faces. I believe him. He's got a collection of knives. And a shotgun.' She retched, but didn't vomit.

'Oh, Jenny! Why do you stay there?

'Where else can I go? I can't afford anywhere else and at least Grainne and Ron let me be myself, or try to be.'

'Ron hardly does, Jenny. Making you do that to him is *not* letting you be yourself.'

'No, it isn't really, is it.' She let out another little tinkling laugh. 'I think Grainne will leave him soon anyway. They're always arguing. She's twenty four now. He's twenty nine, and she's earns more than he does! She can look after herself without him.'

'Then what would you do?'

'I don't know. Nothing really matters if I can't be who I am. I really don't care about anything else. I want to, but I really don't.' She wrinkled her nose and let a more personal, less victimised tone enter her voice. 'Sometimes when I am doing it for him I try to imagine he's someone else, you know, someone I love! And I imagine my body has been fixed so we *can* have proper sex if we want to and that I'm only blowing him because I've chosen to. For love. And then it's alright. I don't mind so much. This evening I could even feel myself liking it. That's what was upsetting me when I saw your fire. I just don't want to feel anything like that. Not the way I am. He washed himself first tonight and he was in a good mood. Because it was my birthday, he said. He stroked my head and told me what a lovely girl I was as he came. He's cunning. He knew saying that would please me and make me feel happier about it. And it did. But afterwards when I came out here I felt confused. *Because* it had, you know? Of course it had. And that's not what being a girl is about, is it?'

'Jenny, you've got to get away from him.'

23

'Yes I know, and live happily ever after in a magical land with the three bears, or better still, my handsome Prince Charming!'

A mad impulse on what was turning out to be the maddest day of her life suddenly burst open like a rare red flower in the desert of Rose's aching breast. She had once had so much to give as a mum, her whole self in fact, and for these last five years had had no-one to give it to. The feeling hadn't gone away though, nor even lain dormant. Just burgeoned within her. She could feel it intensely right now with this – this girl. Over the last five years she had been so full of denial about Luke being gone that she'd completely ignored the feeling as it continued to grow and grow within her, entangling her in its leaves and shoots as she pretended to herself that it wasn't really there.

Listening to this strange child now, she finally allowed herself to recognise it. A large, if not the largest part of why she had wanted to die was the lack of a little one to look after. Of all her reasons for wanting to kill herself it was undoubtedly the most overwhelming.

Why hadn't she realised this before? Because it was selfish? Maybe. But it was also true. Her whole sense of who she most truly was, was still absolutely predicated on this need to nurture; to look after and to love, irrespective of who she was directing such feelings towards. Since Luke had gone and Richard left, that need had grown like the giant beanstalk in the children's story which Lukey used to enjoy so much when he was little, bending and twisting and spreading in her barren sterile emptiness, enormous in its hunger for someone to look after and care for again.

'No, better than either of those. Come and live with – with your fairy godmother!'

They both laughed. Then 'Jenny' stared at her blankly.

'You mean you?'

'That's exactly who I mean,' Rose said. 'You have saved my life and I want to save yours. In return. Come and live with me. Milly can come too! I will look after you and pay for whatever pills and surgery you need. And you can start straight away. You won't need to take up prostitution. I've got more than enough money. And it will have the added benefit of getting you away from Ron. It is the very least I can do. You can be – I don't know – you can be like my god-daughter or my niece. Nobody need know that our true family tie,' she held up both forefingers and wiggled apostrophe's around the word 'family', 'is that we both wanted to do away with ourselves. And if you don't like it, why you can always leave if you want! Just as you can now '

Despite the darkness Rose could see the young transsexual's overly made-up eyes fill with disbelief and hurt. She nodded her head at her. 'I mean it, dear. I'm not lying or trying to upset you, I promise. Let it be my birthday present to you for saving my life!'

'You're teasing me, you must be. Either that or you're mad! You really shouldn't play games with people's feelings, you know. It's not nice.'

'I am not playing games at all. I do really mean it. I promise. I know it's sudden and unexpected and everything. And that we've never met before. So it may seem mad to you, and maybe it is, but I don't care. As long as you believe me! It is wonderful to feel impulsive after so many years of being controlled. I am many things, but never, ever impulsive. It may be crazy, but it is what I want to do. My offer is deadly – No! Not deadly – livingly! It's livingly serious, if you will only accept it. An hour ago I didn't plan to be alive anymore, but now I do. And it's because of you. I want to return the favour. Please let me. You can have the spare room, or maybe even Lukey's old room if you'd like it, and in return I will help you in whatever way I can to do whatever you need to do to become yourself and feel alive too.'

The child was shaking her head.

'I can see you don't mean to play games with me,' she said. 'I mean, I can see you mean it, but, oh dear! What am I doing with all these 'means'? It's just that what you are saying is so – so shocking! I mean, you don't even know me! ' Rose watched her give up resisting the appeal of her offer. 'It's just amazing. So amazing and so kind that I can't believe it!'

'I give you my solemn word, dear, I do mean it. I want to help you. But it's selfish too! It – you – will give me something to live for. Someone to care for I mean. And believe you me, I really am desperate, absolutely desperate to have someone to care for again. I need to. For my *own* mental health. If I can't ever be a mother again, it would please me so much – so much – to be able to be a god-mother. Or an auntie.' Her voice faltered, lost its middle-aged authority for a moment. 'I don't have any nephews or nieces,' she faltered. 'So if you are interested, it would make me so very happy if you would be my god-daughter or my niece. I'd ask only one thing in return from you. I'd like to call you Lucille. 'Jenny' is nice, but I think it would be more authentic, more *you*, if you had the name your mother would have given you.'

'They call me that at work and at home anyway. I don't allow them not to! But, I don't know you!'

'Well, now's your opportunity!'

They looked at each other, smiling. Neither of them really comprehending what it was they were both nodding and shaking their heads about.

Then just nodding them.

'Good. That's settled then,' said Rose. 'You won't regret it, I promise you. Happy Birthday!'

The fit of uncontrollable giggles they then both burst into made the woods ring.

Chapter 2.

Rose wondered what on earth she had done. At the same time she was elated. She didn't care. Whatever else it was, it would be a change to her otherwise meaningless personal existence. For the last five years she had sought respite from grief by immersing herself in her work. Every time her mind drifted back to Lukey's last dying days, his wasted little body and his hacking muddy cough, she would devote more energy to whatever task she was attending to, give it her all. Which was always more difficult alone at home. There were only so many times you could plump the cushions or hoover the carpets when you lived on your own, before they were very definitely done. Then she would collapse on her sofa and just stare into the past going over every single memory of him from every single angle until eventually all she was left with was the unbearable pain of his absence in her lap, heart, breasts and hands. Everywhere. A long silent scream would then well up, but she would suppress it with the cold light of reason, telling herself grief was a process with a defined beginning, middle and end, and you just had to let time go by and in due course your loss would become more bearable.

She knew about these things. She was the consultant family therapist at the local office of the Institute for Family Welfare. She met troubled people every day. Just occasionally there were even cases of children with Cystic Fibrosis on the referral list. As the manager of the centre, Rose always made sure these were allocated to somebody else. They were so rare the other staff didn't notice, and even if they had, they would not have minded. They were a lovely bunch. But what she understood professionally and academically made little or no difference privately and personally. If anything it made matters worse because knowing how she should be behaving and feeling just made her reproach herself more for how she actually felt and behaved.

She had tried to find interests to take her mind off her bereavement but had had to continually re-motivate herself as they were never interesting enough to take her out of herself for very long. She had learned Spanish in an adult education class for two years, but hadn't visited Spain. She had tried embroidery but found she was stitching her emotions and invariably losing her way with her pattern. She had tried going out more, making friends, but people would sense the forced, brittle quality in her and find excuses for not staying in touch.

She had even, once or twice, found men showing an interest in her, but despite her conscious intentions to try not to discourage them, had actually found that all her non-verbal signals were making it crystal clear to them that she didn't want to know. There had been a trainee on placement with her at work who she had found very attractive, but he was nearly ten years younger than she was and she had eventually realised much to her annoyance that he was deliberately flirting with her in order to get a good report. She had given him one anyway. He was a good therapist.

She was forty one years old and beginning to lose her figure. Not because she ate too much, but because she drank and took no exercise. The truth was she did not really care. All she cared about was her work. She needed to believe that if her own feelings about herself were stuck, at least she could help other people in crisis to find a way out of the problems besetting them. If they could never fundamentally alter, they could at least change the relationship they had with the circumstances they found themselves in. Even, sometimes at least, change the circumstances. That was her belief and that was what her training had taught her. She knew she was good at her job. But it was scant compensation for the emptiness she felt inside.

She had arranged to pick up Lucille this afternoon and help her bring her things over. On the way down the wooded hill two weeks ago, with both of them between laughter and tears as she supported Lucille back to her car, Lucille had accepted her offer. They had agreed that she would need a couple of weeks to work her notice at the salon so she could get a reference for another job closer to here. Her Italian boss had not disapproved of her, she had told Rose, he actually felt his clientele liked a nice sissy-boy, as he called her, with a girl's name. But he thought they would feel discomforted by an out and out sex-change. So he had insisted on her working for him in her male attire. When Rose came to pick her up from Ron's flat they had agreed she would leave every article of male clothing behind to mark the beginning of the end of her nightmare. Rose would have felt uncomfortable if Lucille had said anything else. She would help her find a plastic surgeon and Lucille would look for a job locally because she wanted to be able to pay her way and give Rose some rent.

Since then Rose had felt some trepidation about what she had done, but at the same time the sense of purpose in her life completely obscured all thoughts of suicide. It was exciting to be making such a radical change in her lifestyle after all these years of living on her own. And such a responsibility. Lucille's strange journey towards harmonising mind and body was going to require a lot of emotional and financial support. She would need to be stable and strong and reliable. Like a mother again.

It was a dull Saturday afternoon. Rose got out of her car. She was wearing jeans and a jumper under her duffel coat which still smelt vaguely of wood smoke. She must remember to get it dry cleaned and maybe it was time to stitch some patches on the elbows. She walked past what looked like a dismantled motorcycle up the pathway to the Carshalton council house where she had dropped Lucille after making her mad offer.

What on earth was she doing? She knew she must be crazy, but somehow that just didn't seem to matter enough to stop her. She adjusted her coat and pressed the front door bell.

It was opened by big greasy man with an incipient beer belly, and a black goatee beard on unshaven cheeks. His arms were blue with tattoos. His large hands filthy. Ron.

'Come on in,' he said affably, 'you must be Rose. Lukey-Lucie's told us a lot about you'. She was slightly disarmed by his friendly manner. 'I'm Ronald Symes,' he said, holding out a hand.

'Thank you,' she replied avoiding it. 'Yes, I've come to pick her up.'

He invited her to sit down on a threadbare sofa in his linoleum floored front room. The lino had holes in several places. Milly was lying on her side on a rug by the gas fire and wagged her tail lazily at the sight of her. Rose had forgotten about Milly. Oh well, in for a penny, in for a pound. Milly was going to have to come too of course.

'Lulu, it's time to go,' Ron called up the stairs. 'Your auntie's arrived to take you home with her.' He made it sound at once sleazy and innocuous. Auntie? Well, that would do.

'I won't be a minute,' came the reply. 'I'm having a bit of a struggle with my case. Could you offer Rose a cup of tea please, Ron, and come up and help me,' she called.

Rose declined the tea saying she had had one just before she came out. In fact it had been a glass of wine.

'I suppose I better have a forwarding address for any mail Lukey-lu gets,' said Ron with an over-familiar grin.

'Lucille. From now on she will *only* be known as Lucille or Lucie. She's going to have an operation to put her right.'

Rose gave him her address and telephone number which he printed along the margin of yesterday's Daily Star. There was an awkward silence between them. She looked around the room. A large American Confederate flag was pinned over the false chimney breast, and a small tropical fish tank stood in the corner. In the other corner a very big television was flickering with the sound switched off.

'I hear you're going to pay for his – I mean her – operations and that,' he said, scratching his stomach and staring at her breasts. She crossed her legs ignoring him, then modelled politeness, giving him a small smile and a curt nod. She looked away at the door feeling uncomfortable.

'Best thing for him. Her, I mean. Not a proper bloke at all. Grainne – that's my er, partner – gave him one of her best dresses as a leaving present. I told her don't, but she said Lulu looked better in it than she does cos it's got too small for her. I said I like women in tight clothes, but she wasn't having none of that. Wanted to give it to Lu. Nice of her, weren't it?' He flashed dirty, yellow teeth at Rose and said, 'I think I'd better go up now and see if I can help er – her – with the case.'

He lumbered up the stairs and Rose heard him asking Lucille through her door if she was decent. She didn't hear the reply, but heard him laugh and say, 'Never mind, I'll come in anyways and give you a hand.' She heard the sound of a door opening and closing.

Rose shuddered.

Five minutes later she heard the trill of Lucille's voice and thought she must be telling him off about something. She certainly sounded aggravated anyway. Shortly afterwards he came down again, looking both a little confused and smugly satisfied, Rose thought. She suppressed a shudder. What a dreadful man.

'Sorry about the delay,' he said, 'Lulu's in a bit of mess.' He grinned, 'with the packing and that.'

'Shall I go up and help her?'

'Nah, here she is now.'

Lucille was struggling down the stairs with a large suitcase and a sunny smile for Rose, who got up to help her. In the daylight Rose noticed that she had inherited some of her father's North African complexion. Her skin was a light golden brown. With her delicate features, and what must be her mother's green eyes, she was a pretty enough girl. Though full, her case was not heavy. They put it down together, looked at one another for a moment as if each were offering the other a last chance to change their mind. Then they embraced. As she disengaged Rose felt relieved. Since their meeting a fortnight ago in the dark of the woods, one of her many slight anxieties about her hasty offer had been whether in the cold light of day, unmistakable, embarrassing signs of masculinity might be perceptible which would be difficult for both of them. Despite her liberal politics, she didn't want it getting around that she was living with a teenage drag queen. Well, she need not have worried. There was nothing to give any clue at all that she wasn't exactly what she seemed, poor thing. The sooner the offending bits and pieces were surgically removed the better.

Despite what Ron had just said, Lucille was wearing a skirt not a dress. She looked nice, cosy and definitely if unremarkably feminine in a dark blue woollen jumper, a short, but not too short, black skirt and black tights. If she was wearing a shade too much make-up so did many girls her age. Everything would be alright.

'Oh Rose, this is so wonderful,' said Lucille in her gushing, lilting manner which was if anything, overly feminine. But that was understandable under the circumstances, thought Rose. Such girlish timbre, the varied pitch and intonation of her voice would have been utterly out of place on a boy. Rose felt herself glowing with the certainty that what she was doing was right. 'I've been on a high ever since I saw you,' Lucie went on. 'I sometimes thought I had dreamed you, but you really exist! I'm so happy you haven't changed your mind. I *knew* you'd come really. Thanks for ringing me and reassuring me you weren't just a dream' She embraced her again. 'How are you?'

'I've fine, and no I haven't changed my mind at all. Of course I haven't. I've thought a lot about it and the more I've thought, the more I've thought it's the best thing for both of us. Are you ready? Shall we go?'

'Yes, yes and I'm so glad. This is the happiest day of my whole life. I'm sorry I took so long.' She glared at Ron. 'I had to change at the last minute. My dress got messed. Well Ron, my dah-ahling, this is where we say goodbye.' She held a delicate, slender-wristed right hand out towards him, dangling it with an expectant look on her face. He appeared a bit taken aback, but moved forward to shake it. She removed it with a smile just as he was about to grasp it and offered him her cheek instead. Confused, it took him a moment to follow what she wanted. Then he bent to kiss her. Before he could do so Lucille spun out of the way, picked up her case and in her sweetest voice said, 'Fuck off, Ron,' and opening the door swept out. Rose looked at him with a raised eyebrow, shrugged and followed her. The door slammed behind them.

They put the suitcase on the back seat of the little Peugeot. Rose started the car and they set off.

'That's a very full suitcase,' said Rose.

'I know. You wouldn't believe how many lovely things some women throw out. I'm a charity shop junkie. Nearly everything I've got in this case, except for underwear, of course, has come from Oxfam and Scope and places like that. I'm not ashamed. I've got some lovely things, really. Designer skirts. Liberty scarves. I'm very choosy. I'll show you when we get in. I just can't believe how lucky I am to have found you,' said Lucille in a voice throaty with passion and gratitude.

Rose smiled. 'Who knows? Maybe it will all go horribly wrong. But I don't think it will. Obviously we'll have to get to know each other, but at the same time I think we'll both need space too. Don't you agree? I've been living on my own for a long time, you know, and I'm more than twice your age. Certainly old enough to be your mother. You might find some of my little ways get on your nerves, and sometimes I might find you a little, I don't mean to offend you, dear, a little strange too. But we must continue from where we started, don't you think, and be honest with one another. Honesty is very important to me. And, honestly, I have never met someone like you in all my life.'

'And I've never met anyone like you! I will try to behave myself and fit in with you, Rose, truly I will. I would do anything for you. I really would. What *you* are doing for me is unbelievable, amazing.'

'You were wonderful with Ron. I don't think I'd have dared speak to him like that under the circumstances.'

'It was great, wasn't it? After you arrived he came up, of course, to do his thing with me, but I managed to pull away. But now,' she gave a little choke, 'I am afraid I may have made a bad situation worse by hurting Grainne. I know she's been dying to leave him for weeks but I shouldn't have done what I did. I just felt so angry with him.'

'What are you talking about? What did you do?'

'I returned the dress with his stains all over it to the front of her wardrobe with a little note in the pocket saying goodbye and telling her how they got there, what he made me do and what he threatened us both with if I didn't.'

'Oh Lucille. That's terrible! Poor Grainne when she finds out. And like that! Awful.'

'I didn't know what else to do. I felt so mad with him. But I spose it wasn't a very nice way of letting her know about him, was it?'

'It certainly wasn't!' She concentrated on the road ahead as the traffic lights changed. 'Not very kind at all.' Not wanting to hurt Lucille's feelings or set their relationship off on the wrong footing, she added, 'But then I don't know what else you could have done.'

It was a lie and Rose frowned, screwing her nose up with distaste at the squalor of what she had just heard. Once again she wondered what she had let herself in for. Lucille was not going to be easy to live with at all. Young, hot-headed, possibly amoral, and about to undergo gender reassignment – that's what they called it, she'd read up on the subject over the last fortnight. Not the most stable combination of qualities. Definitely not.

'What would you have done?'

'I ? I don't know. I don't think I would have had the presence of mind to think of anything! I'm the slow thorough type who can never make up her mind even when I do know what the choices are.'

'You made up your mind quickly enough about me.'

'I know, but that was an extraordinary situation. And I don't regret it, Lucille. Not for a moment. I've been anxious and worried about how it will work out between us, but I've never once felt that we shouldn't be doing this. And I don't now. But what you did just now was wrong.'

'You're so sweet to me, thank you again Rose, from my heart. And you're right about Grainne. She'll be so upset. Can we turn round and go back? Do you mind?'

Rose looked in her rear view mirror in order to pull over and turn around.

'Oh my God! Milly! I left Milly behind, as well. How could I? We must go back. We've got to turn round and get her, Rose, right now. We *must*! I'm so sorry. But at least it'll give me a chance to get the dress while I'm at it and write Grainne another note.'

'What about Ron? He's going to be a little put out, to say the least, after the way you left him just now.'

'Oh that doesn't matter. He's often like that.'

Rose turned the car around. Within five minutes they were back outside Ron's house.

'I'll go in with you,' said Rose. 'Perhaps he'll be less likely to give you trouble if I am there too.'

They got out and balancing it on her knee, Lucille delved into her ancient-looking handbag for her key, which in her hurry to leave she had neglected to return to Ron. Before she could get it out, Ron opened the door. He looked at them both without speaking.

'I forgot Milly,' said Lucille.

'She also forgot her dress,' added Rose. 'You know,the one you were telling me about. The one that Grainne gave her.'

'So?'

'So she'd just like to pop upstairs and get that as well, if you don't mind.'

'I do mind. I'm not having no perverts back in my house ever again.'

'Oh come on, after everything I've done for you. Ron, please.' Lucille implored. 'Can *you* get her then? Her lead's on the table.'

'I said, no.'

'Would you object if I came in and got her then, Mr Symes?' Rose asked. 'I can get the dress at the same time. I'm sure I could find it.' She turned to Lucille and playing up the maiden aunt role said, 'Where did you say it was dear? In Grainne's wardrobe, wasn't it?' She turned back to Ron as if he couldn't possibly refuse. 'I wonder if you could show me where it is, Mr Symes?'

'No I fucking couldn't. I'm not having some old tart coming into my house neither, looking through my girlfriends things. No.' He looked at Lucille peculiarly. 'Your mutt's asleep. I put her down. She's in the bin.' He made a simple cut throat motion with his hand and shut the door.

Rose stifled something between a gasp and a scream. Lucille didn't. 'You fucking bastard,' she shrieked, 'you bastard.' She banged on the door with the back of both fists, then leaned her head on it before pulling it back as if she wanted to bang her head against it Instead she collapsed to the ground and sat on the doorstep sobbing. 'My baby, my poor baby,' she cried. Rose sat down beside her with her arm around her shoulders. After a minute or two Lucille asked her if she had a tissue.

'I've got some in the car.'

They got up and walked slowly back to the car. As they did so they heard the sound of an upstairs window opening and the dress came flying through air and landed soundlessly on the ground, followed by Milly's lead. Rose went back for them and picked them up. She felt inside the pockets of the dress. The note wasn't there. She looked up and saw Ron slowly and deliberately hold up one fat finger at them both.

Chapter 3.

Grainne O'Riordan got home at ten p.m. She felt exhausted and tired. It had been a long hard shift and when it was done she had felt no desire whatsoever to return to a house which she was sure would feel as good as empty now Lucie was gone.

Two years ago when Lucie had kindly helped her up off the soggy grass to sit down on a bench after she had slipped on some mud while out walking in the park, she wouldn't have dreamed that the pale slender boy with the shaven head and the big frightened eyes who told her he had been sleeping rough in the bushes for the previous two nights, would have ended up staying with her and Ron for so long, and eventually leave with an auburn mop of crimped hair looking even better in her clothes than she did, for god's sake! She could not have imagined that the simple offer to put him up for a few nights would have led to a friendship that had come to mean so much to her.

At that time she had only been living with Ron for four months. He had changed so much too. Back then when she was twenty two and Ron twenty seven he had seemed so glamorous with his dark hair and black beard, his leathers and his Triumph motorcycle. He hadn't had a paunch then either. She used to love riding pillion behind him on sunny summer Sundays, huddling down away from the wind, her cheek against his back and believing he was the kind of man and this was kind of life she had always dreamed of back in Belfast where everything was smaller and wetter and colder. It just wasn't fair or funny how adolescent dreams could trick you into embracing a reality which actually turned out to be worse than the one you were trying to get away from.

As she struggled to put her key in the front door, she dropped the plastic bag containing the chips and doner kebabs she had bought for Ron and herself. She cursed, feeling almost hysterical. She hadn't had a period for two weeks. Earlier, in the middle of the day on her way to work she had stopped off at a chemist for a pregnancy testing kit. Over the next eight hours she had hardly been able to concentrate on the patients at work at all, bustling about mechanically in a thick soup of dread. No-one had seemed to notice. They were all too busy. One or two of the patients had remarked she wasn't her usual cheery self today, but she attended to their clinical needs perfectly and politely, had not let herself be drawn into responding. She had had to resist the urge to take the test there and then for fear of a result that might have left her feeling unable to cope. She hadn't wanted to let her two colleagues down, one of whom was still a student. The ward was too full and too demanding for her to go off sick in the middle of a shift.

But she didn't want Ron's baby and she just couldn't have an abortion.

It was as simple as that. In principle and in the pub she was right on and progressive about a woman's right to choose, but in practice she felt that for her at least, there was no choice at all. To have an abortion would not be against her moral ideology in any way, despite her Catholic upbringing, but it would be to go against all her own natural feelings. You just didn't hack into your body because you didn't like how it was or what it was doing, especially when it involved another little human being.

She let herself in, hoping Ron wasn't going to pester her for attention. He had become more and more strange recently. And even his sexual ardour which had used to be fairly incessant had dropped off over the last few weeks. But damn, damn, damn, the last time they had had sex together they had both been drunk and stoned, didn't remember to use contraception until it was too late. And it had happened right in the middle of her cycle. Since then there hadn't been even a hint of a period coming on, either physically or emotionally. Usually, almost without fail, she would find herself moody and irritable for a day or so just before it was due. But now she was two weeks late and – nothing.

She took her coat off and hung it on the hook behind the door. Tatty, and too small. Even if she wasn't going to turn out to be pregnant. She and Ron ate crap food all the time and drank too much beer. She was a size sixteen if she was really honest. She had bought the coat two years ago when she was still a twelve.

'Uh, hello Grainne,' Ron called from the front room having heard her come in despite having the telly on loud enough to split her headache in two. 'Lukey-Lucie's gone. Off to his or her new life.'

'Her new life. And her name is Lucille.' Grainne shouted back, and leaving the chips and kebabs still in their plastic bag on the kitchen table, she ran upstairs with the pregnancy testing kit hidden in her handbag.

'Dinner's on the table,' she shouted down to him, 'can you keep mine warm for me. I'll be down in ten minutes.'

She went into their dingy bedroom and shutting the door behind her got out of her uniform. She had to put some wee into a test tube. If the transparent window on the side didn't change colour she would be alright, not pregnant, just late. If it went blue then that was it. She would be pregnant and her life would be changed for good unless she was to miscarry. She crossed the landing to the loo in her underwear as if she was walking underwater. She really did not want to have to be doing this at all. She pulled down her knickers, sat on the loo, removed the tester from of its sterile inner wrapping and followed the instructions carefully, as if she wasn't a nurse at all and as if collecting samples was something she had never done in her life before. The result would take a few minutes to show. More than half of her just didn't want to know.

34

She left the test tube on the sink and went back to her room and looked at herself in the mirror. She looked five months pregnant already, she thought, trying to ignore the great folds of flab under her arms and over her hips. She pulled her tummy in, ignoring the livid long cuts she had deliberately made on it because she hated it so much. She had also taken to cutting her thighs which she felt were just as gruesome. And as for her gargantuan cellulitic bum, it just didn't bear looking at.

So she never did. Every time she took a bath recently she would shave her legs with Ron's old fashioned razor, and then to punish their pink, white and freckled grossness she would take the blade out of the razor and slice a series of long horizontal lines across the front of her thighs. Not deep. They would heal up. They usually didn't even need a steri-strip, let alone sutures. She knew what she was doing. She was a nurse. Nobody could see them, except Ron and when he had tried to remonstrate with her she had simply told him to shut up – it was her body and it was none of his business. He had always done what he was told. She was a classic pear, or would be if she wasn't so bosomy. Small neck and shoulders beneath an almost tiny freckled face and pale ginger hair, but breasts which looked ready to feed a baby right now, and great handfuls of rippling fat around her tummy and hips – enough to feed a whole army of babies. But worst of all was her bum which she tried to avoid ever looking at all if she could possibly help it. Especially at times like this, in her bra and knickers or naked. Men seemed to quite like it though. Ron was forever trying to stroke her or pat her on it, which was more often a nuisance than it was welcome, but perhaps it meant she was not as unattractive as she felt. Then again, she knew what men were like. They'd fuck anything. So she only discouraged him half the time.

She looked at her watch. The test would probably be ready now. Then she saw what looked like a small lilac envelope half hidden under the cupboard she used for a wardrobe. What was that doing there? She bent and picked it up and saw her name written in Lucie's handwriting across the front of it. It must be a goodbye note probably. That was sweet of her. But how come it had found its way down there? She'd open it in a minute. First she had to get the result of that test. That fucking test.

And test the result of their fucking.

No, on second thoughts she wouldn't. She didn't want to know for as long as it was possible not to.

'Are you coming down for these chips or what?' Ron called from the bottom of the stairs.

She put on a dressing gown, went back to the bathroom and picked up the tester without looking at it. Later, after she had eaten would be better. She placed it together with Lucie's note on the small high table in the corner of the bedroom between her make-up bag and mirror. After she had eaten there need be no distractions. She could just concentrate on her feelings. She went downstairs to join Ron.

He was already eating, straight from the paper like an animal.

'Couldn't you have got some plates out?'

'I haven't had time to wash them up yet. They're all in the sink.'

'Been busy then? Doing what?'

He did nothing when he was home nowadays, except slob about. Lucie had done everything around the house for them. She enjoyed it, she'd said. And it was true. She'd loved playing at being the little housewife. Grainne couldn't blame her for it. Stereotypes could be such a comfort to those that needed them. Grainne certainly hadn't complained about it. It was great having someone who actually enjoyed doing the washing up and the tidying.

'Sorry. I forgot. I was too tired.'

'Did Lucie leave alright? Or were you sleeping at the time?'

'You pissed off with me or something? You're always pissed off with me.'

'Ron! That's not fair. But I can't be bothered to argue with you. You've got a bit of onion in your beard.'

What had she ever seen in him?

'That woman who said she was her auntie said she was going to take her under her wing and help her every way she could. Lulu was looking very happy. Never stopped smiling, neither of them, even when they was getting in her car. They had to come back though, forgot that dress you gave her.'

'What did she look like, the aunt?'

'I dunno. Average. Posh. I dunno. Anyway what's it matter?'

'It doesn't matter. I was just interested that's all.'

'She was wearing an old duffel coat. And jeans. You couldn't tell she was posh, but I knew, just from looking at her. I'm getting really good at knowing what people are like, Grainney. Even though I don't see much other people at work all day. Good isn't it, Grainney? Maybe I should change jobs, become a psychologist! Trouble is I'm getting tireder and tireder at work. Too fucking tired to do anything. I fell asleep with me blowtorch on today. Carl, the foreman, got so pissed off with me he said he'd sack me if I did it again. But I don't even notice I'm dropping off no more. It's like suddenly I'm just gone. Maybe I should see a doctor.'

'You ought to do more exercise, get fitter. That's your trouble. You're just letting yourself go.'

'Yeah. I gotta get rid of me beer belly.' He patted it complacently.

'You're making me feel sick.'

He wasn't really. She was well used to him, but she needed an excuse to get away from him, go and look at her result. She ate the last of her chips, got up heavily out of her chair, crumpled up the paper their food

36

had been wrapped in and threw it into his lap. He looked at her blankly. He had been giving her more and more of those vacant looks over the last few months. Like he was going soft in the head or something.

'You could tidy up a bit, Ron, that would give you some exercise. Anyway you're going to have to do more around the house now Lucie has gone. We both are.'

'Uh, oh yeah. It was good having, like, a maid around the house.' He laughed.

Grainne snorted, went back upstairs straight to the loo. Without having to put her finger down her throat she bent over the toilet bowl and silently vomited her doner and chips into it. She was getting quite good at this, she thought with some satisfaction. She had only started doing it a couple of months ago after the sight of herself in the mirror had revolted her so much that she had a revelation. She decided that she would kill two birds with one stone, eat to excess but maybe lose two or three stone in the process! She might actually become what Ron so sexistly called her already, a nice looking bird. Which she wouldn't mind, if she was honest, she just didn't want to have to diet to do it. It wasn't as if she didn't actually like food. This plan allowed her to eat as much as she wanted. Or even more, because she could always sick it all up afterwards! She could continue to enjoy the pleasures of eating and drinking without any of the flab-forming consequences.

So that's what she did. At first only in the evenings after her tea, but recently she had taken to doing it mornings as well. Disappointingly she had not seemed to lose any weight though. In fact last time she'd dared to stand on the scales she had actually put some on. She couldn't believe it. It had had to be water. It couldn't be the Mars Bars and Twix she had between meals. She only ate one or two of those at most each day. But anyway, it didn't matter, because she was going to start taking laxatives now as well. That would make the difference. Her weight would soon come down. Then maybe could she look for a way to start a new life.

New life.

Spare her from having conceived new life in her belly. She never prayed anymore, but she found herself doing so now to a god she didn't believe in as she cleaned her teeth to get the taste of the vomit out of her mouth. She didn't want to be a milch cow for somebody else, even if it was her own little somebody else.

She just wasn't ready for motherhood.

She went into the bedroom and picked up the test tube.

Blue.

Right.

Bright blue. Impossibly bright blue.

Alright. So what? It didn't matter. She couldn't have an abortion, but she could miscarry couldn't she? Especially if she was eating and drinking and making herself sick everyday. Yes, miscarriage – That was the answer. It would be important to pre-empt any possibility of morning sickness by continuing to induce vomiting herself. She wouldn't be able to bear pregnancy making her feel sick. That would mean everything was working normally down there and that the baby was growing healthily. She couldn't have that. She would take up smoking, eat and drink far too much, make herself sick and sick and sick until the foetus pressed the abort button itself.

In fact it could be a wonderful challenge! Pregnancy could be the perfect excuse for doing everything to excess until such time as she became un-pregnant again.

She picked up Lucie's lilac billet doux and lay down on the bed.

There was her mother to think about too. Nice Catholic girls from Belfast still weren't allowed to have babies without being married, unless they wanted to be isolated from their whole family and live somewhere far away in ignominy and shame. Her mother didn't even know she and Ron lived together, let alone slept in the same bed.

She felt tears beginning to trickle down the sides of her cheeks, wiped them away more in astonishment then anger. Lachrymal secretions, that's all they were. She never cried. Not worth a penny, crying. There was a lot her mother didn't know. Her mother didn't know about all the tears she couldn't cry about what her brother Uncle Jack used to do to her every time he came to baby sit when she was a little girl. Her mother didn't know he told her he was a member of the IRA and if she ever told her Ma or Da what he had been doing to her, or that he was an IRA man, he would save a bomb that would be better used on the fucking prods and blow them all up instead. All of them, Ma, Da, her little twin sisters Aislinn and Siobhain, and her. Even though it would break his heart to do so.

She had only realised he was bullshitting by the time she was fourteen and he had been doing his disgusting thing with her for six whole years. She been able to tell him where to go after that, but she had never told her mother what had been going on for the shame of it, and the fear that it would upset her so much she might never get over it. That was why she had eventually decided to come to England. To get away from always having to pretend in front of Ma, always having to work to keep her happy. She had 'nerves' Ma did. Always had, ever since she first became pregnant with Grainne when she was twenty four.

Mary Mother of God, as Ma would say! I'm the same age she was when she was pregnant with me.

Ron was coming up the stairs. She jumped up off the bed and ran over to the table with the pregnancy test on it and hurriedly palming it, stuffed it into her bag. When he came into the room she was brushing her hair.

'You look good enough to eat.'

'Fuck off, Ron.'

'That's what Lulu said when she left. 'Fuck off Ron'. 'Fuck off Ron'. It should be written on my gravestone when I die, that should.' He laughed.

Then he lay on the bed which creaked beneath his weight, and patting the space beside him beckoned her to join him.

'Come on, darlin. You look fucking gorgeous. Let's have a bit of nookey.'

As a seduction technique guaranteed to turn her off immediately, it ranked down there with his unashamed farting and ball-scratching. It was a wonder she had never had thrush.

'I'm not interested in having sex at the moment Ron. I thought you weren't either. We haven't had it for the last three and a half weeks. What's made you suddenly come over all randy?'

But he had found Lulu's note lying on the bed beside him.

'What's this then?' He said picking it up as if to open it.

'It's mine. From Lucie. Leave it alone. I haven't read it yet.'

He leered at it her.

'I'll read it to you.'

He made as if to tear it open, but didn't do so. He was teasing her, inviting her to come and get it. She gave him an exasperated sigh.

'You can hardly read anyhow,' she said. 'But be my guest. Feel free. Invade my privacy. Open my letters. Go on.'

His face fell. That wasn't what he had wanted. Good. He put the little envelope back down on her pillow. She put down her brush, walked over to her side of their bed and reached out to take it. He grabbed her wrist. She yanked it away angrily and he looked downcast again. She put it under her pillow and sat down on the bed.

'I'm sorry Ron, I'm just not in the mood for games.'

'You're too good for me, Grainney, and you're too brainy. It's not working between us anymore is it? There's something wrong with me. I'm not who I was and I don't do it for you anymore, do I?

Well that was true. But his saying it made her soften. She bent and kissed him on his forehead thinking at least somebody wants me. He put his arms around her and she let him pull her down beside him. Not just for old time's sake. Perhaps sex would jog the foetus into changing its mind. She would incite him to give her a little bit of rough. After all, that was part of his charm in the first place. Not too much. She hated pain unless she was inflicting it on herself, when she somehow managed to detach herself from it. But if he could overcome his tiredness sufficiently to fuck her energetically enough, you never knew, it might trigger a miscarriage. After all, most miscarriages occurred within the first few weeks of pregnancy, so she knew it was well worth a try.

39

She felt his hand work its way beneath her knickers and grab hold of her left bum cheek. She would encourage him by making appreciative noises and showing an interest in his penis. He yanked a breast from out of her brassiere and started sucking on it. She reached underneath his belly trying to get her hand down his trousers to his dick, but he was so fat that there was no room between his belt and his barrel-shaped stomach. She voiced her frustration.

'We're both too porky, Ron.'

'You're not,' he said, tugging at his belt and undoing his button.

She reached down, and unzipping him took hold of his sex. It felt a bit sweaty and even from up here beside his undeodarised armpits, it reeked.

'I wish you would wear underpants. You are so unhygienic, Ron. I don't like it. It's not nice.'

'You're not,' he said again, 'not not nice, I mean,' he added before returning his mouth to her breasts.

He was not a good lover in the sense of being attuned to her needs in any way, but he was passionate and they had been sexual partners long enough for him to know she preferred plenty of clitoral attention before letting him enter her so that she could try to get used to the idea of intercourse. All too often his sexual greed meant that he was in too much of a hurry and she wasn't ready for him physically either. His penis was not short and penetration always made her feel uncomfortable and sore. She often still felt sore and bruised for days afterwards after he was done with her. Which invariably brought back memories of Uncle Jack.

So she rarely, if ever, enjoyed full sexual intercourse, but right now she didn't care about that. She just wanted him to get it in as deeply and as roughly as he chose.

'Come inside me. Rough me about a bit. Don't really hurt me, mind. Not badly, I mean.'

She dug her nails into the base of his penis to encourage him.

He started to mount her immediately, still in his T-shirt and trousers. The weight of him and the smell of his unwashed body had, as usual, to be grimly ignored. Her vagina was dry and tight and, also as usual, she lacked any feeling as he entered her. Once he was in and she was no longer so dry, she settled her hips and cervix down around his penis as much as she could and moved beneath him responsively so that his ardour would be excited and increased. Grinding as he bumped.

For ten minutes or so he had the energy to thrust in and out like there was no tomorrow. As he did so Grainne ignored all the terrible old childhood feelings of being violated again. Instead she was praying once more. This time her prayer was that his dick would set off the miracle of spontaneous abortion. After all there would be some justice if he was to be the cause of her miscarriage given that he was the one who was responsible for having fertilised her in the first place. She didn't know if her mother used to pray during sex, but she found herself desperate for her as he banged away, and in some peculiar nameless manner felt joined with her in praying now.

Once he finally came she pushed him off immediately and went to the bathroom to wash. She wanted his sperm out straight away. After she put the towel back on the rail she took hold of the razor lying on the side of the sink and gave one tentative superficial little slice to herself just above her pubic hair. Not enough to draw more than a thin red line, but just sufficient to feel the sensation of the blade passing through her skin. Although it wasn't sexual it gave her much more satisfaction than Ron's lovemaking had done. He was in the middle of the bed snoring when she returned to the bedroom. She nudged him awake, told him to get undressed properly, move over and get under the bed covers. He grunted but didn't stir. She started trying to push him over to his side of the bed so that at least she could get in under the duvet herself. Eventually he woke up enough to struggle under it too, still in his clothes.

His habits and behaviour were becoming more and more antisocial.

Lying on her back Grainne stared at the ceiling and listened to him snoring. What kind of life was this? Something had to change.

But a baby was not the kind of change she envisaged at all. Definitely not. In fact she didn't actually have a vision. Not like Lucie, who had always known exactly what she wanted and had now gone off to get it. Good luck to her. She would miss her. They had had a lot of laughs together. Why couldn't she be like her? But she wasn't.

Grainne only knew what she didn't want. She didn't want any of this. She didn't want to be sharing her life with a somnambulant lump whose only interest was in occasional sex. What had happened to his motorbike? He had dismantled it alright, but had never put it back together again. He went to work every day on the bus now! Where was the proud bastard whose tongue used to be as sharp as his dick was long? Gone somehow. Was it her fault? Had living with her done this to him? If so, that was a reason to leave him in itself. He needed to get his act together. It was almost like she wasn't his girlfriend any more, so much as his mother, looking after him. Perhaps that was why she had been thinking about her own mother while they had been bonking. Maybe he was developing CJD or something, the amount of burgers he put away. Whatever, since they had been living together his physical girth had increased as his personality had diminished. There was no question of it, mentally he was now a sad shadow of his former self.

So even if she had wanted it, there was no way he was adequate to the task of being the father of her child. She prayed again. Please God, Mary, Joseph and all the saints, may my body reject this fertilised egg.

It felt curiously, if satisfyingly strange to invoke all this long-abandoned Christian iconography. Not so much because she didn't believe in any of it anymore, but because it was a way of connecting with her mother again, with the need to feel safe, looked after and cared for. Even as she knew it to be a delusion.

She took Lucie's note from under her pillow and used a finger nail to open it.

'Dear Grainne,

I want to thank you! For everything! For letting me live with you these last two years. For being so kind. For being so understanding. For being so much fun. For being such a good friend to me. I hope we can go on being friends forever. You are the best friend I ever had. Ever! Except for my mum. I love you like I love her, with all my heart!.

I have to tell you something that I couldn't tell you to your face. I was too frightened. Of him and of what it would do to you if I told you. He said he'd cut my face if I ever did tell you. But I've got to now or I wouldn't ever be able to be your friend again.

This is it. Take a deep breath, darling: Since the end of September when you went away on that training weekend, Ron's been forcing me give him head whenever he gets me alone. I'm so sorry, Grainne. I never wanted to. He made me, said he'd hurt both of us if I didn't.

There. The truth isn't between us anymore, and our friendship, which means more to me than anything, can maybe go on !!!???

I'm so sorry. Please forgive me,

with loads of love from your friend,

Lucille xxx.

p.s. I will ring you in a few days. If you can bear to talk to me. Luv

L.

Grainne let the note fall to the floor beside the bed and found herself staring at the ceiling again. Her hands knotting together on top of her tummy as the contents of the note sunk in. She felt herself getting angrier and angrier.

With Lucie more than Ron. Why hadn't Lucie trusted her? She should have told her. She should have. Of course she should have. All that lovey-dovey stuff in the letter was so much shit. If she was her friend then she really should have told her. *She* would have, if it had been the other way round. And if she couldn't tell her before, why bother telling her now? In a letter. What was the point? Because she couldn't say it to her face? To get it off her conscience?

In that case she had probably enjoyed it.

Yes, looking back on it, the way they had always talked about men together, of course she had enjoyed it. She had always claimed to be as frightened as she was attracted by the very idea of a man, but in fact she was always talking about them. Always. In that irritatingly coy yet blatant way of hers she actually loved the idea of a dick, didn't she? As long as it wasn't on her. In fact she had wanted one so much she had gone and helped herself to hers. Cowardly little bitch. Bitch!

Well, that was that then. She didn't want to have anything more to do with her.

Grainne started shivering even though sweat was pouring from her. She felt like she was made of stone and jelly at one and the same time. Because overriding everything was the terrible and terrifying fact of being pregnant.

She got out of bed again and staggered to the bathroom. She wanted to swallow all the pills in the house. Not to kill herself. To get away. To make the foetus fail. To punish Lucie and Ron. To have stomach cramps and poisoned blood so that the sensations in her body were the same as her feelings. But she couldn't do that. Not now anyway. She had to get away. She was on a late shift tomorrow. She would spend the morning packing her things and go and find a room in the nurses residence block at work until she could find another job and another place to live.

She screwed her hands up into fists and started hitting herself in the tummy and lower abdomen. Systematically and as hard as she could. She didn't notice the tears streaming down her face because she was too busy punching. Then she picked up the razor blade and this time very deliberately pushed it in to her tummy button; keeping the pressure on, she cut a deep line out towards her right hip. She found herself smiling and whimpering as she did so, but the great thing was her mind was on nothing else as she did it. She was completely focused, exquisitely diverted from everything, absolutely everything, except the sensation of her skin splitting open. She took a deep breath as the blood took a moment to well up and start seeping. At the sight of it she felt a granite satisfaction then dabbed at it with cotton wool for a minute or two before almost regretfully steri-stripping the cut together again.

She was so efficient from start to finish.

Chapter 4.

Eighteen months later, Lucille was going to see her mother. It was her first visit since her final surgery seven weeks ago. She had arranged it for an evening when Papa was out at a work leaving do. She hadn't seen him for well over three and a half years, and didn't want to either. She had tried to see Mum at least two or three times every month over the last year finding the thought of losing their secret closeness almost unbearable. It had been awful having had no face to face contact with her for more than two months, but Mum had used her smallest most frightened voice on the telephone to say Papa wouldn't allow it. Lucie understood. She and Mum knew each other's suffering. They always had. As a child Luke had been very clingy and looked just like her. People often used to remark that they were like one person which had always pleased both of them to the point of absolute smugness.

Wanting to look her best, Lucille had spent almost as long getting ready as she used to do in the days before her body had been altered to fit the shape of her mind. At that time she had been so anxious about being found out that she would spend literally hours on her face and hair and clothes until she could be satisfied no-one could know she was not what she seemed. But now that she actually was, or as much as she ever could be, she only took an hour or so getting ready in the mornings.

Today she had taken advantage of getting her hair done for free at work first thing, and then spent the afternoon bathing and pampering herself. Baths had always used to be a nightmare because of the inescapable horror of what was between her legs and the frightening flatness of her chest. Now they were okay. She could lie back with the hot tap running slowly, enjoying the feeling of the water gently swirling around her, luxuriating in the unremarkable normality of the fit between her nakedness and her natural sense of self. Normal. Just like anyone else. It was in the bath over these last few weeks that she most felt as if she had finally woken up from a horrible dream.

Now, on the train to Mum in Morden wearing a demure, but still stylish, dark blue Katherine Hamnett suit with a flared three-quarter length skirt and a close-fitting little jacket, which she had bought second-hand, but still perfect, from the local hospice charity shop, she felt a sense of closure, of her childhood having ended. In strappy heels and the Prada handbag she'd proudly bought to celebrate going into hospital for the last time, she felt she looked a little bit older than she was. But that was alright, it made up for the fact that actually her womanliness was only seven weeks old. But it didn't really matter how old she looked, she knew her mother would approve of her. That was the important thing.

Walking from the station to the terraced house she had lived in till she was sixteen, she savoured the sensation of just being an ordinary, attractive young woman going home to see her mum, and looking her best. She didn't want there to be anything more or less to her than that.

'Hi Mum.' She held out a little pot of African Violets she had bought her on the way.

Emily Farouk, nee Shaw, was a small white woman with broad hips, short, dyed blond hair and world-weary eyes which briefly lit up after she opened the door before reverting to their customary heaviness. She had turned forty-four this year and looked her age despite her neat appearance and the large amount of foundation she covered her face with. Dressed in a brown knee-length skirt and a dark green jumper, Lucie felt proud of her. She was still pretty and still looked after herself despite her lifelong addiction to prescription sleeping pills and anti-depressants. If she would never have the posh husband or the Country Life mock-Tudor pile she had once dreamed of, she could still look the part. She took the flower with a smile and stepped back to stare at Lucie before letting her in.

'You look lovely, darling, come inside. No. Stop looking so worried. He's not here. You know I wouldn't do that to either of you without proper preparation.'

Her mother put the kettle on and got out a cake from the fridge.

'So how are you? No! Don't tell me. I can see by the look on your face you are fine.'

'I'm me now, Mum. All over.' She wiggled her hips, patting them proudly, eyes shining. It might mean nothing to everyone else to be themselves, but for her it was everything. A dream come true. A dream which only her mother had ever really understood.

'I'm so glad, Lucie. And you look so happy. I never could bear the sadness in your lovely emerald eyes when you were little. And now I can see that it is finally gone. I'm so happy for you, darling. You'd have made a terrible man!'

They both laughed.

'I always loved you for knowing that, Mum.' She kissed her on both cheeks. 'I always loved dressing up and dancing for you so much, pretending I was your little girl. Just so you could see that everything could be alright. Well now it is, It finally is, and I am your little girl.'

The pride and satisfaction in her mother's eyes as she looked at her vindicated everything. They squeezed hands for a moment.

'Yes, you make a lovely young woman! Not that you weren't a beautiful child, mind you! But it was such a shame you were always so sad behind your smiles when you were little. I'm sure it was because you were depressed that you never did as well as you could have at school. '

Lucille didn't want to go there. As far as she was concerned she had been unhappy, yes, but only about her gender, and that was all. It was Mum who had been depressed. It was just that because she loved her, Lucie had always found her sadness catching, as if it was her that had caused Mum to be depressed. So it had always and without fail made her somehow feel anxious and depressed that Mum was anxious and depressed.

'But I did alright, Mum! I did like drama. And history and French. I did do well at all of them. Do you remember the shows I put on for you when I was little?' She said, trying to lighten the mood.

'I do! I do indeed. In fact just now I was reminding myself of them, knowing you were on your way. The tele's just been fixed, you know. The repair man left just a few minutes ago. And I couldn't help remembering that time Papa got mad with you when you were – I don't know – you must have been five or six. It was after school. You were in that nice Mrs Woolsey's class at the time. He was mad because you'd taken a kitchen knife to the box his new telly had come in. You made some kind of theatre show with it. Do you remember? With all your Barbies? And you'd borrowed one of my scarves, made it into a little skirt and drawn Barbies with great care in thick felt-pen all over the outside of the box. Dream Barbie's Magic show, you called it, or some such silliness. Papa found you with it under the kitchen table and got so angry. His brand spanking new telly wouldn't work and he was worried he'd have to take it back to the shop in its original packaging or they wouldn't swop it for him. But he didn't want to. Not with Barbies all over it! He was so embarrassed. The silly man!'

They both laughed at this, but Lucille really had no recollection.

'I had to do it myself in the end. What a day that was. I wonder what ever happened to Mrs Woolsey. She must have retired years ago, I dare say. I was late picking you up from school and she took advantage of getting me on her own to tell me about your interest in dolls and drama and dressing up!' She laughed. 'And how the girls all liked you, but the boys didn't. As if I didn't know! Perhaps she thought I was stupid or something. She also had the effrontery to tell me not to worry about you because it was probably just a phase you were going through. Little she knew! And do you know, I hadn't actually *been* worried about you at all until she said that. I was proud! After that, I must confess I did worry for you when you were out of my sight sometimes. Ah, well.'

She cut the cake and the old magical mother and child silence worked its way between them, holding them together like it always had. They smiled at each other, saying nothing, just feeling it, Lucille basking in the pleasure of her mother's gaze. It was what she had always liked best as a child. More than anything.

'How is Papa?' She eventually managed to ask. If there was one thing she could not understand it was why Mum hadn't turfed him out or left herself long ago.

'More bad tempered than ever I'm afraid, always finding something else to work himself up into a state about. He never mentions you, I am sad to say. But I tell him anyway. And do you know, inspite of himself he always listens. Silly man,' she said again, almost sounding fond of him.

Lucille tried to understand that. Somewhere deep within she could probably still find some love for him herself if she looked very hard, hidden in the little nooks and crannies of her past. But he was more than a silly man, they both knew that. He was a violent man when he was drunk, and too often veered frighteningly between sentimentality and aggression. The silences Mum had shared with her as a child had not only been companionable in a gentle sense. They had often been ones of stunned shock after Papa had hit one of them.

Some things they hadn't shared. Mum would never know what had prompted her to run away, aged sixteen, and stay with Ron and Grainne. Papa had unexpectedly gone into her bedroom one morning to look for some scissors and found her – him as he was then – asleep in curlers and an old nylon baby-doll nightie Mum had thrown out. He had pulled him out of bed and told him to take it off. When there was no response, just a dumb insolent glare from beneath tackily mascara'd, overly shadowed eyes, Papa who was himself wearing only the top half of his pyjamas, roared and started trying to pull the nightdress off him, still holding the scissors in his hand. How Mum hadn't heard she never knew. They had ended up on the floor with Luke underneath and Papa straddling him holding the scissors up in the air as if to stab him. Perhaps it was his rage which had caused his father to have an erection. To be fair to him, when he realised the state he was in and what he was doing, he got off immediately and left the room, scissors in hand and big black member rapidly detumescing, without saying another word. Neither of them told Mum, who had been downstairs at the time. So all she ever knew was that later on that same day when Luke had dressed, Papa grabbed him by his naturally wavy, shoulder-length hair and pulled him screaming out to the car. Then he'd driven him to the men's barber shop he went to himself, with a red and white spiralled cylinder out the front, and ordered what he called a proper army haircut. Luke ran away that night and two days later moved in with Grainne and Ron. Mum secretly paid the rent out of her savings till Luke found a hairdressing job.

'Tell him I would like to see him one day, Mum, please. I mean I'm not Luke anymore, am I? Even though I do still have nightmares about it sometimes. No! don't tell him that. I don't want to upset him. Just tell him that I'm happy to be me and it would be nice to see him again one day.'

Hearing herself saying this it seemed quite unbelievable. Nevertheless, at the same time, a tight little ball of pain, as hard and heavy as lead, which had been lodged in her tummy for as long as she could remember, suddenly evaporated into nothing. Like sherbert on the tongue. Pfft. It completely disappeared. The sense of release made her light-headed as she noticed one of Papa's pipes sitting in an ashtray over the fireplace and found herself wishing he was here to hold her and tell her everything was alright now. She gave Mum a dizzy smile. Mum nodded her head and patted the back of her hand seeing something had happened, but seeing too that she was alright. Lucille turned her hand over and held Mum's tight for a moment. Mum had always been able to see her.

'Oh I'm so glad!' said Emily Farouk. 'You are growing up, aren't you, my darling? It makes me so sad the way you two haven't spoken to one another. If he could just accept you now, he would be proud. He'd have to be – you're such a lovely-looking girl,' she repeated. 'Lovely.' Mum peered over her glasses at her, wrinkling her nose in that characteristic way of hers and beaming with a bright desperation, like the sun in November.

'Do you think he might want to see me?'

'Of course he would. He just doesn't know it, that's all. But I'll tell him and eventually he will know I'm right and see reason. We both realised you were, unusual, as soon as you began insisting on wearing my shoes as a toddler. We did talk about it sometimes. He of course, was very disturbed by your girlishness. As I was not. You were only being yourself. In fact the more disturbed he was about it, somehow the prouder I felt about you. But I think – No! I *know* that in his own way he did agree that children need to be loved and accepted. But he didn't agree with me that you can't change a person's nature. I think part of the problem is he resents me because you have proved me right by doing what you've done. And like all men – as I am sure you will find out – he hates being wrong. And to be fair to him, he did actually buy the flowers we sent you when you were in hospital being, er, you know.

'Being repaired, Mum.'

'Mm.Yes, exactly. So who knows what he's made of you in his own mind! He knows how *I* feel: I am proud of you. I truly am. You've finally found your inner peace. I can see that in your eyes. Your true self. You always needed my help to connect with *that* when you were little. You had to have your little things out of my bottom drawer when he was out, otherwise you'd get all mopey and miserable about being like *him*, and then you were impossible. Absolutely impossible.'

'I want to let the past go now, Mum,' Lucie replied frowning, even now feeling uncomfortable at the very mention of having once been like her father. Her mother caught her glance, changed the subject.

'Everything is in working order, is it? Your body, I mean.'

'Yes, Mum. Thank you. I mean I think so,' she added, needing to share the touch of uncertainty she still felt. 'You know.'

Mum nodded.

'Is there a man? I mean a boyfriend? You're pretty enough. Although so you should be after all that cosmetic surgery.'

For a brief moment Lucie again felt the crushing shame about her body which had characterised her whole life before Rose had taken her in. She glanced down at herself for reassurance, looked up again immediately with a happy smile, said, 'If you'd had no proper boobs till you were nearly nineteen, you would have too. You would, Mum, you know you would have.'

'I wasn't talking about your breasts, you silly thing.' She reached over and gently tapped Lucie on her nose and chin. 'I meant your face. It was pretty enough already, if you ask me. But don't worry, it's still lovely. I mean lovelier still, I suppose.' She arched an eyebrow at Lucie. 'Well?'

'No, Mum. I haven't got a boyfriend.'

'I suppose you want one of course. You haven't done what you've done not to have a man, have you?'

'Mum! I didn't have operations just to have sex! You know that.'

'And you certainly didn't have them not to have it, either. You won't fool either of us if you pretend otherwise. You're not going to tell me that after everything you have been through, you're one of those lipstick lesbians now, are you?'

'No, of course not! But there's no-one at the moment. I'd love it if there was, cos I won't, you know, really *know* everything's alright till I've actually got a boyfriend. But I'm quite happy, at least I'm me now. So I've got everything I want in this world, really.'

As Lucille spoke she saw two large tears welling up into the corners of her mother's eyes. A moment later they proceeded to roll down her powdered cheeks in a slow, almost stately manner.

'You're a little monster, Lucie. I don't mean to upset you, but you are. Here you are finally yourself. And I am proud of you, I really am. But you're a little monster as well, you know. Because nobody can have *everything* they want in this world without being one. Nobody. And people who've got everything they want always upset all the rest of us who haven't. So be very careful, my darling. Especially of men. Men like chasing monsters.'

The tears dried up as soon as they emerged, but Lucille's bubble was pricked and without knowing why she found herself wanting to weep too. But much as she might want to, she never cried if she could help it, it always made her face all puffy and blotchy. She got up, took their cups and plates to the sink and began compulsively washing up. She'd learned that from Rose.

'I was always going to be a monster, Mum, whatever I did,' she said, taking time with the suds, going over and over each item she washed, not wanting her mother to see how wounded she felt. 'And I couldn't live with the monster I was. So I didn't really have a choice when it came down to it, did I?'

'I know dear, I know. You don't have to tell me. But that's not what I mean. Let me tell you something. Being able to have sex with a man and being able to have his babies are two very different things; a woman's ovaries keep her in touch with the important things. For all the trouble they bring, and just by being there, they – I don't know – they make you careful. At least, I always thought so anyway. Because the future matters more in a funny kind of way, knowing what can happen if you're not careful. But I'm never going to be a grandma, because you are a not a real woman inside that perfect little female exterior of yours. Oh no! No, hen, this time I *am* sorry. I didn't mean that horribly at all. Please don't be hurt. You're my beautiful daughter now, of course you are! I just meant you will never be able to have children, that's all. And you may not know it now, but that *will* matter to you one day, and when it does you will be in less danger. And less of a danger to others. Till then, as your mother, I fear for you.

'There's always HIV and AIDs to worry about too, of course.'

'Mum! Please. I'm not interested in having sex with gay men! Not at all. And I'm sure they wouldn't be interested in me. Maybe before. But certainly not now.'

'No dear, I quite see your point. But it's not just a gay disease anymore, is it? But anyway that's not what I am trying to say! So don't distract me. What I am trying to say is if you ever do find a nice man one day, when you are older and want to settle down with him, it will be hard not being able to have his children.' She shrugged. 'That's all.'

'Well I can adopt some then! A little boy, a little girl, and maybe, a little tranny!'

'You're being facetious now. Stop it please, Lucille.'

'She or he would have a mother who could understand. Like I did! But seriously Mum, it does matter to me. It matters right now that I can't have children. It always has and it always will. I'd have given anything to be able to be a mum myself one day too, of course I would have. You know that. I wonder if they'll be able to do a genetic transplant one day. Wouldn't it be wonderful if I could have some of your eggs!'

They laughed at the notion and Lucie felt she was pleasing her mother again because the delicious little sigh of contentment that making Mum happy had always given her, was making her heart and cheeks glow in the familiar old way once more. She closed her eyes for a moment, basking in it. Then the plate she was doing slipped into the washing-up rack with a clatter. 'Whoops. Sorry, Mum! It's alright, don't worry, nothing's broken. And you mustn't worry about *me*. I'll be alright, really I will. I've never been so sure of it in my life!'

'I hope so, my darling. How is that woman you're living with, Rose?'

50

'Oh she's fine. I think she's feeling a bit like you, if you really want to know. Sort of happy and sort of sad. Sad that I don't need her in the same way as I did before. It was kind of like she adopted me.' Wanting to get back at Mum for calling her a monster just now, Lucie tried to make her feel just a tiny bit jealous of Rose, said, 'Anyway she's been like a second mother to me, really, letting me stay with her and paying for all my treatments and everything. It cost her nearly half her savings! Just for me.'

For some reason she didn't want to tell Mum about the coincidence of the names.

'I wonder what she wants back from you.'

'I don't know. Nothing. And it's not like that! She just wants my friendship, that's all. And she's got that. Forever.'

'Hmm. She's nearly my age, isn't she? I wonder what's she was doing befriending a – a child who wasn't one really anymore, and a boy who wasn't one really?'

She didn't add 'to make a girl who isn't one really', but it was left unspoken between them. And it stung.

It was like she was nothing. Lucie couldn't understand it. Having finally achieved her correct gender, something which both of them had always wanted for her, was Mum finally saying, or if not saying then *feeling* things towards her which she never felt before when she had still been a boy? It just didn't make any sense. Especially not when all her life Mum had done everything she could to encourage her femininity.

All her life.

Like when Mum found her on the bathroom floor wincing and busily trying to remove the frightening and hateful testes with her little gold sewing scissors. She couldn't have been more than five or six years old. Mum had swooped down, whisked her up onto her lap and wiped away the blood with cotton wool balls. It had only been a little nick and Mum whispered her understanding; told her she understood, promised it could happen one day, 'but you have to let doctors help you, dearest, when you're older. In the meantime I can buy you pretty dresses which you can wear when Papa is out and we can grow your hair long so that you can feel like a girl. Everything will be alright, chick, everything.' And again when she was a desperate, frightened thirteen year old, scared witless by the prospect of the irreversible changes adolescent maleness was about to bring, Mum let her start taking her contraceptive pills. She'd remembered they contained female hormones that dreadful day when the people at the Tavistock Clinic interviewed them both and then said there was nothing they could do to help until she was older except offer her counselling. Mum shouted and swore, told them that wasn't good enough, but they had been adamant. Afterwards when she was trying to stop herself from weeping and Mum was wiping her nose for her under the trees in the square outside, she shushed her and said she had a plan.

And as far as Lucie was concerned it had saved her life. A dreadful day became a wonderful day thanks to Mum. She was quite happy to rely on the rhythm method from now on, Mum told her, Papa being too drunk to want sex more than once in a blue moon, so Lucie could use her contractive pills as hormonal precursors until she was old enough to have a proper prescription. She was as good as her word, placing a pill on her tongue at bedtime each evening after that when she came in to her bedroom to kiss her goodnight. To some extent her plan worked. The contraceptives were probably responsible for her voice not breaking, and her remaining slight of stature, delicate of build, and very slightly, but definitely and very proudly breast-budded by the time she was fifteen.

Lucie felt herself frowning as she reminded herself of all this in the face of Mum now laying into her, almost telling her off just because she couldn't have babies. Perhaps she should be pleased, now everything was done, to be treated less sensitively by Mum, but it didn't actually feel very pleasurable. Not just at the minute. It felt odd and discomforting, as if finally living in the same sex and gender as her mother, she had also and confusingly dissolved the very tie that used to bind them together – the shared wish that this was how she should be.

'Look, Mum, I'm sorry, but this is beginning to upset me. Why are you going on at me? Would you like me to go?'

'I'm only trying to understand, Lucie, that's all. Come and give me another cuddle. I'm so lonely without you. Me and Papa have hardly said a word to each other since you went away. I really don't mean to be unkind! I know I am, but I do not mean to be. Do you understand? I'm saying sorry to you, hen.'

Mum narrowed her eyes in that way that Lucie knew meant she might be sorry, yes, but she wasn't ever going to back down.

'What you have never realised,' Mum continued, 'is that I have always fought for you, fought for who you are and what you want because I love you. Don't think for a moment that I didn't want a son. I did. I really did. But you were you. From the moment you were born I knew when they said you were a boy that they were wrong. You definitely had a girl's face and you've always behaved like one, since the day you could smile.'

'I'm sorry too, Mum. I do wish it all could have been different. I suppose.'

She shrugged, trying to suppress her shock. Mum had actually wanted a boy! And never told her! Not in all these years. It was hard to believe, and oddly hurtful too. She put down the tea towel and gave her mother another brief hug, 'I love you, Mum,' She made a show of looking at her watch, delved in her bag for her lipstick. 'But I've got to go now. I'll come and see you again soon. I promise.'

Trying to concentrate on fixing her lips in the hallway mirror, Lucille ignored the return of her mother's slow dramatic tears in the reflection behind her. Popping the lipstick back into her bag again with a brisk flourish, she gave Mum a big bland smile followed by another hopeless little shrug. After yet another hug, acknowledging Mum's long drawn-out look which said they both knew she didn't need to be going *just* yet but they both somehow wanted her to, they kissed formally on each cheek and Lucille left.

As she walked down the street she turned round and saw her mother still standing there watching her depart. She waved at her, waited for a belated wave back, then turned a corner, trying for all she was worth to blink back the tears – she didn't want her make-up to run, certainly not now out here where she might draw unwanted attention to herself. Instead she smiled bravely to herself like a child whose mum could actually still see her and who needed her not to be upset.

As she passed through the old familiar streets back to the station, all she could think was I'm not a monster. Just cos you wanted a boy. I'm not. Just because I can't have children. Just because I'm different. I may be different but I am not going to *behave* any different from anybody else. I only want to live a normal life from now on, that's all. I don't want to do any harm to *any*body. I'm not dangerous. Specially not to men. That's so ridiculous. How can she say things like that? I don't understand.'

But she did really. She had always understood her mum. If you wanted a normal life it probably meant you hadn't got one.

Preoccupied with these thoughts she took no notice of a swarthy, moustachioed middle-aged man with a beer belly, fifty metres ahead and slowly walking towards her along the pavement. Then she noticed not only that he wasn't European, there was something familiar about his shuffling arrhythmic gait.

Oh my god! Papa!

She stopped, frozen. Would he recognise her after all this time and all her changes? He got closer. She pretended to look in her bag for something, and actually did bring her compact out and quickly dabbed the corners of her eyes. Then, very deliberately, she put it back in her bag, closed it again and looked directly at him as he shambled towards her.

She wasn't going to pretend to be what she wasn't. She was who she was. She wanted to look at him. And she wanted him to look at her and see her for who she was. She wasn't going to pretend to be a stranger. He was her father after all. She continued walking towards him, proudly exaggerating the swing of her hips and feeling a peculiar mixture of childlike longing to be recognised and at the same time a terrible fear of it. She didn't take her eyes off his face, longing for him to recognise her, longing to fall into his arms. As they got closer she noticed he was swaying a bit in that old familiar drunken way of his, and despite everything, she couldn't help feeling a deep glow of love.

Rashid Farouk had actually noticed her now, but was looking her up and down the way men did on the streets all the time at young women, with a slight leer and without any recognition of her as a person at all. Likewise, now they were actually within sight of each other, she found herself responding in kind, she couldn't help it: she kept her eyes down and directed towards where she was going, like women do all the time when they are out amongst men. Unless they want something.

But she did want something: she felt herself flushing, burning with the need for him to recognise her as they came within spitting distance of one another. She wanted to look at him in directly in the eye, but it would have felt brazen, wrong somehow. So she just glanced at him, needing him to see *her*, not someone brazen; to see her for who she was without having to catch his attention.

But he stepped to one side making way for her and they passed each other by like total strangers.

Lucille felt close to tears again; angry, hot ones. They *were* total strangers. They always had been. She had always been a disappointment to him. She had tried to like boys' things when she was a child. She really had, learning to speak French and to be proud of her Moroccan ancestry, and listening to his stories about the Foreign Legion, wanting to please him and get his approval. She just wasn't that interested in soldiers or trains or any of the other things he had tried to involve her in. She had tried to be. To be 'a good sport'. To be his good sport. She remembered her shock at seeing the sadness on his face when she was maybe six years old. The year of Dream Barbie's Magic show probably. They had been going for a walk, just the two of them in the park. A rare event. They held hands all the way there and she had been feeling very happy even though she hadn't been very good at catching the tennis ball he had brought along and he had been a bit irritated with her. On the way home she had asked him if boys could ever grew up into women because, she told him with the naïve straightforwardness of a small child, she was going to be a woman when she grew up and she wanted to marry a man just like him. She couldn't understand how cold and distant he immediately became. Not violent or horrible on that occasion. Just remote. She remembered feeling as scared of that as she was of his drunkenness and aggression. It was like he just went away from her then and she couldn't remember ever feeling close to him again. Just wanting to. Talk to your mother, he'd said. So she had, and Mum had shut the door and sat her down on her knee, said it was time she learned that that there were things that the doctors she had mentioned before could do to help her and then she told her about sex change operations. Immediately she became happier again and said she wanted one there and then. Secretly, forever after that, she consoled herself that one day Papa would like her better, maybe even love her again if she was properly a girl.

Now, when she got on the train back to Colliers Wood she tried to put all thoughts of Mum and Papa out of her mind. Perhaps prompted by the way he had just looked at her, she thought about sex instead. Again. The doctor at the clinic yesterday had said the best thing for her now was to be sexually active. If she wasn't, he had told her, she would have to continue to dilate herself because of the minute risk that her vaginal cavity might otherwise close up again.

The very idea was horrifying, but she didn't have anyone to have sex with. She glanced surreptitiously at some of the men on the train, then kept her eyes focussed on her reflection in the window. She *was* attractive. She knew she was. But she was so inexperienced. She had never really been interested in anyone sexually before she had moved in with Rose. Not really. She had thought that because she preferred the company of girls she might also prefer them sexually when and if it ever came to it. But back then being penised had been so completely mortifying that no sexual fantasies could be allowed in case the awful thing did what all penises do when their owners are excited. The fantasies would come anyway, but the reluctant boy she used to be always censored them, except when he was asleep and had no control.

With a shudder of revulsion she stared at the dirty floor of the train trying not to remember the unbearable night-time sense of shame and confusion her previous self had once or twice experienced in early adolescence waking up from a sweet enough recurring dream of being properly a girl and being kissed by a boy. Confusingly and unrealistically the boys she dreamed about always seemed to have the faces of the bullies at school who used to tease her for walking and talking like a girl, not realising or caring such comments actually made her feel proud. She would emerge out of sleep into the waking nightmare of finding a horrible wet pool on the sheet evidencing the hated masculinity. She – he – used to feel sick with shame.

Suppressing a frown, Lucie shook her head and crossed her legs, pulling nervously at an earring for a moment. Thank heavens that would never happen again! Just thinking about it now was embarrassing. Similarly, when the gross Ron used to give her his dick to suck just over a year ago, his dim personality and the sheer physical stink of him had made the whole experience of a man not entirely pleasant, to say the least. But, as she had owned to Rose in the wood that night, not completely *un*desirable either. Certainly not. She had delighted in the small sense of power she felt in arousing him by looking like a girl. And under the circumstances actually seeing to his arousal orally had felt the nicest and most natural thing in the world. But afterwards she often used to cringe because of what it said about what she was at that time – not the real girl she felt herself to be, just a little teenage travesty compelled to

55

swallow semen in much the same ambivalent way as she enjoyed the occasional sticky Amaretto with Mum at Christmas.

So now her body had in fact been corrected and she did have the feminine wherewithal, she could and should, at the very least, let herself have fantasies about men. She was stupid, she knew she was, or at least ignorant, after so many years of suppression. 'Imagine you're honeymooning with your favourite pop star, or actor or someone,' her Specialist Nurse Counsellor, Sarah, had said to her at the clinic yesterday with a broad hen-night leer, reminding her that the biggest of the three dildo things she had been given for dilation purposes on discharge from hospital two months ago, was now the only one she should be using. 'It's a vibrator. It's no good pretending it isn't. In case you haven't noticed it has a battery and a switch, and you do need to use it if you're still shying away from men. So for heaven's sake turn yourself on,' she'd said, making Lucie smile with none of the embarrassment the doctor had made her feel earlier. 'Make sure everything works. At least until you've got yourself a real man. After that you can lie back and think of England, if that's what you want. Although I always prefer Corfu myself!'

Not just being given permission, but actually having been ordered to do so, she had taken herself upstairs last night determined to excite herself. At first it was bizarre trying to make pleasure out of an activity which till then had felt horribly like self-inflicted frontal constipation and which she had previously performed squatting in the bathroom each night gritting her teeth as she lubricated and inserted the hateful thing to get it over and done with as quickly as possible. But she knew Sarah was right so last night she lit a candle, took the vibrator and gel to bed and took her time. Her surgery must been successful because she had definitely brought herself to some kind of climax without it hurting too much at all as she closed her eyes and imagined being seduced and tenderly ravished by a strange, but stunning composite of every man she had ever secretly fancied, all rolled into one. Whoever he was, and his face kept on changing, he entered her as lovingly as she could have wished for, with an appendage that from a distance she had imagined to be as big and beguiling as a bull elephant's.

Afterwards though, as she lay there glowing, no longer scared of her dilator, there was still something missing of course. Relationship. Sex with herself was alright, but it was not something she would want to do for any longer than she had to. Not just because it was lonely and ultimately unsatisfying, but because it wasn't grown up. When she was younger she had noticed at school that it was always the more immature boys, the ones who got into fights or who thought it was cool to be bunk off school, who tended to call her or each other tossers. Masturbation was for teenagers. Grown ups had relationships. They had proper sexual relationships with other grown ups and, she thought, with just a little more confidence than she had ever felt in her life before, she would very much like a bit of that too. She was, after all, going to be twenty soon.

But in the real world there just weren't any boys or men in her life. Certainly none who looked like her fabulous fantasy man, whatever the length of their willies. There were none at the hairdressers in Wimbledon where, after getting help from Rose with deeds and documentation, she had been working unquestioned as a female since early last year. The boss was a man, but he looked like a poisonous toadstool with his white spotty head and his shoulders which were almost as wide as he was high. The other three women were all, well, women. She got on with them alright, but only one of them was her own age and she was already coupled. The other two were married, had children and lives of their own. They were all nice though, they had a lot of laughs together when they weren't too busy; but men were just not a part of her world.

Chapter 5.

Slobodan and Saddam, Mary's two Red Setters, never came when he called them. At least fifty percent of the time anyway.

Such were Richard McElvey's angry thoughts as he strode towards the park gates. Putney Bridge road was already filling up with traffic even though it was still only six a.m. Those wretched dogs always seemed to make a special point early in the morning of dawdling as far away as possible from him. Especially when he was in a hurry.

He needed to get home, have a shower and be at work promptly by nine today. An eminent colleague and her Specialist Registrar were coming down from the Queen's Medical Centre in Nottingham to conduct a second opinion on a particularly bizarre, permanently twisted colon. He wanted to make sure he was in on time to welcome them.

Mary's two older children were still only eight and ten, but were already behaving like teenagers. They had lost all interest in accompanying him to the park to walk the dogs. And it was them she had bought the damn things for in the first place. It was ridiculous to have such athletic animals living in London. He himself had never had an affinity for dogs. So why on earth did he do this every morning? Why didn't he persuade Mary to give them away or have them put down? Their need to expend energy come rain or shine, bounding about each morning and evening was phenomenal. And phenomenally dull. Mary had bought them as puppies for Harry and Sarah for Christmas two years ago to give them something to do while she turned her all attentions to her new born baby. Little Robbie had been the product of a last attempt to repair her marriage to the children's father. After a brief and abject, if fully fertilised failure to restore their relationship to its former glory, Mary had wound up with three extra mouths to feed, what with the dogs and the baby. Four, if he included his own. But she never grumbled. When he first met her she was a part-time technician at the MRI unit at work. He'd had passing words with her almost every day when she had first caught his eye. Gradually he'd started swimming in her bright uncomplicated smile and her simple positive approach to life. What he hadn't realised at the time was that after a while you always need to get out of the pool again.

She'd certainly been a pleasure to know at the time. After Rose. And after a few years of living on his own and dwelling on his failure as a husband and father, he couldn't help it: he had fallen in love. He knew at the time it was madness. He'd loved her lump as much as anything. All that female fecundity. After Luke and after the daily grind of ulcers, stomach cancers and twisted guts, seeing a healthy female belly swelling up so beautifully each day had been uplifting, inspirational. Even if the child wasn't his own. So when their relationship reached that point where flirtation must either develop or die, he threw caution to the winds, conducted a whirlwind romance with her and within in a matter of weeks had moved in. The children's father, an accountant now living in Kent, saw the kids every fortnight.

Madness. That's how he saw it now. Living in another man's house. Being married to another man's wife. Robbie at two was a demanding handful. With his tight curly hair and stocky physique there was no doubting that the boy was most certainly not his own, but he still called him Dada. If he was going to end his relationship with Mary, who was wilfully oblivious of his true feelings, he better get on with it soon. Robbie might otherwise be emotionally damaged. Harry and Sarah were different. They would cope. They always talked about their father in glowing terms and spent all their time when they weren't down in Maidstone watching television and practicing sarcasm. Richard knew he meant little or nothing to either of them despite all his attempts over the last few years to make them feel special.

An accident. That's what it was, him and Mary. He had just not realised it at the time. He really should leave her. Soon. Trade her in for a younger model, like that girl here in the park yesterday with the baby who'd asked him if he had seen the baby's bottle lying on the ground anywhere.

She obviously couldn't have found it because Sodp-'em and Slob were fighting over the thing right now.

But if he left Mary there was nowhere to go to, and no-one to go there with. He would be confronted by the fact of who he was, and despite having committed no crime that he was aware of, his sense of the fact of who he was, was completely untenable. The truth was he had no motivation to do anything with his life anymore. Having reached the top of his career ladder and along the way lost his first wife and son, he now felt curiously empty with a second wife, three ready-made children and two dogs he neither wanted nor cared for.

He tapped his toe in an urgent tattoo and reluctantly put his lips to the dog whistle for what was probably the seventh or eighth time. It was supposed to be inaudible to humans, but it gave him a piercing headache each time he blew on it. He was coming to the conclusion it was inaudible to Red Setters. They looked at him briefly, as if he was stupid, then continued to chase each other around the plain trees lining the bottom of the park down by the Thames.

He didn't want this at all, he thought, as he hurried down to the riverside to get them. Children and animals. How was it possible? But there they were, all around him. His whole life just seemed to have happened to him like a series of accidents. Even including his medical training and his career, if he really thought about it. He didn't feel responsible for any of it. Not a thing. Just like he hadn't been for Luke. In fact he felt like a phoney, a complete charlatan behind his magnificent facade. He'd felt like a phoney ever since Luke was first identified as suffering from Cystic Fibrosis. He had always tried to be positive, both at home with Rose and with Luke himself, and at work where he tried to always smile at people, the knowledgeable, wise, and benign Consultant. But inside, where previously he had always known who he really was, the death sentence in his son's genetic make-up had killed his own authentic feelings. So he didn't know who he was at all inside anymore, just that he was at best inadequate and at worst, because of his failure to get it right with Luke, plain bad. In fact if he had been simpler or more psychotic he would have been the type of person who turns himself in at police stations, convinced he was the perpetrator of every crime.

He was going to see Rose this evening for the first time since the autumn, and it was already nearly spring. He could never actually see her nowadays without feeling all the old pain and loss between them. So he avoided having too much contact with her, always tried to keep the conversation between them light. They had to meet occasionally though. There was too much between them that would always be there, and which he needed to revisit two or three times a year just to stay true to their past. After all, he himself hadn't really wanted to part from her in the first place, had still loved her in a way, despite all the slings and arrows Outrageous bloody Fortune had been so free with. It was she who had been insistent about ending it, implacably said they had to separate and divorce or neither of them would ever again want to move forward in life. She'd been right. She'd known she'd been right. He had known it too, without buying into the same rationale as her. But eventually he'd done as he was bid and left her, had 'moved forward' anyway, still not knowing what that really meant and still somehow regretting it. He'd not been used to failure. In fact he couldn't remember ever failing before, but knew he had nevertheless finally managed to do so resoundingly, both as a husband and as a father. Rose had tried to say that like their marriage, their divorce could be seen as a choice which each of them made freely. He had been too depressed to argue with her about it, but he didn't believe in choice. Life, and moving forward in it, or backwards for that matter, just happened. Like death and accidents.

'Come on, Slob, good fucking boy,' he said between gritted teeth, trying to suppress his frustration as the animal seemed more intent on waiting to see whether it would have more fun bounding away from him again, having first picked up the torn and broken baby's bottle just as Richard was bending to attach a lead to his neck. Perhaps Slobodan picked up the mood he was in, because after appearing to consider it for a moment, the dog clearly seemed to think twice, deciding against further misbehaviour, as if he knew Richard's bark and bite would be a far worse fate than simply carrying the bottle home. When Saddam saw what was happening, he trotted over too and let himself be tethered alongside

Slobodan. 'Thank you, Sad-oh, well done,' he said to the other dog, patting them both with a gratitude he resented and setting off purposefully for the gate again. Dogs! Jesus Christ, whatever was he doing with dogs?

He bundled them into the back of the car and set off for home which was five minutes away in Disraeli road. In fact sooner than that he was already starting to pull into it across Oxford road.

There was a sudden screech of brakes from his right. An ancient Ford Sierra ground to an emergency stop within a hair's breadth of his driver-side door. He jammed on the brakes too, stared at the other driver glaring at him from across a matt brown bonnet. Damn. He hadn't looked. But the other guy must have been driving far too fast to have had to stop like that. Surely? Surely! Richard pursed the corners of his mouth and frowned, then shook his head theatrically. After counting to ten, he lifted the clutch and proceeded slowly across into Disraeli road. He heard another shriek of tyres. Clearly exercised, Battered-old-Sierra Man was having the effrontery to follow him. More than that, had turned on his headlights and was tailgating him. Richard ignored the brute, found a space to park and heard the other man pull up beside him in the middle of the road. The driver's side window of his car rolled down in angry jerking movements.

'Stupid Fuck,' said the bald, beer-bellied driver with all the mindless righteousness of the road-raged. Richard shrugged, continuing to ignore him as he got out of the car and went round the back to let the dogs out. He would not give the other man the satisfaction of even another glance. Nevertheless when he heard the screech of the Sierra's tyres driving off again a moment later, he felt angry with himself for heaving just a little sigh of relief.

Letting Slob and Sad in first, he followed them into the house. The radio and television competed with Mary's yells and the children's moans as he shut the door and hung the lead back up on the hook. He went into the kitchen where Mary was souping some baby slop into Robbie's mouth, and flicked on the kettle.

'How are you this morning?' Mary asked with her customary earth mother jollity and her usual friendly smile. He opened his mouth to reply when the door bell rang.

'Alright. Late again, I fear,' he replied, walking back down the hall to open the front door. 'The dogs will have to go if they won't be trained to come when they're called.' He saw the outline of a large man through the stained glass panelling of the front door. The gas or electricity meter inspector, probably.

As he levered down the handle of the door and opened it, a very strong, very large hand reached in at the speed of light and gripped him by the collar. He had a glimpse of Sierra Man's head as three hard right-handers pummelled his ribs, stomach and mouth in that order. Then he was unceremoniously let go of again, dropped. The door was slammed closed.

'Who is it?' Mary called from the kitchen as he sank down onto the doormat, holding his head and leaning against the wall.

He was seeing stars. Even so, he began berating himself for not being more careful and was overcome with a desire to get up and chase his assailant down the street. The reality was that he was winded and unable to move.

'Who is it, Richard?' he heard Mary call again from down the hall with a little more stridency. He tried to reply, but his mouth did not obey. Out of control. Like the dogs. His nose also seemed to have a life of its own.

What the fuck did he need to have done that for? His left nostril felt as tight as a drum filling with blood. Gingerly he touched it with his thumb and forefinger. Not cut or damaged at all, but it was definitely about to bleed. Then it burst like a hot dam, seeping down his upper lip into his mouth. He was dimly aware of Mary coming to the kitchen door, then running down the hall to see to him.

'Richard. Richard. Are you alright? Oh, my God, you've been hurt! Oh, my God!' She repeated. Bending down, she gently removed his hand which was now cupping the blood pouring from his nose. She hastily returned it to his face, said 'Come with me right now into the kitchen. If you can make it. You need a wet cloth. Oh my God. You poor thing. This is dreadful. I'll call the police straight away.'

She escorted him to the sink, followed by an enthralled procession of children and dogs. She ran the cold tap, pushed his head down. He felt her competent arms and big breasts and smelt her perfume, almost sinking into an inviting oblivion.

Instead , he stood upright, holding the cloth she'd given him to his face.

Accidents. He'd had another accident. Or another lapse of judgement to follow all the others. His nose felt alright. His mouth had received the worst of the blows and it was his mouth, his lips and front teeth which felt the most sore .

'I'm alright,' he said, gesturing her away. 'I'll be fine. Just get me some ice, please. Don't call the police. There's no point. I'll have a quick shower and then spend the next half hour with an ice pack. I'll be fine.'

'Of course I'm calling the police. We cannot have someone just come to the door and hit you like that. He might do it to other people as well.' She went back to the front door and slipped the latch on.

'He probably does. But I've got no time to talk to policemen. I *need* to put ice on my mouth, Mary, to stop it swelling up, and then I need to get to work.' If his upper lip looked anything like it already felt it would be huge in next to no time. Fuck. Fuck. Fuck. Whatever would the people from Nottingham make of him? He inched his way through children and animals, all of whom were yapping, and went slowly up the stairs. Mary followed him, radiating saintliness and helpfulness.

'What was that all about? Why were you attacked, Richard? Who was it? You poor thing.' Her voice became more urgent. 'You better be careful,' she said. 'Hold on to the stair rail or you'll fall down the stairs.'

There was no danger of that, but he leaned forward anyway as he trudged up the carpeted steps.

'I'm going to have my shower. That'll sort me out. Keep bringing me more ice, please,' he said. 'I hope we've got enough. With any luck it'll stop me looking like I've been stung by a swarm of bees, which is what it feels like at the moment. As to who it was, I don't know. It was a man I inad–' he winced as his lips, teeth and tongue seemed to fight painfully with one another trying to say 'vertently'. He started an again, 'a man I cut up just now on Oxford Road. He'll be long gone by now. So there's no point calling the police, even if I did have the time to speak to them. I'll call them later, give them a description. But right now what I need is ice.'

'I'll get it straight away,' Mary said behind him. She didn't know the meaning of the words 'straight away', and instead raced solicitously ahead of him on the upstairs landing and ran into the bathroom. She turned on the shower.

'My poor, poor love,' she said, as if talking to one of her children. She reached forward to help him take his sweat shirt off. He lifted an arm to signal it was nothing. He didn't need her help. It was just one of those things. An accident. He was a man not a child.

'Ice,' he mumbled from beneath his enormous old-fashioned shower head, as some of the water ran pink down his chest. 'Please.'

'I'll get you that ice,' she said, all solicitousness and understanding. 'I'll be back in no time.'

* * *

Two hours later he was at work. His nose felt crusty, his smile only slightly out of kilter as he poured the Prof and her toy boy registrar a cup of coffee from the machine outside his office. He looked fine. The bag of frozen peas Mary had supplied him with had done the trick.

When he'd gone out to his car again to go to work an hour after being punched, he'd felt oddly disappointed that his assailant wasn't still out on the street to greet him, affording him the opportunity for revenge. Not that he was the macho type, nor in proper physical condition for violence, but his anger at the ignominy of what had happened to him had wanted an outlet. It didn't get one. Instead, the street had been car-lined, but still relatively empty except for freshly deodorised commuters hurrying along the pavement towards the station. Birds had still been singing as if nothing had happened, forsythias still shining in the early morning sun as they had done every day during this fine spell of weather. There'd been nothing to suggest he'd been punched in the face earlier, only if you really looked hard would you have noticed anything. So he'd been lucky. His ribs hurt now, more than anything. In his car on the way to work, wincing every time he turned left or depressed the clutch pedal, he found himself rehearsing all the obscenities he would have liked to have delivered to Sierra Man at the time if only he had been more alert to what had been about to happen. It reminded him of how he used to pointlessly rehearse all the things he would have liked to have done to prevent Luke being the way he was. Pointless.

'It is a very interesting case, actually,' he said, trying not to lisp, but having decided on the truth if he was asked. He wasn't asked, and felt faintly miffed that he was not therefore going to get any more sympathy either. He would have rather enjoyed being the patient for a change.

He did the best he could to talk about the case, highlighting the complexities that had prompted the woman to ask for a second opinion. The Nottingham people were polite, but bored, clearly wanting to read his copious notes in peace themselves before examining the patient who was already waiting to be attended to for sedation by the anaesthetist. He left them with the file and the use of his office to do his ward round. You had to keep up appearances as a consultant, appear to lead the troops, even if everybody nowadays knew it was managers who were really in charge.

By mid-morning he was speaking normally again, and by the end of the day he had stopped worrying that one of his front teeth would fall out, but his head was still splitting. He was partly ketotic as well, he imagined, having not been able to eat all day for the tenderness in his teeth and gums and the soreness inside his upper lip. Before he left work he examined his face in the mirror again. His upper lip was not even slightly discoloured, and there was no swelling at all by now. Remarkable.

He decided to stop at the supermarket on his way home, buy himself something sloppy and easy to masticate for dinner. He wasn't in any kind of hurry to return home to his kindly buxom wife and her awful menagerie. Shopping would provide a delay. Perhaps Mary would have taken the dogs out already, perhaps the kids would be up in their bedrooms doing their homework.

The car park at Sainsbury's was relatively empty for seven o'clock on a Monday evening, but he couldn't help doing a discreet, if genuinely fearful check for old brown Sierras as he walked to the trolley park and pulled out a trolley.

For nearly an hour he wandered round the supermarket, idly filling it with items that took his fancy, but mostly just watching his fellow shoppers religiously traipsing the aisles with the forlorn faces of the imprisoned, a lot of them clearly as tired, aching and bored as he was himself. He might work with people all day, he thought, but it was never as their equal. It made him feel artificial, fake somehow, always being bowed and scraped to, or despised. He was never the same as anybody else. His status meant people – patients and staff alike – treated him differently. Very rarely did he get the time or chance to feel anonymous, as he did now buying tins of soup he knew he would never actually cook for himself.

He glanced across at the loud couple waiting at the next check-out. They were trying to pacify a fractious school-age child who should have been at home hours ago. The boy looked about ten, but was behaving like a toddler, refusing to return a chocolate bar to the racks of the things piled up beside the till. The mother, lank and underweight, lines of poverty etched prematurely by excess cigarette consumption into her face, was shouting at him. The more she did, the more the child refused to give up the bar. Her partner also lanky and long-haired looked around in an embarrassed unfocused way, trying to avoid people's eyes in the queues behind and beside him at adjoining tills. But they had nothing else to do. Eventually the woman grabbed hold of the boy, raising her voice and her other hand to hit him. The man intervened, trying to pull the boy away. 'Cool it, Tasha,' he drawled, as if he was on the set of some old cowboy film. 'Cool it. I'll deal with him.'

Richard found himself catapulted back into the past as he watched them struggle with the child. He could quite clearly remember something very similar happening between Rose and himself one horrible Saturday afternoon. Luke had been resisting her fraught, angry insistence that he come with her to the Supermarket's toddler-changing facility in the ladies loo to let her give him his hated physiotherapy. He had to have it four times daily, a dreaded combination of chest and back pummelling and massage to loosen the mucus clogging his already badly scarred lungs. He'd been due to have it over an hour before that afternoon, and Rose had become hysterical, frightened that he would be so much more vulnerable to the influenza bug prevalent at the time for which they had still not got him inoculated. Richard felt embarrassed, he recalled now, because he had stupidly been unable to understand why Rose needed to be so obsessive about subjecting Luke to his physiotherapy just then and just there, while they were out shopping and very nearly about to go home. He'd tried to remonstrate, persuade her to wait until they got home, but she had threatened to start screaming at him then, telling him he didn't understand how important it was to keep to the clock if Luke was to have any chance of leading a normal life. As Luke continued to resist – he had been nine years old by then and only a matter of months away from slipping into the very last stages of his life, but nevertheless understandably sensitive about going into the Ladies even if he didn't look a day over five or six physically – Rose had grabbed hold of him, threatened to give him a smack. Richard had known then that she was finally losing it. Not in all his life had she ever once smacked Luke.

Instinctively he'd reached out to take his son away from her, and for one horrible moment they were pulling him like a piece of bubble gum, till Rose let go, and ran off sobbing leaving him to deal with both the shopping and Luke on his own. Later he had found her sitting in the car, her face set as she apologised to both of them for behaving in such a way in public. He'd been aware that he and Luke had both wanted to placate her, soothe her, help her feel better, but she'd denied that there was a problem any longer, blamed herself for the whole incident.

He'd gone on to do Luke's physiotherapy himself. Luke actually asking him to do it, an unheard of request from the boy, who like him had been eyeing his mother sideways with a worried look on his face all the way home. When Rose herself noticed this, she squeezed his hand, said everything was alright, she shouldn't have done what she did. 'It's alright, Mum,' he kept repeating. 'It's alright.'

Richard watched the lanky couple now swear under their breath as they filled their plastic shopping bags and ignored their son whom they had deprived of his chocolate. He was visibly smarting from the smacks across the side of his head both parents had suddenly and simultaneously given him, but did not seem upset in the slightest, taking their blows for granted.

Richard grimaced, as he started piling up his own purchases onto the checkout. After giving Luke his physio that day, he had played with him on the floor, reassured him that Mum would be alright, that even adults get upset sometimes, it was only natural. He remembered making sure to convince Luke it really wasn't his fault Mum was so upset. Just like it wasn't his fault that he had been born with CF. Luke had relaxed eventually and then they had drawn and coloured a home-made board game on a large sheet of paper together. Treasure Island. He could remember it vividly with all its Pieces of Eight spilling out in a yellow and orange apology for gold from the Treasure chest he had inexpertly drawn in the middle. Like Snakes and Ladders it was, using dice to get to the treasure, except there were pirates attacking you and sending you back to earlier squares instead of snakes, and you were always at risk of having to walk the plank – Luke had drawn them everywhere – before you went back with the treasure to your ship and sailed away, the winner. They'd spent hours on the floor together colouring the squares sea-blue and drawing fierce-looking cut-throats and sad-looking swabs. They had both been very proud of it. He couldn't remember that they had ever played the game more than once. But later that same day, in the evening, Luke had designed a little treasure map himself. 'It's not really a treasure map,' he said. 'It's *like* a treasure map. I'm going to hide it under the loose floor board in my bedroom cupboard and get it out if I ever need it again. Or if Mummy does. Or you, Dad.' Richard had smiled benignly at the time, he remembered, not much interested. He hadn't even looked at it, but God, he could do with such a map now. With that map. With that actual map. Fancy remembering it now, after all this time. The amazing thing was it was probably still there. There was no reason why it shouldn't be.

Waiting for his purchases to be processed through the till, with a plastic carrier bag opened and ready in his hands, he noticed a red-haired woman, too young to be a granny yet too old to be a mum, asking the old lady behind her if she wouldn't mind keeping an eye on her toddler for a moment, she had forgotten to get some milk. The baby was fast asleep in its pushchair. He watched her hurry back down an aisle, her heavy shape unused to rushing. The recalcitrant ten year old in front of her had also noticed her go, and with a furtive insouciance he sidled closer to the sleeping toddler. He glanced up at his parents and then at the old woman who was beginning to pile her own purchases up on the checkout belt. Without warning he hit the younger child with the back of his fist across the face. It wasn't a smack. It was a thump. The second vicarious thumping Richard had witnessed in one day, having never seen such a thing before in his life as far as he could recall. The toddler awoke with a scream of pain, but already the ten year old had squeezed past his parents with an innocent, jaunty step. Nothing to do with him. The baby's cries echoed the residual shock he still felt from his own assault this morning. He was debating whether to intervene, and inform on the boy as the toddler's mother came running back with her milk and told her child off for not being patient.

Accidents just happen. They pile up on each other without warning. He found himself hating the horrible ten year old for being alive when his lovely Luke was long dead.

'Er, excuse me,' he said to the lanky couple and their offspring who were now pushing their laden trolley off and leaving. 'Your son just hit that child.'

'Nothing to do with me, mate,' said the father. The woman and the boy ignored him as if he were dirt on their shoes and continued on their way.

It was another five minutes before he was pushing his shopping trolley towards the exit of the supermarket himself. His melon hadn't been properly priced. Like Sierra Man this morning the lanky couple and their unpleasant son would have been long gone. His thoughts returned to his son and his treasure map. Seeing that there was a pay phone by the café area beside the exit, he stopped, fumbled for some coins in his pocket.

'Hello?' A young female voice answered the phone. Not Rose.

'Hello,' he said. 'Who am I speaking to?'

'Who's calling and who do you want?' the woman responded. Her voice had an over-intonated, musical quality to it, reminding him of the girl in the park yesterday who'd lost her baby's bottle.

'Rose,' he said.

'I'll get her for you. Just a minute. Who did you say you were? You sound kind of familiar.'

'Richard. Her, er, former husband.'

'Okay. Hold on.'

He heard the woman calling Rose, and a few moments later she was speaking to him.

'Richard! How are you?'

'I'm okay. Under the circumstances. You know.'

'How's the family?'

'They're fine. I don't want to talk about them, if you don't mind. Sorry. I didn't mean that to sound snappy. I've got a bit of a headache, actually.'

'Still working too hard?'

'Well, no, not really. I got punched this morning after I nearly, but didn't – that's didn't, as in 'Did Not' – cause an accident!' He gave a mirthless laugh, trying to be good humoured , but knew he just sounded petulant. 'The other driver got upset anyway. Hit me a few times. Now I've just seen a child doing the same thing to another smaller, sleeping child in this supermarket.'

'Oh, dear. Poor you. Did you take the day off? Does your head need examining?' She laughed. 'It's always needed examining. What I meant was: were you concussed? Did you need an X ray or, what is it Mary used to do, an MRI?

'Yes. No. None of those. I'm fine. I'm just now on my way home from work. I'm okay, really. Just need a good night's sleep, but first I wouldn't mind coming round and seeing you, if that's alright?'

'You want to see me again? How come?'

'Just, you know, to catch up.'

'But you've never wanted to come back to the house before, Richard, I thought "neutral ground" was important to you? Has something changed?

'That's just it. I'd like to see you at home this time. The house has so many memories. I'd like to revisit them. I *need* to revisit them actually, Rose. If you'd let me? Just briefly.'

'Well I'm not sure. You certainly can't come round now. I'm sorry. I'm going out. I've got Bridge tonight. Anyway what would Mary have to say about it?'

'It's nothing to do with her,' he replied, irritated that she hadn't just acquiesced to his wishes. He'd never asked very much from her. He changed the subject. 'Who's that woman who answered the phone?'

'Lucie? My lodger. She's been here nearly two years now.'

'You never told me.'

'Why on earth should I? Anyway, you never asked.'

'Which room does she use?'

'Luke's old room. Why? What's with all this interest in the house all of a sudden?'

en her emotional and psychological dependence upor
so out of the ordinary, so special.

all, irrespective of what it meant or what it said about
nd it wonderful to be needed again. That had been the
made not being able to get her head around the strange
lly Lucie was artificial, a contrivance, of secondary
needed Rose had, as she had hoped, revisited her
It didn't matter that she felt as if she was both inside
strange netherworld movie. In the comfort of her own
en both producer and actress in a film about the two of
mother' and a 'daughter' and finding fulfilment therein.
harm in it. They had both been so happy in their roles.
d become a memory. Utterly dormant. Well, fairly

was almost unbearable to think that the feeling of being
g to diminish again. For Lucille, their life together had
becoming. But because of being needed, Rose had
ming too. Becoming a kind of mother, a kind of sister
. She certainly didn't want to lose what she'd become
t they had been through together. At the same time,
ts and purposes Lucille was a woman, grown up and
se didn't need to be so relentlessly grown up herself.
f feel *all* her feelings, even childish ones. And she did
at the moment, more and more so recently in fact,
s daily exhibiting little signs of needing her less and
ve her eventually. There could be no doubt about that.
Like her dead parents. Like Richard. Of course she
. There would be something wrong if she didn't. .
t tell Lucie about her dread. She would try to half-say
iggle, as if such feelings shouldn't be taken seriously
she was the grown up one. Lucie would join her in
, would help her to change the subject to something
alcohol brings the best out of a trifle, or how to get
arpets with salt. Grown up things. But the truth was
id indeed stop needing her, then there would be
mpty hole inside her. And that would mean she would
ain.

be untenable.

s she to do? She didn't very often feel she could go
lle anymore. She was so much older, for heaven's
ucille's interests had turned to young men. Tediously.
he went on about at all nowadays, except for fashion
r mother, who she still visited on her days off so long
at home. Of course real mothers and daughters went

'I told you, memories I have to revisit.'

'Well, you're welcome to come round, but obviously you can't go into Lucie's room. It's hers now. I redecorated it completely. She started in the spare room, but it's so small, isn't it? And after I got used to her, I let her move into Luke's old room. It didn't seem to matter anymore, somehow. Perhaps it should have, but it didn't. We have to move on, don't we, Richard? Let the past go.'

He didn't want to tell her about the treasure map. Not if she wanted to let the past go. Anyway, he had nothing of Luke's. Not a single thing. Just some photographs which he had long lost any connection with, not least because the boy had looked so much like his mother. He had to have something of him for himself. So he didn't ask Rose whether she'd removed the built-in cupboards when she redecorated. He'd just have to hope not. He wanted to find Luke's map as discreetly as he could and keep it to himself. It had been Luke's message to the future. What was it he'd said when he put it there? 'It's a treasure map. Well, like a treasure map, but it's not. I writ it for someone to find so that they could know what it was like for me when we were living here. What the truth was'. That's right. Luke had asked him if they would ever move house, and when Richard had said maybe or maybe not, Luke told him, 'I writed it for the people who are going to live here in a hundred years time then.' He'd marvelled at the idea of people being alive in a whole century's time, perhaps intuitively knowing he wouldn't reach eleven years of age himself.

Richard grimaced. It felt like a hundred years already since then. A thousand, since those precious days in which he and Rose had been stupid enough to feel so sorry for themselves so often. But how would he ever get hold of Luke's treasure map if the room was now occupied by Rose's damn lodger? He would just have to find out if the lodger ever went out at all. That was all. Not a major problem.

'Oh, yes,' he said. 'Yes, we have. We've got to let the past go, but it would be nice to see you. Our marriage may be past, but you're not. Seeing you, seeing your changes would really help me let the past go. Some of it, at least. Would you mind?'

'Of course not, Richard. Probably not, anyway. But I'm sure Mary might have something to say about it.'

'So when can I come, then?'

'I don't know. This time next week maybe. How about that?'

'Okay.' He tried not to sound disappointed. A whole week. 'Maybe I could invite myself to supper?'

'Alright, Richard. But something's going on! You're up to something, I can tell.'

'Will we be on our own?'

'I don't know. Yes, I expect so. Lucie's out a lot nowadays. But if she's in I'm sure she wouldn't want to intrude. What are you up to, Richard?

You're being devious, and perhaps, under the circumstances, it actually wouldn't be a very good idea for you to come here.'

'It is. It is. I'll see you next Monday, Rose. Definitely. Perhaps I'll meet your lodger too?'

'Probably not, Richard. I don't know. Do you want to meet her? I think you do, don't you? Is that why you want to come here?' she said, with an irritating knowingness, as if he were still some kind of womaniser.

All he could hope for actually was that this Lucie woman would in fact be out. But he wouldn't let Rose know that, because she would quickly cotton on he was interested in something else if she hadn't already, and being so obsessional she'd pursue her suspicions interminably. So let her think what she liked. In fact if the other woman was in, it could even be a good thing. He'd easily be able to find a way of slipping upstairs, to the loo perhaps, when both women were downstairs distracting one another, and quickly look under the floorboard in the cupboard. If he was found out, he'd have to explain, of course, but he could cross that bridge when he came to it. He wanted the map to himself. It would be the only authentic memento of his son that he possessed, and therefore the only real evidence that he had once been a father. In contrast to what he had now, he had enjoyed being a genuine father. Sometimes at least, when he and Rose weren't both wracking themselves or each other with guilt. He had enjoyed being authentic. And he had loved his son just as much as she had, if less demonstratively.

Now he was a mere cipher. A phoney. A step-father. Someone you either struggled, or didn't even bother struggling to be polite to, if you were Sarah or Harry. Either way, rude or polite, the 'step' they all loathed was always in the way. When the television wasn't on.

He had loved his son, and he had loved his first wife, too. Far more profoundly than his simple affection for the warm-hearted woman he shared a bed with now. Even if she was in fact a lot easier to live with than either of them.

'Rose, there's a part of my heart that's always only yours. You know that, don't you?'

'Don't talk wet! And be warned: if I have any of that kind of nonsense I will be asking you to leave immediately. It wouldn't be fair on Mary.'

It was Sunday evenin
and tidying. As was becoming
her friend's baby all afternoon

Rose liked her home
When she had finished the
obsessionally though. She
again, like she used to be w
would hoover the house
exacerbating his asthma. A
clean everything, including
raw and bloody because sh
sure she was not carrying ar
infection. Richard would be
others he would hold her
uselessness of it all.

He hadn't been a b
Luke died they simply had n

Now as she plump
bins and made the place
become depressed again.
evenings now, leaving her
herself was like being alone
needed to be needed. She

So it wasn't only b
become so closely involve
sex over the last twenty
bizarre, and in principle ar
down her nose at the vanit
– quickly became mundan
patently right. Cases like h
had intuitively known that
been confirmed ever since

For the life of her,
weird facts of Lucille's ide
have been a bit of a 'wee
female, her delicate fra
feminine. Thanks to the
twenty months she had de
though it was ridiculous tl
had at the moment on E
looked fine as she was. I
girl in her late teens.

It had be
her that had been

And all in
her, Rose had fou
important thing. It
fact that biologica
interest. In being
maternal feelings.
and outside some
home, she had be
them becoming a
There had been no
Her emptiness ha
dormant anyway.

Till now. It
needed was startin
simply been about
found herself beco
and a kind of friend
after everything tha
now that to all inter
properly herself, R
She could let herse
feel slightly upset
because Lucille wa
less. She would lea
Like her dead son.
would leave one day

She couldn'
it with a sorry little
because, after all,
laughing it away too
easier, like whether
wine stains out of
that when Lucille
nothing but a deep e
be feeling suicidal ag

Which would

But what wa
out herself with Luc
sake, and anyway L
Often they were all s
and, occasionally, he
as her father wasn't

out together. But unfortunately she wasn't Lucie's real mother, and even if she denied it, Lucie wouldn't want to be accompanied everywhere by her middle-aged friend. Not all the time anyway. It wasn't that Lucie had discouraged her. The very opposite in fact, but as Rose saw it, this was just more evidence that she wasn't really needed anymore.

So just as there was very little for her to do now to help Lucie be herself, she was beginning to feel conversely that there *were* little things that Lucie could actually do for her, to help *her* feel more comfortable with being who she was, for pity's sake; to help *her* feel less lonely and more confident in facing the changes age was inevitably bringing. She didn't like to admit it, but she felt Lucie owed her something.

Somehow though, she just couldn't let her give her anything, as if it was important that their relationship remain unequal and she herself remain a saint, caring and bountiful. And ageless.

She had recently noticed she'd begun developing wrinkles on the back of her knees. She was getting *old*. So dispiriting. When Lucie was around it was so much easier to be diverted from what in her own case was definitely vanity: this lurching slide into middle age. To counter it she was making a conscious effort to stop trying to pull out the grey hairs from her head whenever she was alone with a mirror. But that didn't stop her wanting to. Lucie said they looked good on her, but when she snapped back that she didn't like them and that was that, Lucie had blinked twice then brightly suggested she go blonde and have her hair cut shorter, saying she'd do it for her if she liked. Of course that was sweet of her. Rose should have been grateful. Instead she pretended to be, apologised for her waspishness and refusing Lucie's offer with her kindest, most self-deprecating laugh, said she really ought to be content with becoming grey haired because, as she so often said about all kinds of things, it was only natural. But the truth was both more complex and more prosaic than that. With Lucie beginning to drift off into her own life, insecurity in Rose about not being needed was being replaced by vanity, of all things.

For some reason Rose continually fought shy of telling Lucie how she felt. Why? To maintain the illusion of sanctity? Or was it more likely because she knew her feelings were turning her into a witch? As much as she did want Lucie to know how insecure she was beginning to feel, like a cantankerous and contrary old crone, she didn't want her to know it at all. She had never been vulnerable with Lucie, not even that first night they met in the woods the year before last. She didn't want to start now.

She was using the truth to shore up the lie that they were still as close to one another now as they had always been. She knew she shouldn't be discontented. And she knew she shouldn't be feeling lonely. It was ridiculous to feel lonely when actually they were living under the same roof together. She had lived on her own for the best part of five years before Lucille had joined her, so why have to have such stupid, unnecessary feelings now? They still had breakfast together every morning and it wasn't as if Lucie was out every night of the week. But there it was, from having been the confident enabler of the unfolding and flowering of Lucie's femininity for so long, she was now rapidly in danger of deteriorating herself, into an anxious, insecure and emotionally dependent old bag.

It was almost as if her own identity had somehow been sucked out of her.

How on earth did these things happen?

It was also maddening to feel she was hateful for the minor sin of occasionally envying Lucille her youth and her future. It was just a feeling, after all. Nothing more, and not in itself particularly bad. It was, if anything, and when she thought about it, a sign perhaps that she did in fact care about herself, which in turn was evidence that she wanted to live. All the same, it made her feel uncomfortable that the nicer and happier Lucie became the more of a bitch she found herself beginning to feel. She didn't often let it show. Not really. But it was increasingly what she felt inside. The odd ambiguous remark inevitably slipped out sometimes, although so far, thank goodness, that was all.

Lucille gave her no real reason to feel cross with her. She was easy to live with, helped with all the chores, never stayed in the bathroom too long or left dirty cups around or dishes unwashed. If she was ironing clothes, she would always do Rose's too. In fact she was perfect, neither moody nor insensitive. She was just a bit, well, vacuous if the truth were told. But overall, for someone so young and with such a strange history she was amazing.

So why am I becoming dishonest with her, Rose asked herself. Why can't I be myself?

She noticed she hadn't hoovered the front hall properly. Well, she *had* actually, but since doing so five minutes ago a petal had fallen from the tulips she had bought herself yesterday. No doubt a few grains of pollen would have tumbled down as well, even if she couldn't actually see any. She got the cleaner out again and hoovered around where the petal had fallen, and then for good measure decided she may as well do the whole downstairs again. Why not? It was true she had got some notes to write up for work, but they could wait. If she was ever to become a more efficient manager she ought to be able to find time to do them at work anyway. As an afterthought, she quickly gave upstairs a once-over again too. It did no harm and she was alone so no-one could remark upon it, as Richard used to do.

He was coming round tomorrow for one of his once or twice-yearly 'catch up' sessions, which usually meant him telling her about what he was doing and how the children were, and not saying anything about Mary, his new – well, *newish* – wife. Perhaps there really was nothing to say, but she and Richard used to talk so much about everything when they were married. At least that hadn't changed: he would talk about himself. He was bound to.

If he had time to ask her about herself he would usually try to, before he had to dash. Never one to neglect the little politenesses was Richard. More often than not they met on neutral territory in a restaurant or a pub. The house was too full of history. This time however, he had insisted on coming round. Perhaps because when he rang it had been Lucille who answered the phone. Maybe he was curious about who she was sharing their old house with now. Well he probably wouldn't be able to satisfy his curiosity because, as she told him, Lucie was likely to be out tomorrow evening as well. What would they talk about? Anything, as long as it was nothing too personal. There was so much that could never be said about how they missed their little son, without one of them becoming too upset and the other feeling unable to offer comfort.

But they did have to meet up once or twice a year in order not to say it.

She put the hoover away in the cupboard under the stairs. She just had the bathroom to do. She'd been putting it off, both desiring and fearing the almost erotic charge of becoming attached to the taps again like in the good old, bad old days when having a husband and a child had been the chore and housework had been her pleasure. She had felt an overwhelming need just to clean and clean the taps till she could see her reflection in them. At first in those days it had been so satisfying to make them sparkle. She would take a break from giving Luke his physiotherapy, having resolutely resisted his piteous pleas to be let off just this once from having his little chest and back pummelled, and simply polish the taps knowing that she did have control over them like she did not over his steadily decreasing lung capacity. She used to have to do it to him two or three times a day and he *always* hated it. Each time she would go to the bathroom afterwards feeling she had to wash her hands which had somehow been sullied by all the pummeling she had had to give him to loosen the mucus and pus clogging his increasingly scarred and useless lungs. She knew it was irrational and tried not to. But if she didn't wash her hands she would find herself starting to clean the taps instead. Then she had somehow ended up being unable to get away from them, rubbing and polishing them long after they could gleam no brighter. On more than one occasion Richard had physically lifted her up to get her away from them after she had been at it for four or five hours or more, half-dragging, half-carrying her out of the bathroom kicking and screaming for him to leave her alone, tears streaming down her face. Lukey would cry too, of course, as he watched them. And to her shame that would sometimes snap her out of it.

75

But now there was nobody to stop her and she could take as long as she liked. She didn't have to pretend or invent a rationalisation that what she was doing was sensible, that they did actually need cleaning. She didn't have to convince herself that if she could not get them to shine, they could be replaced.

Unlike Luke.

She made her way back upstairs being careful to keep precisely to the path she always took, up on the left, down on the right, so that the carpet didn't get too worn. With some trepidation she went into the bathroom.

She pulled up with frustration. Forgotten on the floor under the sink lay a pair of discarded tights and knickers. She picked them up. Lucille's of course. She was becoming more and more sluttish recently. There was a laundry basket in the corner from which they filled the washing machine each week, taking their turn; Lucille had never neglected to use it before.

Disgruntled, Rose put the things in the basket and looked at her watch. Her concentration on the task she had come in with was broken. She would have to go downstairs, clear her mind of her annoyance, perhaps have a cup of tea, and come up again in fifteen or twenty minutes time, so that she could give the taps her undivided attention.

She was sitting at the kitchen table sipping her tea, vaguely listening to the radio telling her about cyclamens and wondering whether the veins on the back of her hands were becoming bluer and more prominent, when she heard the front door opening. Lucie. Well, she would have to have words with her. Serious words.

She heard her hanging up her coat and then she came into the kitchen, kissed Rose on the head and flicked the switch on the kettle.

'I've just seen a man who looked like Ron – remember Ron? – with a dog who looked just like Milly on the corner of our block,' Lucie said, taking a pair of clips from her hair, laying them on the table and shuddering dramatically. 'I don't *think* it was him. He was too far away to see properly, and disappeared before I got close enough to tell. Anyway he was far too fat. But for a moment it was scary. No. It couldn't be, could it? Because Milly is dead.'

She gave Rose a characteristically bright bland smile, which always came out when she was nervous or frightened, and poured herself a cup of tea. Then she became more animated.

'Oh, you must see the dress I got today! I'm going to wear it to go to Fabric in tonight.' Before Rose could say anything, Lucille went out into the hallway where she had left her things and Rose heard her delving into a plastic bag. A few moments later she floated back into the kitchen, smiling broadly and fiddling with her hair, wearing a dark red dress with a plunging neckline. It was cut close over the breasts and tummy, but fell into pretty, flowing feminine shape over her bum and legs. It wasn't too short either, thought Rose, which made something of a change. It looked nice.

'What do you think? Not too tarty or too tight?'

Lucille twirled, eyes sparkling, unselfconscious, knowing she looked good.

Rose sighed. 'It looks lovely on you,' she said automatically, yet also meaning it. Hearing how middle-aged the lack of enthusiasm in her voice sounded, she added, 'And you look stunning, Lucie.'

Nevertheless, she felt confused by her compulsion always to be nice to her, even now when actually she was angry.

'I wouldn't exist without you, Rosie.'

It was just that Lucie was so disarming which always left Rose feeling as if she was somehow in the presence of a tiny baby in a grown up body. And you just couldn't be angry with a tiny baby. It wouldn't be fair. You looked after them. It was instinctive.

Lucie sat down, wiggling her legs and feet in the air and smiling inanely. 'I can't believe I got it so cheap. It only cost me fifteen quid in the sale.'

Rose nodded, was about to speak when Lucie stood up frowning, said there was no way she was going to risk marking her dress before going out later, took it off again and laid it carefully over the back of the chair beside her. As usual, Rose tried to avoid noticing the chair was the one with singe marks on the foot of each leg caused by the fire she'd set in the woods the autumn before last when she first met Lucie.

Rose shook her head, tried to ignore both the marks on the chair legs and the memory of what she had been trying to do that day. Lucie sat down again and sipped her tea.

'I'm going up in a minute to get ready. I can't wait for tonight.'

Looking at her sitting there in bra and tights slurping at her tea, as easy and familiar with her as if she were family, the last residue of Rose's earlier anger evaporated. She couldn't help it. It really was like having a daughter. One she had made herself.

'What kind of place is 'Fabric'?' she asked.

'Oh, just a club' Lucie replied airily, as if she went clubbing all the time now. 'I went there with Fiona from work a couple of months ago, when she wasn't speaking to her boyfriend. Don't you remember?' She hummed a tune. 'I'm going with David.' The way she said his name with a distracted little giggle threatened to irritate Rose again. She really was too old for this kind of thing, and most certainly not jealous of it.

'Is that the one who used to be a boxer and plays the piano, or the medical student?'

'Rose! They're both the same person! You know they are.' She laughed, tilted her head to one side in the practiced yet innocent manner of a coquette, and said, 'I think he really likes me. He said he did. But he hasn't even tried to kiss me yet. I don't know what's the matter with him.' She pouted theatrically. 'If he doesn't try it on with me tonight, I'll just have to, to – I don't know,' she wailed. 'I don't know what I'll do.'

'Come back for comfort to your Auntie Rose!'

'I love you, Rosie. But I need a man! It's been over four months since I was put right. Four months and I still haven't... you know. I can't believe it!'

Rose knew there'd been no lack of interest from men, on the few occasions Lucie had met any, but surprisingly, since her operation male interest as often as not made her feel tense and anxious, which had confused her a little. Ambivalence towards men hadn't been part of her plan at all.

She had so much to learn.

'Relax,' said Rose. 'There's plenty of time for that, believe you me. You're only just starting out. Chill out, my darling. Take it easy.' She hadn't mean this yoof-speak to sound spikey and it didn't, because she felt no envy or resentment towards Lucie at all about adolescent issues like this. On the contrary, she felt ever so glad to be past all that herself. Giving Lucie a kindly sympathetic smile, she settled back into her customary, comfortable, wise old Auntie Rose role. Her own anxieties about getting old and lonely could always wait when she was being needed like this. Always.

'I just want to accept myself as I am now, but how can I when I don't know how I feel?'.

'We none of us do a lot of the time. We have to just do the best we can and put up with the pros and cons of being who we are. Don't you worry, it won't last long,' Rose added with the tart certainty of experience.

'What's the matter with me, Rose?' Lucie asked. 'Do I give out the wrong signals?'

'I don't think so,' she replied carefully. 'Except sometimes you sound happy when what you're saying is actually sad. And vice-versa too, sometimes. Men are easily confused too, you know. You're frowning, but it's true.'

'I know. I'm not completely stupid. Even if I do confuse myself.' She shook her head, pushed some hair behind her ear. 'I've always been topsy-turvy. That's what my Mum calls it. But I can't help the way I'm made, can I? I can't help it that some of the happiest hours I've ever known in my whole life – like when I first woke up after my surgery knowing that at last I was normal – I just cried. And I giggle when I'm unhappy. I do! I actually used to laugh when Ron pulled my hair. Do you know what I mean?'

She stood up, picked her red dress up off the chair and put it back on again, going out into the hallway to look at herself in the full length mirror once more as if to reassure herself she looked normal. She wants to feel pretty not crazy, thought Rose watching her. Well, that's okay, that's understandable. Craziness could persist on and off all your life, but prettiness was very temporary and quickly past. She should enjoy it while it lasts.

'Perhaps I'm a bit mad, Rosie. Do you think I am?'

'Of course not! All I meant was you sometimes seem as if what you're feeling and what you're saying are somehow quite separate.'

'You mean, like a man?' Lucille asked with an increasingly nervous, high-pitched edge to her voice. Rose decided to ignore it.

'If you like.'

'I do not like! I don't like it at all.'

*　　*　　*

Lucie flounced upstairs to her room, took off the dress again and lay down on her bed hugging the pink Care Bear her mum had given her when she was ten years old. Life was certainly not turning out to be as simple and easy as she had imagined it would. She glared at the poster on her wall.

I am nothing like a man, she thought, picking at a little bit of fluff from her new dress. Disconsolate, she flicked it away towards her waste paper basket.

Nothing like a man. Not even a little bit. She wiped away a hot tear that had dribbled down the side of her nose. She had always been a girl – well, feminine anyway – even when she was a boy. Always. Always. Always.

In fact a man was what she needed right now to feel better, to feel like a woman. Even if they were a bit scary.

Maybe something would come of her relationship with David tonight. He was good-looking, intelligent, or supposed to be, being a medical student. And big. She liked big men. So she did fancy him. He was the same age as she was, and he blushed and sometimes mumbled which made him sound stupid, but that was okay. It made him less scary. She wasn't ready for her ideal man just yet. Ideal man was at least ten years older than her, absolutely sure of himself and confident in everything he did.

Anyway, she should be so lucky. Such men only existed on television or at the movies, and if they did happen to exist in real life then they always already had women dancing attendance upon them. If they weren't already married. She knew that, even if she had never met one.

She got up and went to the bathroom. If something didn't happen tonight with David she might have to put her scruples aside, try to become predatory. A man eater. But she wasn't keen at all. She wanted a man to eat *her*.

David would be round at eight. She had met him at Grainne's flat a couple of weeks ago. Soon after finding her note – nearly two years ago now – Grainney had quietly packed her things and left Ron while he was out at work. She had moved into a nurses' residence near St George's where she worked as an agency nurse. She got a permanent post a few weeks later, renting a flat which she shared with two other nurses in Tooting. Lucie had found all this out when they'd bumped into one another again a couple of months ago in Wimbledon. Ever since then she had been looking after Grainne's baby for her every Sunday afternoon for a couple of hours, purely out of friendship, no money involved. It gave Grainne a break.

She took off her underwear and ran the bath. As usual she checked her nakedness over in the full length mirror as she waited for the tub to fill. She looked like any other girl her age. She'd been in enough changing rooms by now to know that. But it always helped to remind herself. Feeling more secure she turned off the taps and got in. She settled down with sigh into the water, trying to relax. She had to get herself in the mood for going out, stop being so anxious and uncertain. You only got one life.

David had been a friend of one of the other women Grainne was sharing with, whose birthday it was. Grainne had invited her to the party, said it would be fun, but actually it had been boring. She hadn't enjoyed being a wallflower at all. She didn't know anybody and nobody seemed to be interested in getting to know her beyond the usual party-time small talk. There were very few men there anyway, so David immediately stood out. She had noticed him out of the corner of her eye as she tried to play with Grainne's baby. The baby allowed her to hold him which was pleasingly more than he allowed anyone else to do – even his mother, often enough. Unfortunately the price exacted by the baby for this dubious privilege was that she keep moving. In her highest party heels that hadn't been as easy as she tried to make it look. He started to cry every time she stopped walking around the room or tried to put him down or pass him on to somebody else. Everyone attempted to make a fuss of him when she did so, but he was so clingy in the brief moments between his baleful stillness and his bawling that she was effectively prevented from being able to chat with anyone anyway. And then he had sicked up the big feed Grainne had given him five minutes before over the new top she'd bought specially for the party. Not just a little burp. A great big vomit. It had soaked right through to her skin. Embarrassed and uncomfortable, she had plonked the baby back into Grainne's arms, dolefully deciding to leave early. She sponged herself down in the bathroom first, rinsing her bra and top, stuffing them into a plastic shopping bag to take home with her and borrowing a fresh top from Grainne. Choosing it took them both back to memories of a shared past which now seemed very distant indeed. But even with a clean top on, she was sure she could still detect the distinct whiff of burped-up milk. When she was saying her goodbyes David had said he was leaving too and offered to walk with her on her way back to the station. She tried to hide her delight. Definite male interest at last. Her heart had naturally skipped a beat or two behind her acceptance of his company with a non-committal nod and a polite smile. Thankfully he hadn't noticed her being sicked up on earlier, but she kept a more than discreet distance from him as they walked to the tube so that the faintly sour smell wafting up her nose didn't get up his.

They'd met again since, and he definitely seemed to be interested in her, asking her about her life and family and interests without looking at her like she was a complete ninny when she said she was hairdressing at the moment, but would like to be a teacher or a nursery nurse one day because she loved children. He was nice and as they got to know each other his shyness lifted a little which had helped her confidence too. He actually admitted over a shared pizza that he'd only left the party early that night because *she* had, tentatively stroking the back of her fingers, his voice wonderfully deep and throaty. She'd hid her excitement behind an appropriate mix of modesty, suitably sugared and spiced, she hoped, with stunning, seductive and equally desire-filled glances back at him. Her heart raced for him to make another move between restaurant and home. A kiss on the lips goodbye would have been nice, or a pat on the bum, even another squeeze of her hand. But nothing. She'd kicked her shoes off with frustration when she got in, trying to console herself that at least he had made another date with her. She had mentioned clubbing at Fabric, then found herself purring behind her rocket and ricotta when he said he'd never been himself and would like to go with her.

So at least there was a possibility that something might happen with him tonight. If he did want her, she would be happy to lose her virginity to a boy like him because she could hopefully still have some control. Real men could come later. First she had to be as certain as she could be that she was as good a fuck as any other girl her age. And for that she needed a twenty year old boy like this one.

She got out of the bath and towelled herself dry. She went back to her room, dried her hair and put on her new dress for what was now the fourth time since she first saw it hanging on the rail during her lunch break. Then she put the radio on – 'Crapital' as Ron used to call it – and did her make up. She painted her fingers and toes, trying to relax as they dried and get in the right mood for her evening ahead. She wasn't sure she actually felt very sexy at all. It all felt a bit too much like a project she had been waiting all her life to put herself through. She would have preferred to have felt more natural. Perhaps if everything went okay that would come later. Or maybe it never would. Perhaps Rose was right about her feelings not fitting properly with the things she said. Like coffee from a teapot, or tea from a cafeteria, still warm, still wet, still tasting of tea or coffee but somehow just not quite right. It might be a residue of maleness. This thought was so terrifying and so humiliating that the old envious anger which used to slow-burn in her belly all the time before her operations, reared its ugly head again. She bit her lip. She just didn't do anger anymore if she could help it. It wasn't nice. She always preferred to laugh or cry instead.

She glanced at herself in the mirror again, instinctively widening her eyes and touching her hair. At least she didn't look angry. She just looked like a girl getting ready to go out. No more, no less. Good. She didn't want to think about things like that. Not now. She looked for a pair of tights in her drawer. None. None suitable anyway. Not a single pair. She'd have to ask Rose if she might borrow some from her after she had done her face and hair. If she didn't have any, she'd be in trouble.

'Rose,' she called down the stairs half an hour later, brushing her hair and confident she otherwise looked immaculate. 'Have you got a pair of tights I could borrow? Good ones, if possible. Do you mind? I'll replace them, I promise. I'm sorry, I thought I did have a pair, but I think I must have put them in the wash.'

'You didn't. I did,' said Rose from the bottom of the stairs. She made her way up, went into her lilac bedroom which Lucie knew she'd painted herself after Richard had left, and brusquely gesturing for Lucille to follow her, opened her knickers drawer. She fished inside, pulled out an unopened packet. 'Here you are. Wolford. Eight denier. I've had them for ages. Months anyway. Go on, take them. I don't need expensive tights. Nobody ever comes to take me out!'

Lucille hesitated. The price was still on the back. She made an Oh-I-shouldn't face, then grabbed the packet with a grateful smile and ripping it open, sat down on the edge of Rose's bed and bent to put her toes into them.

'Lucille, we've got to talk or at least I have.'

'What's the matter, Rosie?' Lucie stood up smiling, pulling the tights up over her bottom and smoothing her dress down, looking at herself this way and that way in Rose's wardrobe mirror.

Now was not a good time for this, thought Rose.

'You've started treating me like I was a part of yourself, Lucie, and I'm not,' she said.

'What do you mean? I don't understand. I know you are not a part of me. Of course I do.'

'I need more from you than you are giving me. At the moment it's like we both feel I only exist for you.'

They looked at each other. Both of them knowing this was true.

'Oh Rose. No! I mean, yes! You're right. I know you are. I've been taking you for granted I know I have,' Lucie replied, startled, apologetic, sincere.

Rose softened. Again. Why couldn't she ever resist Lucie's need to be cared for? Instinctively they moved towards one another and hugged. Rose didn't want to let go, even if Lucie did smell like a whore's handbag. She didn't want Lucie to see how pathetic she felt.

It was Lucille who eventually pulled away and reached for a tissue from the box on Rose's dressing table. She glanced at Rose and handed her one too. Oh, well. Never mind.

'There,' said Lucie, moving her hair out of her face, 'Topsy-turvy again. I'm crying and smiling at the same time. Again.' She went close to the mirror and attended to the dark smudges running from her eyes. Rose sighed.

'And talking about yourself again, Lucie. That's the thing, you see, sometimes I need to talk about me.'

'Oh, Rosie! I'm so sorry. I'm going to make a big effort from now on. I've been really selfish. I know I have. I must do more listening, Talk to me now, please. Talk to me now. I'll stay in. I can tell David I'm not well.'

Whether she meant it or not, it was a lovely thing to say. Rose was disarmed. Yet again. All the feelings she had been harbouring over the past few weeks just flitted away now there was an opportunity to talk about them. She would have felt angry about the irony of this had her capacity to do so not gone too.

'Don't be silly! And he'd never believe you anyway, the way you look. There's plenty of time.'

She tried to recover her earlier annoyance. 'You left your knickers and tights lying on the bathroom floor. That's all. It's nothing serious. But *I* was cross,' she added lamely. She had not wanted to talk about tights and knickers. She had wanted to talk about how much she needed Lucille's interest and attention because her old comforter, the idea of suicide, had come to stay with her again and woke her up at four in the morning, every morning recently, to tell her she really would be better off dead. But she couldn't. Not just now, with Lucille all dolled up and about to go out.

The doorbell rang.

'That'll be him now. You better get your shoes and coat on. I'll see you later.'

'I might not be coming back tonight Rosie,' Lucille replied with a mock-innocent grin. 'I'm hoping to be ravished! But we'll talk tomorrow. I promise.'

'Go on, off you go! Good luck.'

The doorbell rang again and Lucille ran to her room for her kitten stilettos and clutch bag. A few moments later she was down the stairs and gone.

Rose took off her own shoes and got into her slippers. She would do the bathroom taps as planned and she would take her time. If she felt sad to be almost deliberately falling back into an old self-destructive pattern of behaviour, she didn't care. There was a mark on the front of her skirt. It looked like bleach. Ah well, it couldn't be helped. Like her, the skirt had seen better days. It was only an old cheap cotton thing. Perhaps she would go through all her clothes later and throw out what she didn't need anymore. If she still had time. Perhaps Lucie would like some of them. Probably not. Too middle-aged for her.

Chapter 7.

At quarter to six the following evening Ron Symes felt the light spring rain wash down the back of his neck as he pulled the collar of his jean jacket up and turned away from the woman in the long dark skirt and business-like, slate-grey raincoat walking purposefully along the street towards him. She was on her way home from work laden with shopping bags. He stared at Milly, whom he had renamed Malcolm, settling down on his hind quarters to shit on the grass verge. He hadn't recognised who the old cow was until just now because she had gone and had her hair done, hadn't she, dyed blonde and cut short and wispy. Hope that she wouldn't recognise him oozed out of every pore in a telltale stench. He was always sweating nowadays. Perhaps it was a side-effect of the medication.

She did glance at him as she re-shouldered her bags and passed him by, but he studiously avoided letting her catch his gaze. It was a year and a half since she had last seen him and then it had only been for a few minutes while she waited for Lucie to come down the stairs and go off with her in her car. And he had put on quite a bit of weight since then, what with the drugs the psychiatrists had put him on. It should be alright.

But it wasn't. She stopped, turned and raised an eyebrow. He felt himself quaking. Like he was up before the headmistress. He let out a silent groan. He always made more of things than they were. He always gave himself away. He could always count on himself for that.

'It's Ron, isn't it?'

He didn't say anything, studying Malcolm intently like he was the object of a vital scientific experiment in canine street behaviour.

'And if I am not mistaken, that's Milly too.'

'Malcolm,' he said sideways, still not looking at her. Rose looked at the animal with what even Ron could recognise as obvious distaste as it stood up and turned round to sniff its own excreta. 'He's Malcolm. Same breed. Mongol,' he said, as if she might be interested.

'I take it you mean mongrel. Lucie said she thought she'd seen you around here. If you're a stalker, you're not doing a very good job. And if not, what may I ask *are* you doing here?'

'I'm not a stalker. I just like walking the dog around here that's all.' He replied. And then with an almost visible brainwave said, 'and my name is not Ron. I'm er, – .' He couldn't think of a single fucking name. 'Robert,' he said, with sigh of relief. He affected a nonchalant pose, staring up and down the street in a caricature of just another member of the local dog-owning fraternity.

'I hope you're going to scoop up that mess,' Rose said in such a loud voice that he thought the whole street would hear her humiliating him, 'and take it home with you, because I know where you live and I will give your name and address to the police if you don't - or if I ever see you around here again.'

The word 'Police' triggered alarm bells and sirens all across the top of his head. His heart started thumping. He lifted his arms up and flapped them, not knowing whether to massage his head or his heart. Two fat tears filled the inside corner of each eye and he felt himself panicking as he imagined the police arriving, tyres screeching, to take him away.

'Don't do that missis, please,' he said reproachfully, feeling like a little boy. 'I haven't done nothing, Me and Malcolm just like walking round here, that's all. I've got a right.'

'We'll see about that.' Her efficient professional manner was confident and sure in the face of his resentful timidity. He knew he was giving himself away as a recipient of a certain type of community care.

She put her shopping bags down on the ground and swinging her handbag round to the front, pulled out her mobile phone. As she did so, she failed to notice 'Malcolm' putting her nose into the nearest shopping bag and lifting out a package of chicken breasts.

'Hey Malcolm, put that down you fucking idiot,' Ron barked.

The dog started to beat a hasty retreat into the nearest front garden together with his prize.

'Put it down, you stupid mutt,' Ron yelled, pulling his belt up over his girth and starting to give chase.

The very next moment he slipped on the wet verge and landed with a sixteen stone thump on the pavement.

'Oh shit,' he said. 'Shit. Shit. Shit. I've fallen in his shit.'

'No, you haven't,' said Rose, pointing at Malcolm's freshly produced faecal offering less than a centimetre away from Ron's be-jeaned hip. He shifted hastily away from it, the pain in his left wrist shooting up his arm to his shoulder as he did so. He rolled and shifted further to the right, groaning miserably, his trousers soaking in the wet grass, his elbows on the pavement. Damp and dirty.

'I think I've broken my fucking wrist.'

'I think you owe me three pounds fifty for providing your dog with its dinner.'

'I'm bleeding.' He moaned, heaving himself up into a sitting position on the kerbside with his feet in the gutter. He looked at the palms of his hands which were grazed and black with grime and wet.

Rose dug a tissue out of her bag.

'Here, take it.'

Ron knew how to respond to compassion appropriately. He blew his nose. She gave him another one for his hands. Looking tiny in them the tissue almost instantly became sodden as the rain became more insistent.

'Never mind about the chicken,' said Rose. 'Just keep away from here, that's all.'

'You are a very kind woman.' He replied, trying to use the tissue on his trousers. 'A very kind woman.' She gave him another.

'For your hands,' she said impatiently. 'Your trousers will just have to go into the wash.'

When he tried to wipe his left hand his wince of pain was visible.

'It's broken,' he said piteously, holding it up with his right.

Rose looked at it. The bone at the base of his palm certainly looked swollen.

'You'll have to take it to hospital to have it seen to then.'

*   *   *

Rose picked up her plastic shopping bags. The rain was going to ruin her hair which rather guiltily she had taken nearly two hours out to have done at lunch time. She normally worked through every lunch period writing case notes and doing phone calls to referring doctors and social workers, and it didn't set a good example to deviate from that habit so obviously. Her staff had all been very nice, as of course they would be, and told her she looked great. She wasn't used to flattery of any kind and had lapped it up. Gracefully, of course, and with not too much obvious delight. After all she was the boss. But she had felt pleased with herself during her afternoon sessions. It was ridiculous at her age to have to rediscover that looking better could also somehow make you feel better, but she had definitely felt more creative with the families she had worked with this afternoon. How odd it was that a trivial thing like a hairdo could make such a difference to how she felt. And how very stupid of her to have forgotten such a truism.

She gave Ron a curt nod and carried on her way, the rain lashing her face. It was such a nuisance she had been banned from driving and had to brave weather like this. On the other hand, to think positively, it was very unlikely that after the dressing down she had just given him, that dreadful man would ever bother Lucille or herself again.

As she opened her front gate she glanced back up the road and saw that he was still sitting on the kerb. Dreadful but pathetic, the way he had shouted at the dog like that. Ridiculous. Just as ridiculous in his own way as she was in hers. He was not even a bit frightening anymore. She vaguely wondered what might have happened to him over the last eighteen months to change him from an aggressive leering lout into the pathetic creature he was now.

She unpacked her shopping and then went straight upstairs to the bathroom to see to her hair. The rain had plastered it down over her face and she looked a fright. She took a hand towel from the rail, rubbed it dry trying to restrain her usual vigour and impatience with little fluffing movements so she didn't ruin it. It wasn't every day you had a new hair-do. When she looked up at herself in the mirror again it took a bit of getting used to. Blonde definitely seemed to suit her though, and shorter hair did seem to take attention away from her incipient second chin. She went to her bedroom, took the hairdryer to it, then put on a touch of lipstick. Lucie might be a bit miffed that she hadn't let her be the one to do her hair, but she was sure to be impressed. It certainly made her look a few years younger. Softer. It was though, a bit strange to be having such thoughts about herself. Maybe Lucie's preoccupation with appearance was rubbing off on her somehow; or maybe she had been so lost in looking after Lucie these last eighteen months that she had forgotten to look after herself.

It was a pity that Lucie needed her less and less, but she would talk to her about it when she got a chance. Their relationship had to change, but there was always something else going on. In particular, her friend's baby with the unfortunate name seemed to absorb so much of her attention recently. Lucie was now looking after the poor little thing every Sunday afternoon, and she had no shame at all admitting how much she loved giving people the impression the baby was hers when she took it out to the park.

It seemed nothing Lucie did nowadays had any reference to anything or anyone other than herself. Perhaps that had always been the case. They had so much to talk about. Tomorrow. Not tonight. Tonight she would be talking with Richard, or rather he would be talking with her.

She changed into a rarely worn black dress. She liked it well enough, just didn't have enough occasion to wear the thing. It had a huge, but subtle dark blue floral print across the bodice and skirt. It must be at least two years since she had last worn it. She hoped she didn't look too old-fashioned because she liked the way it set off her new blonde head. She fluffed her hair up a bit more, then went downstairs to prepare the dinner she was cooking for Richard who would be around in a couple of hours.

The doorbell rang.

It was Ron, dirty and bedraggled in the pouring rain and looking as mournful and self-piteous as his dog looked post-prandial. He had stepped back out into the rain from her front porch as she opened the door, and both he and the dog were dripping. He was still holding his left hand gingerly in his right, like he was tending a day old chick, and Rose couldn't help feeling sorry for him.

'Could you ring 999 for me?'

'Come and stand in the porch out of the rain,' she said. 'I'll get you a towel first and then, of course, I'll phone for an ambulance straight away.' She closed the door while she went up stairs for the towel. She would have to invite him in while he waited for the ambulance. She couldn't leave him out there in that state. But what was she playing at, she wondered, as she got a fresh one from her airing cupboard. More irrationality, no doubt.

She traced her usual path back down the stairs shuddering at the thought of the dirt and rain he was going to bring in with him. At the same time she wanted it. It would give her something to clean up later. And she did so like cleaning.

'You'd better come in,' she said, 'and dry yourself down while I make the phone call. They're not going to hurry to get here for a mere fracture. Possible mere fracture I should say. Cheer up Ron, it may not be broken at all. Come on. In you come. I want to shut the door – it's cold.'

He hesitated looking at the dog.

'Bring Malcolm in with you,' she said, immediately regretting it.

She held the door open and preceded by Malcolm, Ron stepped inside. She shut the door. Malcolm ran straight into her kitchen and shook himself dry spraying the units and the lino floor with a patina of dirty rainwater. 'You'd better follow him, and kindly attach him to his lead. I don't want him running all over the house.'

She picked up the phone and dialled the emergency services and was told an ambulance would arrive as soon as possible – waiting times for minor injuries were currently anything up to two hours. Rose sighed as she put the phone down. Richard would be here in less than that. She'd better accept that her evening had already gone out of her control.

'Don't stand there looking uncomfortable Ron, sit down and rest your hand. I'll make you a cup of tea.'

She poured some boiling water onto a tea bag for him. He asked for three sugars. She spooned them in, put the cup on the kitchen table in front of his right hand, and then started bustling about trying to get her meal started.

'I knew you'd look after me,' said Ron helping himself to another spoonful of sugar, 'like you looked after Lulu. I know what people think and feel. I can tell from the expressions on their faces. And I knew *you* would look after me.'

She hoped he could 'know' from the expression on her face that she was busy, she had a dinner to prepare, necessarily vegetarian now, thanks to his dog. The last thing she needed was idle chatter with an oaf like him. But she found herself adopting a kind professional smile and enquiring how he had developed such a skill as he had shown no sign of it when they had last met. She noted that despite his claim to telepathic-like powers he didn't seem to hear the barb in her tongue, responding only to her kindness and taking her words at face value.

Culinary concerns to the fore, she cut some onions while she engaged him in polite conversation, deciding that, on second thoughts, she preferred to have him talking with her than just sitting there silently, a huge lumpen, alien presence. She offered him a glass of cheap Shiraz and poured one for herself.

'I didn't know things then. It only really started after Lulu and Grainne left me and I had a breakdown, like,' he said. 'Grainne was sposed to be my girlfriend, see. So then I got upset and I couldn't go out except when it was dark. But I watched. I used to watch people from out of my window during the day. And I knew what they were thinking. And what they were saying. Not lip reading, I couldn't do that. But I could tell by looking at them what they were thinking and feeling. That's how I realised they all hated me. So I stayed in doors cos it wasn't safe.'

Rose didn't feel disturbed by this revelation. It was becoming increasingly apparent that her first impression had not been mistaken. His world had become circumscribed by psychosis, just as hers had by depression. That didn't make him more dangerous. Less probably.

She put the onions in a skillet and took her can opener to a tin of tomatoes. The little rotating cutter would not find a purchase to pierce the rim of the tin.

'I can do that for you. I'm very strong,' said Ron.

Despite his size and what she knew about his past he wasn't the least bit threatening, so without a second thought she passed the can and the opener over to him. Wincing he propped the tin awkwardly against his injured left hand and used his right hand to hold the opener. Rose saw the sweat run down his brow as the pain at the base of his hand intensified. She felt mortified, exclaiming that he should give it back to her when his face lit up and the tin started turning with no further need for resistance from his left hand. He pushed it back over to her.

'Thank you, Ron, but I see that your power to read minds and feelings doesn't extend to your own - you really shouldn't have done that for me and I'm sorry to have been so thoughtless as to ask you. Does it hurt very much?'

'It's okay. *You* didn't ask me to open it. But you're right,' he said with great solemnity. 'I don't know what I feel. I've never known that, even before I discovered my powers. I think maybe it's the price I have to pay for having them.'

'How did you discover them?' She poured the tomatoes into the skillet and adding some basil and oregano and a stock cube, she put it on the stove. 'I mean how could you tell what people were thinking and feeling if you couldn't go out and ask them? You know, check it out that you were right?'

He touched the side of his nose with his right forefinger trying to look clever, but achieving the opposite effect.

'I've never told nobody before, except at the clinic, cos you never know what they'll think. But I'll share my secret with you because you're helping me,' he said.

'Please do,' she replied, hoping the ambulance would arrive soon. Some years ago she had worked in a psychiatric hospital and she knew paranoia when she saw it. She also knew there was research evidence that people suffering from it were less likely to feel you were persecuting them if you kept what the researchers called your expressed emotion 'low', meaning undemonstrative. So she would just stay calm and reasonable, as if she was still at work and carry on chatting with him till he was taken away.

'I've got a rare cancer,' he said with a look of idiot pride on his face. 'I don't need to check out with people whether I am right about them. I *know* I am.' He looked at her intently. 'The cancer is in my head.'

'You've got some kind of brain tumour?'

He shrugged, not interested in the cause, only the effect.

'My psychiatrist said what I do is, and these are his own words I swear – I won't ever forget them because at the time I thought it was a curse, but now I know it's a gift too – he said what I do is: I attach too much significance to things.'

Rose poured some water and martini into her cooking, opened a cupboard and took out a packet of Arborio rice. It was quite remarkable the way this man was talking so openly. Despite his beliefs he didn't sound as simple as he was perhaps pretending to be. Just mad. Quite plainly mad. It was clearly a function of his mental condition to be so disinhibited, of course. But it nevertheless lent him a certain gravitas, and perhaps surprisingly it had also quickly created an easy comfortable atmosphere between them. She might have expected rather the reverse to be the case, but it wasn't. She sensed no danger from him at all.

'What's that got to do with cancer?' she asked.

'Don't you see? No. Course you don't. Cos you haven't got it, have you? You're not all fucked up like me.'

'I don't know about that! Got what?'

'Cancer of the mind. Not the brain. It's not physical,' he said, with the pompous pedantry of an expert. 'One of its main side-effects is you get all fucked up.'

'I'm sorry Ron, I don't understand.'

'That's what used to happen to me. I didn't understand why I was falling asleep all the time. I didn't understand how Lulu couldn't be a girl. Or a boy. And I didn't understand why Grainne left me. I mean we weren't getting on, but she never said nothing. And after that I didn't understand why I got frightened of going out in daylight. Nor why they were talking about me on the telly all the time. But I do now. I understand the meaning of everything now, cos of me cancer.'

'Your cancer? I don't understand why you call it a cancer.' She stirred her risotto mechanically, then started chopping up various kinds of mushrooms which she scraped into another pan and poured olive oil on to.

'Because the first doctor I saw said it was a kind of cancer of the mind and soul. And because it spreads. It's very advanced now. That's why I've got so fat. Weight-gain is a side effect of me medication. My psychiatrists told me. I never see the same one, but they all say the same thing. And they're right. I'm much bigger than I used to be.'

He sounded amazed, yet matter of fact at the same time. Rose felt herself becoming a bit impatient.

'How come you lied about Milly, Ron, a year and a half ago or whenever it was, you know, that day I came to pick her up? What was the meaning or significance of that? Lucille was devastated, you know. It wasn't very kind of you, was it?' She was careful to speak gently, with no undue emotion.

'Malcolm. His name is Malcolm. He's a great little dog. We all went to Battersea and bought him together, all three of us. But it was always me who took him out for his morning doings before I went to work ever since we got him. Not Lulu and not Grainne. I didn't want Lulu to take him with her cos he was mine too. She had told me to fuck off for no reason that I knew of. So I just locked him in the shed down the bottom of the garden when I saw you coming back. I know it was bad of me.'

'I'd have thought Grainne might have told Lucie her dog was still alive, unless, of course, she didn't want to. No! I remember now. Lucie told me Grainne was probably going to be very angry with her. About you. Perhaps that's why she never told her.'

'Grainne didn't know nothing about what I done with Malcolm. Anyway she never spoke to me again really, after Lulu left. I couldn't understand it. But I do now, of course.'

'So why was that then?'

'She was jealous of Lulu.'

From what little she knew of their household, it was bizarre enough to be true, but Rose felt intrigued as to how he had he managed to come to this conclusion.

'Why?' she asked, continuing to keep her voice soft and neutral.

'Cos Lulu was always going on about wanting to be a girl, and she – Grainne I mean – was always *moaning* about being one. I think she would have liked to want to be a girl too, 'cept she couldn't cos she already was one and she didn't like it very much. Didn't seem to anyway. Always moaning.'

'You really can be quite perceptive Ron, can't you.'

'Not me. It's my cancer what does it. I didn't get GCSEs or nothing.'

'Do you mind if I ask you another personal question?' She took a large gulp of wine, emptying her glass.

He nodded with a guileless, open smile. He hadn't touched his wine. It was so hard to believe this was the same monster who had hurled Lucille's semen-stained dress out of the window at them.

'Why did you force Lucie to give you oral sex?'

'What?' The astonishment on his face was almost comical, and certainly genuine. 'I never! Not forced. No, never.'

The mushrooms hissed and crackled in the pan, but she left them alone and carried on stirring the risotto.

'Now that's not strictly true Ron, is it?' She wasn't asking him. She took more Dutch courage from her wine glass. 'Lucille has told me all about it, you know.'

'I never. It was Lulu used to dress up all pretty every evening after work, and when Grainny was on late shifts she used to come and sit next to me, nudging up close, you know, touching my arms and waving her legs in front of me. I couldn't help it.'

'You didn't have to force her Ron.'

'I never. I just told you. She would pranny around in her make up and skirts asking me if she looked nice and if I thought she was pretty. The first time we did it she–' he faltered.

'Tell me, Ron, I want to know. You won't shock me.'

'She said she really was a girl. I mean I ain't gay or nothing, but you know what she looks like and everything. You couldn't tell she wasn't. She asked me whether I thought she had a nice mouth, said her lips and her tongue was the same as any other girl's and asking me to kiss her because she wouldn't feel like any other girl unless a man had kissed her.' He shrugged. 'So in the end I did. I kissed her.'

'What about Grainne?'

'I know. But I couldn't help myself. Me and Grainne weren't really doing it together very much anymore. And Lulu was always coming on at me whenever she wasn't in, asking me if I thought she looked nice and that. After we kissed that time she said she needed to see what a real man looked like. You know – wanted me to unzip me jeans. When she saw I was horny she just went straight down on me and sucked me off. After that she wouldn't never let me kiss her again, said I should keep my kisses for Grainne. But she would always give me another blow job if I wanted one, cos I'd been nice to her about the way she looked, she said, and cos she knew me and Grainne weren't having much sex no more, so it didn't matter, but we'd have to keep it a secret. And I admit I did ask her for more blow jobs, but I never forced her. Wouldn't never let me touch her neither. Not that I wanted to, mind. I mean, I knew what she really was underneath her clothes and make up and that. I'm not mad. But she's all fixed now, thanks to you, isn't she, a proper woman now?'

Rose nodded impatiently.

'And the last time? That day I came to pick her up? Why did you mess her dress?'

'I didn't. I mean I didn't mean to. That was her. I went up to say goodbye, like, and help her with her case, and she was all dressed and ready to go. Looking great in that dress, she was. Really beautiful. Just like a woman already, I thought. I told her she did and wished her luck and everything, and she thanked me and sat down on the edge of her bed and told me to come over and stand in front of her cos she wanted to give me a special goodbye present. What she meant was – well, you know. And just when I was coming she stopped, leaned back and held my willy down so that I came all over her. On purpose. Smiling she was as she did it. I thought she was mad. But she looked so happy. I couldn't understand it. I didn't mind. Then straightaway afterwards she started shouting at me and telling me off, which I really couldn't understand at all. Like it was me that had done it to her, not her that'd done it to herself and like she was cross about it after all.' He shook his head. 'I still don't understand that, to be honest. Shocking it was.'

He still looked hurt and confused after all this time, thought Rose. She had no doubt whatsoever though that he was telling her the truth.

'And the next day,' he continued, his voice glum. 'Or the day after, Grainne left me without telling me. And that shocked me too. Even worse. Maybe Lulu told her what we'd been doing or something. Grainne didn't leave me a note or nothing to tell me, but that's what I think. And when I rang her work to see if they knew where she'd gone, the lady I spoke to said they weren't allowed to give employees' addresses out to members of the public. That's what she said. I remember 'cos I said I wasn't a member of the public. I was her boyfriend. And she said well in that case you will know Staff Nurse O'Riordan isn't working here anymore, and she put the phone down on me. My cancer started getting really bad soon after that, so I had other things to think about.'

Rose was icily calm as she cut up a French stick and arranged the slices in a little raffia basket for the dinner table. It was only when she decided to cut the end off the crust that the knife slipped, even as she somehow knew it was going to before it actually happened, and sliced the skin on the inside of her hand where she was holding the bread down on the wooden cutting board.

'You alright? You got to be careful with knives.'

'I understand you know about such things! Hindsight is a wonderful thing isn't it, Ron,' she replied, sucking her palm and peering over at the mushrooms which were still sizzling.

'Looking back you mean? And understanding? Yeah, it is good, but not as good as being able to look into the future and see what is going to happen.'

'You can do that too?'

'It's another side-effect of my cancer. First I see the meaning of everything I look at and think about. And then the meanings all come together and there it is – the future!

'So what's going to happen to my supper?'

'It's going to be good, I reckon, from the smell of it.'

He licked his lips like a child. Rose smiled, allowed herself to feel gratified.

'And what's going to happen to you?'

'My wrist, you mean? Well they're going to say I hurt it, but it's not broken and there's nothing they can do and I should just rest it.'

'Can you do horse racing, things like that? The weather?'

'Nah. It's not like that at all. It only works with people.'

'Alright! What's going to happen to me then?'

'I'm not a fortune teller or nothing. But I would say you are changing and you are getting angrier.'

'That Ronald – by the way, does anyone ever call you Ronald?'

He shook his head.

'Then I will. That, Ronald,' she continued, 'is an understatement. I am certainly angry. But not with you, or even your dog.'

'I don't really know what you are angry about, but it's none of my business.'

Was he being a trifle disingenuous? She looked at him. No, he really meant it.

'I am angry with Lucille, Ronald, for not just being economical with the truth, but for actually lying to me. And, what would be the right word? Conning! Yes, conning me. Never mind,' she added, not wanting Ron to see the extent of her hurt. 'I am sure we can resolve it one way or another. But there's just one more thing I'd like to know, Ronald. Why have you been stalking her?'

'I told you. I ain't been stalking her,' he replied, offended.

'So what have you been doing?'

'I'm worried about her that's all. My cancer's been letting me know she's in danger.'

'From whom?'

'From men and from women.' He tried to look sly. 'I don't really know,' he admitted. I have to go into one of my trances to really see what's going to happen and I don't always remember it when I do. When I come out of it, I mean. It's a bit like dreaming, see. You wake up and it's gone. But I do know she is in danger from men and from women. I do know that. Even if I don't know who exactly. And I feel I owe her, you know? She was good to me before she left. So I want to be good for her in return. Even if she doesn't know nothing about it. I just want to keep an eye out for her, you know. For her own protection. As an old friend. And,' he tailed off, shrugging.

'Yes, Ron?'

'I need to know why she spoiled it with me and Grainne.'

Ah, thought Rose, giving another stir to her risotto.

Not just a guileless fool then. He's also feeling hurt and rejected, has definitely been stalking her, could even be a little dangerous. But not to her. He was no danger to her at all, even if the truths he had just told her about his relationship with Lucie were distressing to say the least.

That false and falsifying little bitch has based her whole relationship with me on lies.

She washed and returned the bread knife to a drawer, holding a tissue to her cut hand while she waited for it to stop bleeding. It wasn't a bad gash. A sticking plaster would see to it alright. She took her mushrooms off the flame, spatula'd them out on top of the Risotto, didn't stir them in. She put a lid on top and switched the gas off.

'I understand you have a collection of knives yourself, Ronald, and a shotgun.'

She didn't need to hear his reply, the confused blank expression on his face said it all.

'I don't hold with killing animals for sport,' he said. 'And what would I want to go collecting knives for? I'm not interested. I used to like bikes, but I don't care about them no more either.'

'Do you want to see Lucie again, Ron? I mean meet her again. Here. You can if you like. Come again another day. Come and see us. We can all be friends together. I think she ought to know that you have been acting as her private security guard. For nothing and purely out of friendship and loyalty to her. What a wonderful thing friendship is.' He nodded his agreement with her, clearly missing her sarcasm.

Rose wondered what on earth she was doing. Revenge of some kind, for having been deceived perhaps. But she didn't really have a plan. She just wanted to get back at Lucie somehow. Was she trying to encourage him to continue to stalk or harass her?

No, not really. She simply felt they needed to meet again. That was all. In front of her. They'd been secret lovers after all.

'Why don't you come round next Sunday to see us? Please do. I would like it very much if you did and I am sure Lucie would too. She doesn't work on a Sunday. We can surprise her. And I think it would be a very good idea if you shaved that silly beard off and perhaps had your hair trimmed a little. That ponytail is frankly, well,' she shook her head. 'Never mind! You need to do something about your appearance, Ronald, that's all. I hope you don't mind me saying so. But you look dirty. All my life, and that's forty two years now, I've never known a woman who could bear a man who was dirty.'

'But I just fell over in the wet,' he wailed. 'I keep myself clean, I do, but–

The doorbell rang. It was an ambulance woman. Ron said his goodbyes and Rose repeated her request that he should visit her again on Sunday, meet Lucie. He nodded assent and she showed him out, offering him her cheek and a smile at the door. He didn't have a clue about social niceties and didn't bend to kiss her. She gave his right arm a squeeze anyway and sent him on his way. She watched the ambulance leave with blue and red lights silently flashing, and closed the door.

Then she lay the kitchen table with a seventies style bistro-chic red and white checked table cloth which she had bought when she was still married. Richard probably wouldn't remember it. She laid cutlery and glasses on it together with the basket of bread. As a finishing touch she lit a single candle and placed it in the middle of the table. She kept the lights on. She didn't want it to appear too intimate. Satisfied, she went into her front room, settled herself in her over-soft, cream-coloured sofa and reached for the remote control to watch television until he arrived.

A loud breathy snuffle destroyed her attempt at self-contained solitude in one shocking snort. She nearly jumped out of her skin.

Oh for heaven's sake! That was all she needed!

Milly or Malcolm was lying sidelong on the floor by the fire, gently wagging her, his or its tail. She took a few deep breaths. There was really no point getting in a tizz about it. No doubt Ronald would be back for the damn thing. In the meantime she would just have to hope that it wouldn't relieve itself on her rug or anything awful like that and just ignore it.

As soon as she switched on the TV, the phone rang. It was Richard. Mary had come down with flu and it was too late to arrange a babysitter. He was terribly sorry. Some other time, he said, it was important not to lose touch. He really wanted to see her again. He really did. He had something he had to talk about with her. Memories he really did have to revisit. Rose didn't want to give him the satisfaction of another date right now, not after all the trouble she'd been to get everything ready. She told him to call her then put the phone down before she could listen to his reply.

How typical of him that was! He had so often been an unexpected let down. He always had the air of someone reliable and dependable. You could rely on him for giving that impression. You just couldn't actually rely on him. He seemed to be one of those people whose public and private personae were two quite separate things. She knew that at work he took pride in being respected for his medical skills and his overall professionalism, was obviously not completely incompetent in his dealings with the external world or he wouldn't have achieved what he had in his life. Nevertheless, at home with her during the years of their marriage he had all too often been forgetful, confused and far too emotionally

97

dependent upon her. Admittedly that was five years ago, but he'd given her no reason to think that he had changed at all since then. Indeed, at the party of a mutual friend a couple of years ago she had sought out a chat with his new wife, Mary, who made it quite clear in that politely non-informative way that first and second wives always use to communicate with one another, that he had simply transferred his dependence onto her.

She stared at the dog who returned her gaze and then rolled onto its back panting. It definitely seemed to have a willy. Malcolm then. She might have guessed. Was that a hair on the rug where he was lying? It was. In fact there were two or three. She couldn't have that. Not in her house, thank you very much. Well, not in her front room anyway. Not in any of her rooms in fact. She would show him up to Lucie's bedroom, shut him in there. After all, it was her dog. If it was indeed the same dog. She still wasn't entirely clear about that.

She wasn't clear about anything anymore. She felt so angry with Lucie she didn't even want to think about it. She got up from the sofa and taking the dog by its damp collar started hauling it up the stairs. It didn't want to move away from the fire and resisted her with an irritating whine. Then it sensibly seemed to realise that if there was one thing she was implacable about in her house it was dirt. And dog hair counted as dirt in her book. Serious dirt. She hussled the animal into Lucie's room and shut the door on it. The sound of its continued whining as she carefully went back downstairs again along her usual invisible route reminded her of how she really felt. Angry yes, about being conned, but equally, or perhaps more, hurt at having been betrayed with lies. That was the worst thing. The betrayal of their relationship, of what they felt for one another, of their mutual trust.

Lucie shouldn't have made herself out to be another victim. That was what she really resented. She shouldn't have. It was so depressing to feel that the whole basis of their relationship over the last year and a half or more, right from the outset, was predicated on a lie about her being Ron's victim. Why hadn't she just told her the truth. She would still have helped her become who she was.

Or would she? Was she now being dishonest with herself? Would she *really* have still taken Lucille under her wing if she had given her something closer to Ron's version of their sexual relationship in the burning woods that night? Or would she have perhaps felt more sympathy for Ron, dismissed Lucie with a slight shudder of pity and revulsion for disgracefully seducing the poor simpleton by pretending to be female?

It was just impossible to say now, because they had a relationship, Lucie and herself. As an ersatz mother and ersatz daughter maybe, but there it was, they had one. The other thing, of course, was that anatomically, interpersonally and socially Lucie now lived the life and experiences of a female member of the human race. That was not a pretence. When Rose thought back to that night in the woods there was no question then either, that the person she had met out there, had somehow actually been a girl not a boy. And that was despite the fact that Lucille had told her what she was right from the beginning.

At least she had done that. And Rose had responded to her as a girl. Girls have feelings and desires, of course they do. And girls can tell lies. Of course they can. And girls seduce boys and men into having sex with them all over the world. Of course they do. They are not all or merely victims, made of sugar and spice and all things nice. Rose had known that twenty five years ago when she herself was a girl. She had always known it. She still knew it now as a middle-aged woman. She wasn't completely stupid.

So perhaps after all, she would not have stereotyped Lucille and turned her back on her that night in the woods. And yet, if she was honest, she might well not have taken her under her wing either, paid for all her treatment and so on, if she had not thought of Lucie not only as a girl, but as a victim too. A victim who had needed rescuing. By her, a professional rescuer of victims.

It was embarrassing what that said about her own view of women as the playthings or victims of men, despite her personal experience to the contrary. That she had actually been conned into fanning the flames of this stereotype was insufferable. She felt so angry she could scream.

Instead she poured herself another glass of red wine and knocked the whole thing back all at once before getting the vacuum cleaner out and hoovering the dog hairs up off the rug in front of the fire. She was so full of her own thoughts and feelings that she carried on hoovering unnecessarily for more than twenty minutes and only heard the phone ringing because she had happened to be cleaning under the coffee table where she kept the phone.

It was Ronald calling from the hospital. He thanked her for looking after him earlier before the ambulance had arrived, said he was very happy, he had got a hairline fracture whatever that was, but he'd just seen Grainne of all people. He apologised for forgetting Malcolm, said he'd come straight round and get him. She replied that with his fractured wrist it would be far better if he just went home to bed. The great lug obviously still needed a mother to care for him. He clearly wasn't very good at caring for himself. She told him she was sure Lucille could manage to look after the dog perfectly well until he came by on Sunday and anyway it would give his arm a rest not to take the dog out for a few days.

As soon as she put the phone down she heard the sound of the front door opening as Lucille let herself in. Noticing her hand was shaking, Rose picked up her empty wine glass, went with it into the kitchen ignoring her. She sat down at her candlelit table, trying to keep a lid on her simmering rage. She heard Lucie hang up her coat on a hook in the hall and tried to take a few deep breaths to calm herself, hold on to what she had just been thinking a few minutes ago before Ron rang.

Lucille followed her into the kitchen looking a bit tatty if not downright tarty in the same frock and shoes she had been wearing yesterday evening, but otherwise irritatingly radiant.

'Oh Rose,' she gushed, 'your hair! Your hair. It looks fabulous. It's just so right for you! You look great! And what a gorgeous dress. It looks lovely on you. You look like a different woman.'

'I am a different woman.'

Lucille didn't seem to notice the hard edge to this reply, too busy sniffing the aroma of the cooking in the air, pronouncing on its deliciousness and how wonderful her dinner table looked adorned with a cloth and candle. Then she looked at the clock on the wall.

'Your husband, I mean ex-husband isn't here yet, is he? I've got so much to tell you!'

Rose blew her nose, nodded her head, but said nothing as Lucie lifted the lid off her risotto, dipped a finger in, licked it, and made appreciative noises. She leaned back against a kitchen cupboard, flicking the kettle switch on. Her eyes were bright with the need to burst into a description of her night out, Rose observed, glancing up at her from behind her tissue. Well, perhaps she wouldn't let her. There was a hole in her tights. It ran down her left leg from the hem of her dress to her knee.

'You owe me a pair of tights,' said Rose, unwilling just yet to look her in the face.

Following her gaze, Lucille looked down at her leg and laughed happily.

'Oh, dear. Yes, so I do! But the important thing is I'm not a virgin anymore and I've had such a wonderful time! I've made it Rosie, I've made it!' she burst out, clapping her hands. 'So they're cheap at the price and—

'And you're a liar and a cheat! And they damn well weren't cheap actually.'

Rose never swore. Never. But the anger she had been suppressing was now unstoppable 'But you are, you little, you little – Oh! I don't know what you are. But I think 'whore' might be one word for it. Selling yourself to me so that I could feel like a mother again. And I've always been paying. ALWAYS,' she repeated. Her voice so loud, she even shocked herself with it.' Her ears were rang with the sound of it.

'Rose! Rosie! What's the matter? Why are you shouting at me? What have I done? I love you. You're my best friend!'

'What have you done? What have you done? Why you've conned me. That's all. From start to finish. And I've been such a – such an idiot! I've been completely taken in.'

'Rosie? I don't know what you mean. What do you mean?' Lucille's confusion made the pitch of her voice rise like that of a terrified child.

Rose watched the tears start welling up into her stupid cow eyes. Good! That's appropriate. So they should! And she looked frightened. Good! So she should be. She should cry and cry and cry, the little slut. For me.

'You conned your way into my life, exploited my grief and taken my money – what little I had I've spent on you – and from start to finish you've tricked me. And you'll trick everyone else. All your life. To get what you want. You are not just deceitful. You're an imposter! Look at you standing there with your tits nearly falling out of your dress and a ladder in your tights. Those things don't make you a woman. They make you a slut. A fucking slut,' she said slowly, but if it were possible, her voice had become even louder. 'So you finally got yourself bonked last night, did you?' She boomed. 'Well, whoopee, but that doesn't make you a woman either. You'll never know what it means to be a woman. Never.'

Shaking her head in incomprehension, Lucille put one hand to her breast and the other to the run in her tights and then brought both hands slowly up to her mouth in shock. Her face, pale already, went white. Then she ran out of the kitchen, and Rose heard her collapse, sobbing onto the sofa next door. Rose was unmoved. This was just another example of Lucille doing the tragic little victim role again.

Rose took a few deep breaths, trying to calm down. It was odd, but in all the time they had been living together, although she had sometimes been unhappy, Lucie had never once really cried. Not howls like this anyway. So was it just possible she really was upset? Well, that would be a turn up for the books. Rose listened to her sobs become more keening, and tried to ignore the small but definite feeling emerge in her heart of wanting to run to Lucille and console her. She also ignored the small nugget of satisfaction she could feel gleaming within her. Certainly, she had never shouted at Lucie or at anyone like this before.

Well, if Lucille's distress was genuine, it would do her the world of good. And if she could feel even a soupcon of remorse or guilt that would be something too, a tiny sign perhaps, that one day she might be able to have a jot of feeling for somebody other than herself.

Somewhat mollified, Rose refilled her glass and followed Lucille into the front room. Feeling as if she was at work, where she often had to do this, she placed a box of tissues on the sofa beside Lucie's crumpled form. The white heat of her anger had cooled a little now, but there was no way she would allow this to end without finishing what she wanted to say. Then she would insist on hearing some kind of explanation from Lucille about her lies. Every one of them.

She sat down on a chair opposite and waited for Lucille to collect herself.

After a few minutes Lucie sat up, the blank, hopeless expression on her face making her look like a cow waiting for slaughter, thought Rose. Well she wasn't going to slaughter her, but neither was she prepared to respond to that kind of pathetic appeal from her ever again.

Lucie wiped her eyes with a tissue. Despite herself, always and ever the mum, Rose couldn't help pointing to the dark streaks of make-up which had run down her cheeks. Lucie licked the tissue and wiped some more.

'Is that alright?' she sniffed.

Rose nodded, but didn't say a word. Lucille stared at her and said nothing either. Eventually Rose spoke.

'All I meant was that what makes someone a woman, or a man for that matter, is the capacity to have feelings, Lucie. And especially feelings for others. If you do have any feelings, genuine feelings, they are only for yourself. You play the poor little victim extremely well, but I won't and I will never be taken in by you again.'

'Why Rosie?' Her eyes became watery again. 'Why do you think that about me? What have I done?'

'You never told me the truth. In the woods that night when we first met. You lied.'

Lucie did not try to deny it. She tucked her hair behind her ears and nodded.

'How do you know?'

Rose didn't reply, but selfish and egotistical as she was, Lucille wasn't completely stupid when it came to reading emotions on people's faces, especially hers.

Lucie shrugged. 'I didn't know you then. My whole life was a lie,' she continued reluctantly. 'A few more lies to a stranger didn't matter. That's what I felt.'

'You lied about Ron. And about cutting yourself. You know it was those things which prompted me into wanting to look after you. Into having you here. Into paying for your surgery' She was becoming shrill again, but now didn't want Lucie to think she could not stay in control. She cleared her throat and lowered her voice. 'I should have realised, of course. I have seen you often enough in next to nothing by now to know that there isn't a mark on your body, but I didn't let myself recognise that that meant you couldn't ever have cut yourself either, despite what you told me in the woods. There would have been scars.'

But she was losing control, Rose realised with a dim sadness. She was talking too much. It was the wine. She wanted to hear from Lucille now, she really did, but she couldn't stop speaking herself because she was getting pissed.

'I *ached*, Lucie. I ached to rescue you from what I have now learned was the absolutely spurious horror of what Ron was doing to you. It was a complete and utter lie, wasn't it! But it made me want to look after you, you manipulative creature. Is that *why* you lied to me? Could you tell even then I *needed* to look after you? But what really hurts – what I really don't understand – is why you've never ever told me the truth since? We were supposed to be friends. You should have told me. I would have understood. There is nothing wrong in wanting sex. But there is in lies. And in pretending to be a victim when you are not one. You should have told me the truth, Lucille. Eventually anyway. Told me the lie about Ron having guns and knives and about his forcing you to have sex. Once we were properly friends. The fact that you didn't is completely hateful to me. It just means that inspite of everything I thought we meant to each other and – I am sorry to have to say this – everything I have done for you, you have never actually trusted me. And that hurts Lucie, that hurts.'

Rose found she was struggling to hold back the tears herself now and she helped herself to a tissue too. She kept looking at Lucie as she did so, not wanting her to get the wrong impression. *She* wasn't going to play the victim. Her tears were just emotional and she wasn't trying to use them manipulatively in any way. She didn't want Lucie's sympathy. She just wanted her to know the facts.

Lucie picked and pulled nervously at the hole in her tights, putting her fingers under it and spreading them to make it larger. Rose took another sip of Shiraz and the old familiar rush of drunkenness took possession of her again. She finished the glass anyway and then poured herself the rest of the bottle. I must shut up now, she thought. I must just shut up, give Lucille a chance to reply.

But Lucille didn't.

'Speak to me Lucie! Speak to me!'

Lucille opened her mouth as if she wanted to, but nothing came out. Instead she shrugged, opened her purse and got out a nail file. She had noticed she had snagged a nail fiddling with her nylons. She buffed it a couple of times and put the file away again.

'I don't know what to say.'

'Don't you understand what I'm trying to tell you?'

'I don't understand how you can know what went on between me and Ron. And that makes me feel like there are things *you* are keeping from me. I feel frightened of how angry you are. And I never know what to say when I am frightened. I think, maybe, you're not really telling me the truth either. If you were, you'd be coming straight out with it, saying you have had enough of me and that you want me to go, and *that's* why you're so mad with me.'

'No! That's not true at all. It's rubbish in fact!'

Lucie gave her one grateful glance, then seemed to need to carry on staring into nothing. After a while she sat up, crossed her legs and looked at Rose through the continuing silence between them. Rose thought she heard the dog in Lucie's room whining again, but Lucie didn't seem to hear anything. Rose sipped at her wine.

'I know I am not very good at feeling for others,' said Lucie. 'and I am not very good at anything really. Because there is no more to me than this – than what you see. I have never felt there was anything inside me. Nothing real. Except my love for my mum maybe. And maybe my dad too if I had known him better and if he hadn't – well never mind. When I was little I used to feel like these.'

She put a finger in the hole in her tights, lifted the nylon up from the top of her thigh for a moment, let it go with a little flick.

'I felt like nylon. Like I wasn't natural. Like I just about existed, but if I was stretched, and I always felt like I was being stretched so sheer you couldn't see me, I would disappear. It was like I wasn't there. Unless I was with Mum. When I felt like a part of *her* really. My mum knew me and saw me, but she was the only one in the whole world who really could.

'My earliest memory, I was, I don't know, three or four years old. Maybe five. I don't know. It was a sunny summer's day, you know?' Lucie sniffed and without thinking wiped her nose with her sleeve like a child. So much for brand new dresses and lady-like manners, thought Rose, but perhaps she was being genuine at last. 'We were in the back garden,' Lucie continued. 'It was a lovely day – blue sky and brightness all around. And I was helping Mum put the damp clothes up on the washing line to dry. She was so beautiful. I can still remember perfectly what she was wearing – a fifties-style polka dot skirt, full at the skirt and cinched at the waist. White with big red spots. And she had patent red heels. She looked so lovely. She was hanging the clothes up and I was at her feet passing them to her from the laundry basket. When I look back on it, it is like I was almost in some washing powder advert or something!' She shrugged, threw out her hands in a gesture of despair at the tackiness of her comparison. 'I know, but that's how it was. The fresh smell of the clean washing *was* so wonderful. I've always loved it ever since. I felt so, so happy. Like I really belonged. Like I was a part of the sunlight and the smell of her and the smell of her clean clothes. Like I was a part of her.

'When I passed her the last of the washing out of the washing basket I remember I touched her ankles wondering at the difference between the little brown bundles I had been passing up to her and the glamorousness of her legs. Then I stood up under her skirt. I felt so safe in there. Like I was in a wonderful white tent. And she laughed and patted my head and held me against her before telling me to come out. And I knew even then that I was nothing without her and that there could never be anything more to me than being a part of her, and that I didn't ever want there to be, because if I wasn't a part of her then I wouldn't really exist. I'd always be as insubstantial as the scent of the washing, or the breeze, or her nylons. I didn't have the words for it then, but that's the way I felt. It's the way I've always felt.

'I'm not making any sense am I?' She shook her head and her hands in exasperation. 'What I'm trying to say, Rosie, is that you are right. What you said: I *am* selfish. Because till now I have been too stretched, too sheer – as a person I mean – to have any feelings at all for anybody else. Except my mum. And except, I thought – I really did – you, Rosie. So when I lied at first, when I didn't know you at all, it didn't matter to me, because I wasn't really a person anyway. And if I wasn't a person then nobody else was either. And if you aren't a person then you cannot really tell a lie, can you? Do you know what I mean?'

She moved both hands up over her thighs, hips, tummy and breasts to her face.

'I had a body which I hated when I met you, and I couldn't be myself inside it like I can now. So lying to you didn't matter. Because *nothing* mattered. Then, when I got to know you, I still felt it would be wrong to tell you the truth because it would spoil what was between us by showing me up to have once lied to you. Because lying did matter then. I just didn't feel I could lie anymore, not to you anyway, not without it mattering. And yet I couldn't tell the truth without, you know, without hurting you and spoiling what we had together. I didn't want to destroy that either. And I thought – well that's it really. So I just forgot about it. I thought you would never find out anyway, and...' She shrugged. 'So that's why you're right. I've always struggled simply to feel that I, you know, exist. I mean enough to actually have any feelings for any one other than myself. But I want to! And I am getting a *bit* better at it, don't you think? If you weren't mad at me I think you'd say I was. So please don't be mad at me!'

Rose shook her head. It *was* maddening that even though Lucie's forlorn pout was so patently both put-on and genuine, she couldn't help responding to Lucie as if she was wholly authentic. She just couldn't help it. She nodded.

Once again Lucille had succeeded in disarming her.

The trouble was she could talk the hind legs off a donkey without Rose knowing exactly what she was saying at all. Yet she could *feel* it somehow. She could feel that everything Lucille was saying was true, even if it was a lie, and somehow because it was true, she could no longer be cross with her.

She still should be, she knew that, but she just wasn't.

'How did you find out I lied to you about Ron?'

'Go upstairs to your room.'

'Wh-what? Why?'

'Go on. Go to your room. You'll understand when you have. Just do it, Lucie.'

Rose would have liked to have followed her up, seen the mixture of surprise, delight, confusion and realisation dawn on her face when she saw the dog in her room, but she staggered drunkenly when she tried to get up off the sofa to follow her, and flopped back onto it again. A moment later she heard Lucie's astonishment and the dog barking in reply. She got up off the sofa more slowly this time, but instead of going upstairs she went into the kitchen and opened another bottle. She would share her dinner with Lucie and perhaps Lucie would have a glass of wine with her herself for a change. In celebration.

Chapter 8.

'I'm sorry about last week, Rose.'

This time, rather than ring her and risk being fobbed off, Richard simply took a detour into Putney and dropped in on her after work. His mind had become fixated over the last two weeks on whatever message Luke had left. He knew it would only contain the mundane and prosaic thoughts of a small boy. Nonetheless he had to have it.

'I dropped by on the off chance,' he said. 'It's good to see you again.'

He bent to kiss her on the cheek which she allowed him to do without making him feel he should be grateful, then stepped back so he could come in. She smelt of red wine.

'I've got nothing for you to eat,' she said. 'But plenty of plonk. Plenty of that.'

She steered him towards the kitchen.

'You've had your hair done differently. It looks good on you,' he said. 'In fact you look better than ever.'

'Don't be silly,' she replied, but she was smiling. A rare event these last fifteen years. 'Your tendency to flatter too freely has always been a flaw.' She almost sounded fond of him. 'But not a major one.'

'And alliteration has always been one of yours! How are you, Rose?'

'You know I never answer that question. That's for others to decide.'

He looked at her, studying the lines on her face, noticing that she was taking a bit more care of herself than she used to. Perhaps it was the influence of her lodger. 'I would say you're alright. You've been better and you've been worse, but at the moment, I think, you're alright. That's good.'

She nodded with clear impatience, not really interested.

'What was it you said on the phone a couple of weeks ago about revisiting old memories?' she asked. 'And why? '

'You're full of questions, Rose.' He covered up the defensiveness she would hear in this with, 'It's good. I'm glad if you're coming out of yourself a bit more.'

Her almost curt nod reminded him, if he needed reminding, that she didn't suffer fools gladly. Stating the obvious had always irritated her. So had being patronised.

'What old memories do you need to come here to revisit?' She poured a glass of wine from an opened bottle, passing it to him with no question that he wouldn't take it. He would have to be careful not to let her get him sozzled, he might give himself away. He had to drive home of course too. Taking a cagey, small sip, he smiled thanks at her as if he had just downed the whole glass in one gulp, and said,

'Luke memories. You know. That's all. Just memories of our little Luke.'

She nodded, unsurprised, knowing, even.

'Such as?'

'Oh, nothing specific.'

Did she hear the lie? She'd always had a good antenna for lies. 'I just need to feel closer to him, that's all.'

'And you thought coming round here would help you do that.' She nodded her head. 'I see.'

Why was he always wary of her? Even if he hadn't been coming here secretly intending to lift a floor board, he would still have been careful about how he was with her. Her direct, no-nonsense manner still intimidated him even now, made him feel guilty, despite having nothing to feel guilty about. Except a little deception to get what was rightfully his. Nothing serious.

'Yes, it will. I'm losing all my memories of him,' he said. 'I remember the obvious things as if they happened five minutes ago. I remember his bravery every time he caught another infection knowing it could be his last. I remember his coughs and my own way of suppressing my feelings about them and what they were doing to his lungs. I remember how pinched and tiny he was. I probably remember everything that happened, but I have forgotten the little *person*. I cannot really remember who *he* was at all,' Richard found himself almost shouting. He collected himself, concluded, 'So I needed to come round.' He forced out an apologetic smile. 'Sorry. I didn't mean to raise my voice like that.'

'It's alright, Richard. You were a good father. And husband.' She spoke softly. For a moment the gulf between them was bridged by a tenderness which had been excised by their hopeless struggle to maintain some quality in their son's life. The attrition of it all had seemed endless at the time. Now when he looked back on it, the ten short years of Luke's life seemed to have shot by so swiftly, he felt as if he had somehow blinked and missed them.

'To tell you the truth,' he said, and for a change this phrase did not presage a lie. 'I used to be frightened of asking you how he was when I got in from work, for fear such a stupid question would only add insult to injury. There was so much I couldn't ask you, or tell you for fear of hurting you.'

It was aggravating, ridiculous that even now he felt he was taking a risk by naming this fact between them. Nevertheless, from his side of their relationship, fear of hurting her was definitely one of the main things their marriage had foundered upon.

She pursed her lips and brows in that characteristic frown he'd often feared, but which he used to love so much too. Still loved, in a way, as he watched her shaping her reply.

'You're still a patronising bastard, Richard,' she said, knocking back some more wine. 'But we've only got one life, haven't we? So you really shouldn't have worried about hurting me.' She looked at him with a hint of contempt, making it plain she knew what he had actually been afraid of was hurting himself. 'I am grateful for your good intentions though, truly I am, Richard. Even if they did just pave our road to hell!'

And you are more pompous than ever, he thought. As drunks so often are. Her self-importance had been further inflated by her marriage to alcohol.

'I wouldn't want to discourage you now – or then – from saying what you like to me,' she continued. 'Certainly not now. I'm contemplating retirement.' She laughed. ' A lot of the time I find the only thing I want is to join him. On the plus side, nothing hurts me anymore. Not much anyway.' She stroked the stem of her wine glass. 'I suppose I enjoy distractions,' she mused, glancing across at him with a look which acknowledged she had a problem with booze, but defying him to challenge her about it. She took another slurp. He didn't rise to her invitation. They weren't married anymore. It wasn't his business.

'And I'm just a charade, Rose,' he said. 'A fake. I spend all day looking after people, trying to make them feel better about their lives, or their deaths, without letting who I really am show at all. At home it's the same. I'm the husband and step-father, I fulfil my function as breadwinner. Wherever I am I'm an absolute expert at concealing what I really feel.'

'We learnt together,' she replied. 'Cheers.'

She knocked back her wine, reached for the bottle to refill her glass. He left his untouched. While they were still married this conversation would have been impossible. They would have sought to look after one another, soothed one another's sad and sorry brows, even though they had nothing left to give. Either that, or they'd have guiltily shied away from doing so. In the process further bricks were added to the wall between them. Neither of them had wanted to be building it. They'd done it to protect Luke from having to cope with anything more than he had got already. It had been a mistake. Richard had known that at the time, although he had been too weak to say so. He knew it now.

'We had no choice,' she said.

He had a choice now. He could – he should tell her what he had come for. Share his secret. She wouldn't begrudge him. She would let him have the map, recognising it was more his than hers in so far as Luke had drawn it after they had made and played their Treasure Island game together. And in so far as he had been the one to remember it now. Surely she would.

But he didn't want to tell her about it. It was as if a secret shared would be a secret halved. On the other hand a secret unshared would also lose its preciousness because of the tarnish placed upon it by lying and evasion. Having immediately fallen back with her into a genuine sharing of their true feelings together, he would feel uncomfortable if he actually hid the main purpose of his being here this evening from her. He sighed inwardly. As ever, whatever he did, there would always be a down side to it. He would always be ambivalent.

'What's the matter, Richard?'

His tongue felt swollen into wordlessness with all the answers that question evoked. In response he cleared his throat, articulating the shape of his broken heart as clearly as the sound of a cracked bell.

'Tell me about Luke,' he begged. 'Tell me what you remember.'

'I can't. Like you, Richard, I can't remember him properly anymore. I haven't really thought about him in ages. I *feel* him. I feel him all the time in here.' She put a hand to her breast. 'But I'm not sure anymore that I can put any actual words to the feeling. Can you? Not without still hurting too much.' She arched an arrogant brow at him. 'So, please, do, if you can, tell me about the boy you knew.'

'I *have* told you already. All I can tell you, anyway. For the rest, no, I can't either.' He stared at her, filled with an empathy and compassion he was a little shocked to find he still possessed. 'We've both forgotten him then.'

'No, not forgotten him.'

'No, you're right. Not that.'

They might be agreeing with one another, but they had immediately become as maudlin as they used to be in the dog days before they finally parted. He tried to change the subject.

'Being a stepfather's not much fun. You're always trying.'

She nodded, clearly not very interested in that. She was right. He didn't want to go there either. Not now. He had come to find Luke.

'I didn't have to try with Luke,' he said. 'Not in the same way anyhow. Do you meet him here sometimes? In your mind, I mean? Like a ghost?'

'Of course, but Lucie, my lodger, has done a lot to help me exorcise that.'

Instinctively he found himself disliking the lodger then.

'Is she here?'

'I don't know. Why?'

He shook his head. Just asking.

'She doesn't always tell me when she's going out. Not anymore. But, hey, as she herself might say, I'm not my lodger's keeper.'

'I want to look in Lukey's room .'

'There's nothing in there of his, Richard. Not anymore. And I was lying. She is in. Upstairs.'

He would just have to go for the Secret Shared option then. On balance it felt better than the Tarnishing it with Lies one, now he knew she was just as disconnected from memories of Luke as he was.

'Remember when Luke and I made a board game together?'

'No. You're a bit discursive this evening, Richard, are you alright? Have you had another bang on the head?'

'Well, we did,' he pressed on. 'We made our own board game. And afterwards because he'd enjoyed the idea of maps and buried treasure so much, he wrote a map or some clues, or a message to the future or something for himself – I don't really know *what* it was exactly. I wasn't overly interested at the time, so I can't remember, unfortunately. But whatever it was, I think he put it under the loose floorboard in the fitted cupboard in his bedroom. And I want to see if it's still there. Would your lodger mind if I had a quick look?'

'She might well. It all depends.'

Rose went to the bottom of the stairs.

'Lucille!' she called.

There was no reply. Then a muffled female voice replied, 'I'm in the shower.'

Rose went upstairs and he heard her talking briefly through the bathroom door to the lodger.

'She doesn't mind at all,' Rose smiled from halfway back down the stairs again. 'If you can excuse the mess. She only just went in the shower. She'll be at least another ten minutes. It shouldn't take us a minute, should it, to look under a floorboard?'

She beckoned him to follow her up.

Everything up here was changed, except for the old slightly worn carpet which led up from the stairs. That was still the same. The walls had been transformed from Magnolia to light Magenta. The doors had all been painted pale verdigris. He didn't recognise it at all. He didn't like it either. Rose crossed the landing straight into the second room. He stood at the doorway and looked in. At least he recognised the view of the houses opposite. The room itself was now shockingly different: pure white with a bright red bedside lamp and a red woolen rug on the floor in front of a mirrored dressing table draped with a red hat and scarf. Articles of feminine clothing were strewn over a small red rattan armchair. There was absolutely nothing about it that remotely reminded him of his son. Gone completely were the green walls with the huge Jack and the Beanstalk mural he had painted at Lukey's excited instruction when he was four or five years old. The mass of toys and games in coloured plastic boxes on the floor had been replaced by a few pairs of women's shoes and a little red rattan waste-paper basket, matching the chair.

He shook his head, and tried to block out the room's irritating and disorientating differentness.

He was glad to see that the fitted cupboard, now looking tacky in the same white gloss as the door and the window frames, was still there between the chimney breast and the outside wall.

They both went for the cupboard doors at the same time. Delving down through hangers with more female clothing, and moving aside yet more shoes, he lifted up the small loose floor board at the back. Rose quickly got down on to her knees beside him and pushing past him reached in. He stood up still holding the board so it didn't mess her dark blue cashmered shoulder. She looked up at him, her face puffy and red with the wine and exertion. She shook her head.

'Nothing,' she said. 'Just dust.'

'Let me try. I've got longer arms than you.'

She shook her head again with that old characteristic wilfulness, reaching in deeper, her newly blonde head almost disappearing into the cupboard. He felt a curious, slightly disorienting sensation of still being married to her, as if all these years of separate lives were as nothing.

'Got it,' she said, sitting up on the floor and brandishing a tattered, yellowing bundle of paper tied up in string. She didn't pass it to him or allow him to help her up off the floor, just beamed with delight and with a triumphant, shared glow which felt almost conspiratorial they both went back down stairs to the kitchen. She took a pair of sissors from a drawer, cut the string and carefully unfolding the bundle, laid their dead son's pictures out on the kitchen table. There were twelve of them.

* * *

[Interlude – words for secret pictures, never to be spoken or heard.

I am lucky to be ten now becose I'v got an illness and I need fizzio every day and now I have to have oxygen every day too. I didn't need it last year when I went to France. I just took my pills and my nebulisers with me, that's all. I know how to spell fizzio properly. I'm good at spelling. I just like spelling it with an f. It would be great if I could live till I'm twelve. I don't think I will becose of my CF. But I don't mind if I don't become a teenager like Jills and Robair. I don't know how to spell their names. These pictures I drew are from last year when I was nine. If I'd had a camera on that day I would have taken these pictures with it not drawed them like this.

My first picture is called Clown. I like it because it looks a bit like my dad. I don't like it too because he looks sad. Mummy says he is good at clowning around. I writ 'Daddy happy' undernith it after I done it because I wanted him to be happy. That's why I didn't tell him and Mummy what realy happenned on my French exchange holiday and that's why I hidd these pictures. I love my mummy and daddy. I put that red upside down moon in for Daddys mouth to make him look more happier. It didn't work.

My next picture, Picture Number Two, is smudged, but I still like it. It took too long and I tried to get it right but it went rong. Its called My Family, but Mum looks too messy now and not pretty enough and Daddy is too strate.

112

But it dosnt matter. They still look good. I'v drawed myself too small in the middle between them. I didn't meen to and my arms are too short like a babys, but if I made myself bigger it wood make it even messier and you woudn't be able to tell that I was the child. Realy I can reach their hands easily if I walk between them when we go out for a walk together. Even if I am the smallest boy in my class so what. When I was little I liked them to swing me. But we don't go out walking together now because I might catch a cold Mummy says. Aniway I'm too old to hold both their hands like that.

My next picture, Number three, is full of lots and lots of things, insects and Madame de Lansquenet and the airplane I flew in. Mummy taught me how to spell her name when she helped me write my thank you letter after I got back home again from France. Mummy taught me loads and loads more French too before I went away because we only do it once a week at school and I didn't know enough. I call this picture En Vacance because it was about going on my French Exchange holiday near Bordeau. I know that's not how you spell it propaly but it doesn't matter nobody is going to know. The de Lansquenet family were all horrible to me over there. I don't know why. I missed Mummy and daddy. That's my suitcase with all the stickers on it. I drawed it too big. Madam de Lasquenet who is beautiful but smells of cinnamon and cat poo said the yellow flower which was outside my bedroom window and all up the side of her house is called Callifornian Glory. Those yellow dots I done everywhere are its dust which was all stingy. Madam's children, Robair, Isabelle and Jills put it in my pyjamas and my bed one night and locked me in my bedroom. I hate them now. I was was itching all over. I got it in my eyes and it felt like glass and I cudnt see. It felt like the sun exploding in my eyes. I culdn't sleep all night with it and I cried and cried but nobody came and I cudnt open the door. Even when it was morning again and birds were singing I still cudnt see. But it slowly got better after that. The insect in the corner of the picture is my butterfly. You can tell by the wings. It landed on my window sil. They made me pull its wings off becose I kissed with Isabelle and they sed it was disgusting. I made that other butterfly underneath it look just the same as the one with wings becose it is the same one exsept it hasn't got wings so its sad. See? I made its face look sad. I'm rubbish at faces becose it looks like my face which is wrong because its not. It is a butterflys face. I was sad in France and I wanted to go home but they took my letters away and Madame de Lansquenet had told Mummy not to ring me becose she said I would only get more homesick and I was only going to be away for a week.

This one, Number four, is called Le Chateau. I don't know why they call big houses cat waters in France. I didn't like it at all their house but my drawing of it is quite good. It looked a bit like a pallis with terrises and lots of little gardens with little walls round them and it had woods and orange groves and vine fields all around it like these ones in my picture. The window I'v drawed up in the corner above the yellow callifornian glory was my room. I hated it.

My next picture is called Ma Soeur et Mes Freres cos Isabelle and her brothers Jills and Robair were pretending to be nice to me and I thought they realy were nice and Isabelle was very very kind to me at first and I felt very hapy staying with them for the first day of my holiday. Like having two brothers and a sister. Isabelle is very beautiful but I havnt drawed her very well. She said she wanted me to be her boyfriend because she was only a little bit older than me. She is eleven. That's why I drawed us holding hands. I drawed Jills and Robair too small. I didn't mean too. They are _very_ big boys. Jills is thirteen and Robair is fourteen and a half. Madame de Lansquenet their mummy lets them play all day long every day without keeping her eye on them like Mummy does with me. They are sposed to be old enuf to look after Isabelle but I think she looks after them even though shes the youngest.

Picture number six is me and Isabelle in front of a realy real medieval fort with some fishes. There was nobody living in it. It was small and round but it was still as big as a house. It had a tower and turrets and everything. And it had a draw bridge over a moat which was full of green water and realy scarey realy big fishes. You could see hundreds of them swimming in it. Robair and Jills said they were pikes and held me by each arm and leaned me right over them and said that they would throw me in the water and feed me to them if I told anyone about what they were going to do with me. They said pikes eat every last bit of you so nobody would know. They were cross with me cos Isabelle told them she kissed me. They said they were going to punish me. So we all had to go out for a walk past the fort to the woods. And that square box thing I drewed in front of her is sposed to be her day camera. She called it that. She said it was invisible so I couldn't see it and now I know it wasn't realy there, probly, but I'v just drawed one anyway. Isabelle said we all can have an invisible day camera on if we like. She said we use them in the night to video our dreams and that you can play them back again in the day when your awake by pretending the dreams are really happening. She kept on saying put your day camera on, Lukey, put your day camera on. And then she kissed me again. I didn't believe in her camera but I felt a bit like I was being hypnotised. I did feel like I was in a dream. So I spose I must of did put my day camera on, cos Robair and Jills didn't like us kissing again and threw pine cones at me and it was like a nightmare.

114

My next picture, number seven, is full of fir trees and those pointy dotty shapes are loads and loads of pine cones flying through the air. They hurt a lot so I knew it really wasn't a dream. I tried to run away but the ground was all soft and sandy and I couldn't go very fast becose of my lungs and I didn't know where I was or where to run to. I was frightened. The trees were even spikier than Iv drawed them. I bumped into one and fell over so they caught me. I call this picture Le Bois. I am top of my class in French now.

Then Jills and Robair and Isabelle too they all made me dig a deep hole in the middle of the woods with my hands. It took a long time and they were angry with me and when I finishd they made me get into it and kicked and pushed the sand back into it on top of me up to my neck till only my head was sticking out like I have drawed here. That's why I called picture number eight, Sad Head. I wasn't frightened so much. I mean I was but I was more sad. My drawring of myself does look a little bit like me. What I was frightened of was the red ants. They were big and dark and their nest was a hill and it was nearly as big as me exsept it looked even bigger cos I was burried up to my neck beside it. Jills and Robair were still throwing pine cones at me even when I was burried and one of them hit me and cut my forhead. And a ant climbed up my face and I screamed becose I thought it was going to drink the blood coming out of my forhead so Isabelle told her brothers too stop and brushed the ant off me with a bit of branch from a fir tree.

Then Robair and Jills said they would protect me from the ants by building a ring of fire around me and they did. They swept up pine needles with their feet and picked up cones and twigs and broke off bits of branches and lade them down in a perfect ring rite the way round me. Robair smokes cigarettes even though his mum dosn't know. He used his matches to light the circle. You cant see me in this picture which is number nine becose I am behind all those orange and red flames and that black smoke Iv drawed coughing. You cant see the big boys either becose after they lit it they ran off. I could here them larfing far away.

Picture number ten is called Mes Freres sont Mauvais. Isabelle said that to me after the fire futted out. Her brothers were gone but when the fire went out there she was sitting in front of me eating a pomagranit. She is very pretty. I drawed her head too small but you can see the ringlets in her hair and that is not suposed to be an orange or a ball she is holding in her hands it is her pomagranit. I still love you she sed and put pomagranit seeds in my mouth and they were so nice I didn't mind being burried in the sand. She said she wood let me marry her when we gruw up and that her brothers were jelas and bad. I sed we cant get marrid becose I wood not be alive probly when I was grown up. I sed I had got CF and my lungs don't work propaly and I always get infections. She cried. I sed I didn't mind I wos more afraid of dying slowly over the next ten years then dying suddenly from an infection. She sed she loved me so she wood help me die more quickly if I wood like her to. I sed I wood. I don't know why.

I did picture eleven carefully. It is a picture of lots of different pots. Isabelle sed she wood run home and come back with a kitchen knife and cut off my head. She wood bury it with Basil at the bottom of a big terracotta pot on the terris outside her bedroom like in the story she been told in school. She said there were loads of pots on her terris and it was a true story so it cud be done. Even though it was disgusting she wood do it for me becose she loved me and becose it was what I wanted. It was not what I wanted. I had only said it was becose she was so beautiful and she had sed she loved me. I have drawed lots of pots and a big sharp knife with blood on it all the way across the top of all of them. The pots have all got heads inside. You just cant see them. I did desines of them on the outside of the pots becose you cant see through the clay. Cats heads and dogs heads and snakes heads, goats heads and my head. I copied my head from looking in the mirror. I writ who is Basil over it becose I didn't have time to ask her who he was before she left to get her knife. I waited ages and ages for her to come back but she never did so I got myself out of the sand by myself and went back through the trees folowing the way she had gone past the fort and moat to the de Lansquenet chateau even though I could hardly breathe so I walkd very slowly. It was getting dark and the stars were coming out and wen I saw them I knew the stars were ded peple and the spaces in between are for the living. I went on my nebuliser for an hour when I got in. At dinner Monsieur and Madame de Lansquenet and Isabelle and Robair and Jills all carried on as if nothing had happened. So I did too. The next day when I asked her Isabelle sed she had changed her mind on her way home. She didn't love me after all so that's why she had not come back with the knife. Becose if she didn't love me she cud not kill me. She said killing people is rong and I was bad trying to make a murdrer out of her.

My last picture is number twelve. It is a drawring of my last morning in France. I new I was getting ill again. It was brekfast time and Isabelle and me had alreddy eten. We were sitting on the window sil. There was plenty of room. Sunshine was streeming in through the open windows onto the coffee and cwassonts and jam on the table. That is what I have drawn. My chest was sor but I was stil brething very well. Robair and Jills wer stil upstares in bed. Isabelle was angry with her mum who hadn't come downstairs yet eyther. She wisperd in my ear that her maman was a witch becose she was letting me go home the next day and she hated her becose she did love me realy, she'd been lying yesterday when she said she didnt and she akshuly didn't want me to go away ever. It was her horrid brothers who had told her to tell me she didn't love me animore she sed, but it was a lie. She sed she didn't want to cut my head off animore eyther becose it would be too messy and upsetting. I still felt fritened of her, but my brething was fine. Isabelle had a spoonful of jam in her hand as we sat by the open window together. She was smiling like a queen and waving the spoon around in the fresh air out the window until a wasp landed on it. And then another and another till it was cuvverd in them. Her mother came in and sat down at the table. Isabelle went back to the table too with the spoonful of wasps behind her back and dropd her napkin. While she was under the table picking it up she smeered the inside hem of her mother's skirt with the wasps and jam. I watched from the window sil but didn't say anithing and my brething was stil okay even though I knew now I was defnitly getting another infection. I cud feel the stikiness in my chest. Then Madame de Lansquenet went all wite and stood up and screemd and fainted. She had to go to hospital. When Monsieur de Lansqenet came back on his own later he said she wud have to stay in hospital for a while because she was seveerly alergic to wasps and cud have died. Isabelle sat on his lap and smiled and said she thought it was my folt her Chere Maman had been stung becose I was cross with her becose I didn't want to go home so soon. Monsieur larfed and said to me that if this was so he wud like to congratulate me as he cud not stand his wife animore and was considdering leeving her for the housekeeper who made the brekfast every morning.

When my plane landed at Heethro I had a tempriture of 103 and I cud hardly breethe. I was taken by ambulants to hospital in an oxijen mask. I didn't mind. Mummy and Daddy came with me and they wer so worrid I cudnt tell them anything ever again.

By Luke McElvey aged 10]

*   *   *

Richard's hunger for understanding and connection with his son was overpowering. As he stared at his drawings, taking in the directness of what they were communicating without understanding them at all, his frustration was immense even as he relished them. The 'Daddy Happy' clown made him feel understood and connected with by Luke, but it was curiously frustrating. He didn't need to be understood by by his dead son. He wanted to understand him. But it was a connection. At least it was that. As he and Rose looked at the pictures together each seeing that the other was smiling yet choked, delighted yet disturbed, he had to resist wanting

117

to give her a hug as if their son had just been born rather than long been dead and as if they were still married. The one entitled 'My family' was somehow lovely despite how scribbled and messy it was. It connected them both with him and with each other. Luke had clearly been right to save it. Richard wiped away a tear.

'Some of these are from his week away in France with the de Lansquenets,' Rose said. 'It says, 'En Vacance'. Look at this – a suitcase, an aeroplane, a chateau. What else could it be referring to? I don't know about some of the others though.' She pointed to the picture on which Luke had written 'Sad Head'. 'That one's rather disturbing, isn't it? Anyway, I'm sorry Richard but here doesn't seem to be a treasure map of any kind.'

'Even before he left for that holiday I was worried he was incubating an infection,' Richard said. 'How could I have let him go in such a state?'

'And on his own' Rose replied. 'But he so insisted on it and it was only week. How long was he in hospital for? Well over a month, as far as I remember. It was horrible. All he wanted was to be back home, having already been away for a week already. Poor little darling.'

'I can remember *nothing* at all about what he said happened in France,' Richard said, holding up the picture entitled 'Mes freres sont mauvais'. He felt so angry with himself that the word, 'nothing', came out somewhere between a grunt and a shout. 'Sorry,' he said. 'I don't mean to bark.'

'He didn't say anything, Richard. He delirious, out of it, with his head on my lap in the back of that ambulance all the way to the Brompton. And once he was settled in hospital and the antibiotics were beginning to work he didn't want to talk about France so I didn't insist.'

'I still feel livid with Robert's mother. The bitch never once gave him his physio despite assuring me she understood his condition and promising beforehand that she would.'

'Yes,' Rose replied, studying the picture of a large bloody knife with what looked like a row of shields or perhaps they were pots underneath it. 'Why we didn't get him a mobile phone, I'll never understand. And I will always, always regret letting Madame de Lansquenet fob us off about ringing him.'

'He was too young for a phone,' Richard replied, wanting to soothe her. 'Anyway, they weren't so readily available in those days, and – stupid of us though it was – we did actually trust the de Lansquenets, you know. We had no reason not to.'

'I was so upset about his letters,' Rose said, putting down the knife and pots picture and picking up the one entitled 'Sad head'. 'It looks just like him, doesn't it?'

The smile he now shared with Rose was bitter. 'What about his letters? What letters? You never told me.'

'Yes, I did. I must have.'

'Tell me again then because I've forgotten.'

'What little I did manage to wheedle out of him a few weeks later in the Brompton – because he didn't want to talk about any of it, Richard – was this: He said he wrote to us every day. It was only a week, but for a little nine year with frail lungs a week was a very long time to be away from his Mummy and Daddy for the first time in his life, so he *did* write to us every day. Every morning after breakfast he would give a letter to Madame de Lansquenet which he'd written to us the day before for posting, but her daughter – I can't remember her name just at the minute. Oh, yes, I can - Isabelle! That's right. Isabelle kindly informed him on his last day there, that her mother had in turn given his letters to her oldest son each morning to take to the post office in the village. Robert, I think his name was. He was supposed to post them and pick up any incoming mail. He did nothing of the kind. Nor did he tell Lukey that he hadn't posted them, or picked up ours. I sent him one to reach him in the middle of the week. In fact on his very last morning just before the de Lansquenet man took him to the airport for the flight back to Heathrow, Lukey said Isabelle told him what had happened to his letters and Robert brandished them all in front of his nose, scornfully reading out the bits where he begged to be brought back home and laughing at him. Then he tore all the letters up into little bits in front of him. Horrible.'

Richard caressed the back of her head and she didn't try to stop him, but looked into his eyes with all their shared sorrow. If Compassion was her middle name, Solace was his. It had been his middle name in their marriage and it was in his professional life too. It had stuck to him all his life, like glue. Richard, the great consoler of frightened, breaking souls. But right now their hearts were genuinely going out to each other and he somehow felt happy even as he felt the deepest sadness looking at her looking back at him feeling their grief.

'It's no wonder he only lived another nine months.' He bent to touch his forehead on Rose's and held it there for a minute before they straightened up together in silence.

'I came looking for a treasure map,' he said eventually, loving the close-up smell of her and admiring the lined, flaccid softness of her middle-aged skin. Close to, her eyes shone like a girl's whilst her skin was crumpled, lined and thin, ancient like Luke's paper in front of her, and beautiful. 'I came looking for Luke,' he said. 'And, sad as it may be – sad as it is – I'm glad to say I've found him. I think, for our sake, he pretended to want to live in those last nine months of his life but actually all he really wanted after that was to die. When I think about him now, that's who I recognise, a little boy who really did not want to bother with oxygen cylinders and respirators and endless cocktails of cutting-edge antibiotics dripping into his veins, who was just doing all that for us. He'd had enough.'

Rose nodded.

They stared at each other sharing a renewal of their bereavement so deep that all their was and all there could be between them was silence.

Just then the young woman whose room they had raided while she was in the shower appeared in a towelled dressing gown. She was drying her hair. Did her face light up with recognition? She looked friendly enough, and vaguely familiar, but he really couldn't be bothered with politeness and social niceties. Not now. Rose blew her nose and as soon as she had finished introducing them he quickly made his apologies and left, the picture of his son's Sad Head snug in his jacket pocket over his heart.

Maybe it *was* a kind of map.

In a way.

Chapter 9.

'Staff Nurse O Riordan, you have formally chosen not to have a representative from the Royal College of Nursing for this hearing, and I have to say between you and I that I think you made the right decision. As Assistant Director of Human Resources for this NHS Trust I am not in the business of persecuting staff because of their poor sickness record. On the contrary. But as you know, when the figure of more than ten days off sick at any one time appears on an employee's record, or three separate instances of sick leave occur within the space of one calendar year, then of course we have a duty to do an investigation in order to help that member of staff in whatever way we can. If the Trust can support its staff in helping them to stay well, then the Trust itself is helped to provide a better service to its patients and everyone is happy. Isn't that so Sister Salmon?'

The ferret-faced woman from Occupational Health simpered her agreement with the unctious, grey-suited director who seemed to be continually adjusting his collar. Perhaps it was a nervous twitch to counterbalance all that suave self-assurance he was emanating.

Grainne looked down at her fingernails. They were bitten to the quick, although she was not aware of actually being nervous about this interview at all. She would have to train herself to leave them alone, but since she had given up smoking two months ago she had found that her fingers almost automatically went to her mouth without her even noticing it half the time.

She knew how this was going to go. The interview would end up with her being given a formal warning that her health record wasn't good enough, to be followed by a written reprimand and an admonition to improve it over the coming months or else they would have to reconsider whether she was in the right job. She would be reminded that her contract gave her little or no employment protection rights and that the best way of ensuring she kept her job was to come to work every day. She suppressed a yawn. She did not want her disdain to show and complicate the proceedings. They all knew they were just going through motions, and Grainne wanted to get it over with as quickly as possible.

'Now let's see,' said the assistant director, 'you started working for this Trust in January of last year working Monday to Friday with only one late shift a week, on a Monday – a package tailored precisely to your needs as a working mother, in line with the government's 'Come back to Nursing' initiative. But before the month was out you suffered from influenza which necessitated your taking two whole weeks of sick leave. It must have been a very bad attack. Do you remember that?'

Grainne nodded. She remembered very well. She had been three months pregnant at the time and trying to get out of the enormous

Orwellian nurses residence block she had moved into after leaving Ron's flat back in November of the year before. She had kept her promise to herself to try and binge the baby out of her body and the Christmas period had been a long, lonely, boozy attempt at doing just that. She had put on twenty pounds in that time and became a size eighteen in the process, these joyous tidings being imparted to her when she was being fitted out for a uniform for work. She had carried on hitting herself in the tummy and making herself sick. But as if in revenge the baby had just carried on growing. She had taken too much paracetemol both prophylactically and otherwise, but nothing had seemed to stop the remorseless determination of the foetus to develop and thrive in her womb. That 'flu' he was talking about had actually been a reaction to a particularly fierce attempt to deprive herself of all goodness by starving herself, existing on an apple and water all day, and vodka in the evenings. The pounds had quickly started coming off again, but she had also started fainting and having dizzy spells and had just felt too weak to work. So she reluctantly added a carbohydrate in the form of a banana to her diet because she couldn't use the loo without laxatives anyway. After that she seemed to do remarkably well. She thought so anyway.

Needless to say the baby seemed to do remarkably well too, and had continued to grow.

'Then of course you suffered from blood pressure problems as a complication of pregnancy and had to take a substantial period of sick leave – forty working days to be precise – before becoming formally entitled to statutory maternity pay when your child was born. But I think in all fairness we can overlook the problems connected with your pregnancy.' He smiled at her as if he expected to be congratulated. 'So how old does that make your baby now?'

'He's eight months,' she replied, not finishing her sentence with 'you nosey, patronising old git'.

'What is his name?'

'I'm sorry but I'm not sure how relevant that is to this discussion.'

'No, of course. I was only enquiring out of friendly interest.'

'His name is Sean. Sean Lucien. After Connery and Freud, Lucien Freud, the artist. I like his paintings.' She tried to smile at him. It was important not to fuck this up. She just couldn't afford to be out of work. He looked blank, but nodded his head to signal familiarity with Freud. Grainne thought he didn't actually know that the difference between art and a fart was anything more than an 'f'.

'Mmm. Right. You returned to work at the end of October but took another week off within two days of starting back. It says here 'severe back ache'. How is your back now, erm, Grain-ne? Is that how you say it, 'Grain-ne'?'

'I would prefer it, please, if you did not use my Christian name at all, Mr Andrews.'

Why, oh why did she have to be so confrontational? It was so stupid. Ah well, at least she had said, 'please'.

In response he laughed in an oily I'm-sure-you-will-agree-with-me manner, too full of himself to be offended by the likes of her, said,

'Hardly a Christian name, I would have thought anyway,' he drawled, as he looked at Sister Salmon for her appreciation. To her credit Salmon didn't even smile. He collected himself with a clearance of his frog-like throat. 'Very well, Nurse O'Riordan. Your back?'

'Yes? What about it?

'How is it?'

'It's fine now' she said. 'Thank you.'

It had been fine then too. The problem had been Sean. He hadn't been fine. She had been told by the paediatrician that there was some evidence that he might have some kind of learning disability. At that time it was too early to say so definitely, nor to give her a precise diagnosis; autism, or some specific brain malformation perhaps sustained during pregnancy, or possibly brain damage as a result of oxygen starvation, a common complication with breach births, but there was no doubt she would need to prepare herself for the likelihood that his was not going to be a normal childhood.

The guilt had been unbearable. It had been like being thumped from behind in the back and she had taken a week off just to recover from the shock of what she had been told. The trouble was that after all the hatred she had had for him in the womb – and when she had first felt his little feet kicking her, she had shamefully hit back hard, punching her swollen tummy precisely where she had felt his foot, continuing to do so throughout the pregnancy whenever she felt upset – she now knew him as a little person. Whilst she still felt an unbridgable detachment from him, she was nevertheless also aware she loved him now too. As completely as she was able. After the paediatrician's pronouncement she had cried with Sean for a week.

The other two girls who shared her flat had been consistent in their support. They didn't help exactly, or ever offer to take him away from her for a little while, not after the first few weeks anyway, but they never complained about the sound of Sean's endless crying, or the stench of his disposable nappies in the bin, for which Grainne had counted herself lucky. She knew she would have to move out at some point, certainly by the time he was toddling, but for a year or so she could continue to share with them.

No-one back home in Northern Ireland even knew Sean had been conceived, let alone born. There had been a scare at one point when one of her twin sisters had wanted to come over and see London, but Grainne had made it painfully clear over the phone that it was quite out of the question for her to come and stay with her.

Neither had she told the father, as she now thought of Ron Symes. Despite the fact that she had been planning to leave him anyway, she had still felt betrayed by his sexual goings on with Lucie. Initially her anger had been with Lucie, and then with both of them as she tried to shut what they had been doing together out of her mind. But after she packed her things and left, she lost all her feelings of anger, hurt and betrayal in a sea of activity – moving to a different area, signing up with an agency for work, getting a room, and last, but not least, deliberately hurting herself whenever she might have any time to think about what she was actually feeling. But it was really her terrible anxiety about being pregnant which drove her then. Everything else was secondary. By the time she had reluctantly come to terms with the fact that it was an abortion or nothing if she wanted to get rid of it, it was too late anyway, she was twenty four weeks gone and the baby would be delivered whether she wanted it or not.

'In December, one of the busiest times of year, of course, you had another week off sick. With gastritis. A whole week. It must have been a very bad attack.'

'Yes. It was actually. Very painful indeed,' she said with a blithe insouciance which reminded her of Lucie. 'I could hardly move without being sick. I obviously felt really guilty about letting the other nursing staff down, but I just could not have got to work the state I was in, not without passing it on to them, probably. Or even worse, onto the patients.'

'A very responsible decision,' muttered Sister Salmon with a sanctimonious nod from behind her gold rimmed reading glasses.

Grainne could smell his bad breath from across the table as the man harrumphed, sourly agreeing such an attitude was certainly in line with the Trust's occupational health policy. He continued perusing her sickness record like it was a magazine. She felt naked. Illness was such a private personal thing. Her privacy was being invaded.

So she didn't tell them that actually her milk had dried up because she continued to subsist on an apple and a banana a day and therefore continued to lose weight that she had never really put on whilst pregnant. Nor that Sean in turn started to lose weight, expending all his energy at that time in crying and screaming for her tits, and just wouldn't take to bottle-feeding at all. She told them nothing about the fact that she had tried to stay detached from his cries because her health visitor had told her that as long as she provided him with a predictable pattern of maternal care everything would eventually turn out alright, that he had reached an age when it was normally to be expected that a baby has settled into its life and routines, and cries only in distress. She didn't tell them she lost weight at an alarmingly satisfying rate, that by the turn of the year she was on the verge of skeletal, with a body mass index of just under fifteen, and was absolutely unrecognisable from the person she was before she got pregnant. Of course she didn't tell them her 'gastritis' was self inflicted. Nor that she had needed to be reminded by Suzanne, one of the other two she shared the flat with, that Sean was not a part of herself, that when he was upset she could not just sit passively beside him, listening to, yet ignoring his wracking and choking cries. Oh, couldn't she? She said not a word now to Andrews and Sister Salmon about how she would passively wallow in her agreement with the feelings Sean was going through as he bawled his little brains out, very capable indeed of just sitting beside him without doing anything to attend to his distress. It wasn't the business of these two idiots to know how much of a struggle it was for her to get up off her bum to meet his needs – hold him, feed him, cuddle him, console him.

'In January you had influenza again. And again, just for a week, which obviated the need for a doctor's certificate, of course.'

'With all due respect, Mr Andrews, if you are trying to insinuate I was not genuinely ill I would have to consult with my union rep, consider taking out a grievance procedure. I'd honestly have to. My integrity as a nurse and a trained health care professional would be being impugned.' It was as well to occasionally use a long word, just so as he'd know she wasn't going to be anybody's pushover. 'Do you know what I mean?'

'I'm sure Mr Andrews is not trying to imply anything, Grainne,' said the obsequious Salmon. 'This investigative 'Return to Work Interview' has been triggered soley by the amount of sick leave you have taken since joining us. Its only purpose is to ascertain how you can improve your health record and how we can help you to do that. Both for your own benefit and that of the Trust. So I don't think there is any need at all for any animosity, if I may say so.'

Grainne gave this tart admonishment the contempt it deserved.

'Is that what you are trying to insinuate Mr Andrews?'

'Sister Salmon is quite right of course and I er, apologise for any mistaken interpretation you may have put on my words.'

'You are apologising for *my* mistaken interpretation? I don't understand.'

'What I mean is, any lack of clarity on my part.'

'Then you are not actually suggesting that I was *pretending* to have flu in January?'

'I was simply referring to the fact that a medical certificate is not required till you have more than a week's sick leave.'

'I'm afraid I still don't know what you are saying precisely Mr Andrews?'

His discomfort was palpable. She was enjoying this. The shoe was on the other foot. Speaking of which he was no longer looking at her in the face, instead he was shifting his gaze from his papers to her feet and back again.

'My only purpose is to help our employees perform to their optimum.'

'Sorry?'

'Shall we continue?'

'Oh, let's!'

He was definitely looking at her feet and legs. Dirty old dog. Instinctively she crossed them and tucked them under her chair. Since she had lost weight her legs had become more acceptable. She had never liked them before, but they did look alright now, even if she said so herself, and even in regulation black tights and flat shoes. But that didn't mean she wanted smooth old bastards like this one eyeing her up surreptitiously from behind his papers.

She pulled the hem of her uniform further down over her knees. It was like wearing a tent it was so big. She should have 'downsized' her uniform three times since starting at this hospital, but in fact had only done so once, instead becoming adept with scissors, needle and thread. She liked to think of it as downsizing. It was more purposeful and controlled somehow. A sensible economy of scale rather than a mad consequence of obsession. And she should have done so again really. This uniform was a twelve and by now even size tens were far too big and baggy for her when she tried them on. She couldn't ever remember being an eight before, although she must have been once. When she was ten or eleven years old? Maybe. Anyway people seemed to notice her now she wasn't a dumpling. Which was okay. Even though she still felt like one. Rivalrous female glances, when she got them, boosted her confidence and self-respect far more than the lascivious interest of men which she ignored completely, if she got it at all.

She used to get it all the time, even when she had a bottom as big as HMS Belfast. But not anymore thank goodness. Sometimes she thought she saw one or two people frowning when they passed her, like she must have messed herself or something. Their glances would make her feel guilty, as if she had just been sick or been to the loo because the laxatives were working. But she hadn't, because she didn't do those things anymore, putting so little inside herself in the first place nowadays. She had to tell herself that the way they looked at her was their problem, not hers.

'February. In February there were two absences because of sickness. The first from the sixth to the eleventh. Migraine. Continuous migraine you wrote on the form.'

'That's right.'

She had been upset. Not so much distressed as perturbed. Waiting listlessly at a bus stop in Wimbledon with Sean who had been lying in his push chair screaming as usual, her mind had been where it was always was, stuck in a rut of running from the horrors of the past. She had automatically rocked the pushchair back and forth trying to soothe him. There was no point picking him up, despite what the nosey old lady waiting beside her was saying. It was quarter to six, cold and dark apart from the continuous raucous roars, squeaks and grunts from the snarled-up traffic. There was no sign of a bus. She didn't even notice the young woman coming out of the hairdressers opposite, stamping her heels a few times with the cold then doing the collar of her coat up before crossing the road towards her; until she happened to look at her again, felt there was something familiar about her.

It was Lulu.

Looking not much different actually. Her hair a bit fuller maybe, her figure more natural looking. She looked prettier, a little less transy perhaps, more female, but otherwise much the same. She looked so relaxed and natural it made Grainne smile as she struggled to recognise her as the same tortured little person who used to witter on and on about all the things she would never be able to afford to have done in order to be herself. Grainne watched her pass between the gridlocked cars coming straight towards her. But Lulu clearly hadn't seen her yet as she concentrated on crossing the street.

'Lu!' She called when she was just metres away and still hadn't recognised her. 'Lulu! It me, Grainne! Hi!'

Lucille stepped on to the pavement, looked at her with a blank lack of recognition for a moment. Grainne kept on rocking the pushchair and stared right back.

'Grainne? Grainny!'

'Yes, yes its me! You look wonderful. Lulu!'

Lucie came up to her and for a moment they just stared at one another, smiling stupidly, looking at each other. Up and down.

'I can see you're all girl now, aren't you? That's great!' Grainne exclaimed, breaking the spell. 'Just great.'

'Grainny! I can't believe it. I hardly recognise you. You look so different! You've lost so much weight. So much! I can't believe it. And you've got a baby!'

'Well, you look just the same. So there! Except more so. ' It was true and as intended, it obviously pleased her, so Grainne added, 'You're looking good, Lulu.'

Greetings over, Grainne sensed how uncertain they both were of who the other was across the distances each of them had travelled in their lives since those days before Ron, childbirth and weight loss on her part, and Ron and operations on Lulu's, had put an end to their being best friends and parted them. Even as they squealed their delight now in meeting again, they were taking the measure of each other. Grainne was thinking back to when Lulu first moved in with Ron and herself, of how their friendship had been so close and so desperate that they soon made a decision to jointly play at being girls together as they both tried desperately to be normal. Ever since Uncle Jack had spoiled everything Grainne had had to pretend to be normal. But in order to pretend she had to continually learn what 'normal' was by watching how other girls handled themselves. She'd been aware of this pretence all the time. If she'd often tended to be eating as her awareness grew, she didn't mind, it helped her cope to stuff herself. In Lulu she'd had a friend whose search was essentially the same.

And they'd had so much fun together. They'd both adored pretending to be normal with each other, comparing notes and having fun. Far too occasionally, when they were both off work at the same time, they'd spent whole days together dressing up and going out, talking, laughing, window shopping, trying things on. Buying very little, of course, both of them being so low paid, but pretending to *nearly* do so, playing at being chic and sophisticated women of the world, going as far as they possibly could to convince salesgirls who earned no more than they did, that one of them really might just purchase this Dolce and Gabbana belt or that Max Mara handbag.

Yes we had the best of times, you and I, she thought, as she watched Lulu cooing over her baby. He had thankfully cried himself into a fitful sleep, but must be developing another cold, mucus was running down from his little nose into his open mouth. She wiped him. He didn't stir. She and Lulu couldn't say goodbye, not straight away, not with such a close unfinished friendship between them. Lulu clearly felt the same because she didn't try to make her excuses and say goodbye either. They went over to Costas together for a coffee, each knowing the other well enough to see she was lonely, wanted to take a chance on becoming reacquainted.

Grainne sat down as Lulu took off her coat and hung it over the back of a chair before going up to order their coffees. Grainne watched her. If you knew her history you wouldn't believe it.

For the next twenty minutes they swopped stories, each of them trying too hard to retrieve the old sense of being closest friends again and avoiding the subject of Ron altogether. In that unspoken way old friends often use to resolve disagreements, they somehow each managed to make it clear to the other that he was history. Ancient history.

But ancient history belongs to the dead and sitting here now with Lulu who was very much alive, Grainne found herself wanting to feel alive again too.

'It's so strange,' she said. 'I feel like it was only yesterday since we were eating each other up with jealousy! But it's nearly two whole years now since I was twelve and a half stone and so jealous of you being able to get into all my nicest things. I wanted to die of shame. I know! I know I encouraged you. But *really* I was jealous. While you were busy being the bitter little Queen of Sorrows, jealous too – of my boobs and bum and fanny, and ashamed of being a boy. And now I'm less than half the weight I was then – although you wouldn't believe how much flab I'm still carrying! – And you're a woman! Aren't we the lucky ones!'

She raised her eyes to heaven, knowing that neither achievement would weigh heavily on the great scale of things. But she could see from the happy expression on Lulu's face that she, of course, did feel positive about the changes she had made, as she would, and wasn't therefore going to join her in this delicate sneering. If it didn't stop her, it did help remind Grainne not to turn everything into something bad, to try just for once to be positive herself. She nodded away her sarcastic tone with a genuinely grateful smile and said,

'We certainly don't need to be jealous of each other anymore now, do we? Not any more. I mean we *wouldn't* – if we still knew each other, if we were still friends.'

She let that sisterly thought hang in the air between them as Lulu repeatedly nodded her full agreement.

'I want to be your friend again, Grainny.'

'Good, me darlin!' She said, piling on the Oirish. So do I! Now tell me all about the big snip! Did it hurt? Don't you miss your – your thing? I'm sure I would! Are you pleased with its replacement?'

Lulu put her elbows apart on the table, brought her palms together in a prayer of mock gratitude, removed the mock, closed her perfectly painted lids and lashes and went into herself, becoming Lucille, Lady of the Deep Contented Sigh, a role she used to play with Grainne whenever she was happy. In response, as she had used to do, Grainne grinned and stuck her tongue out between her teeth and her lower lip, the Knowing Queen of Fools. They'd loved striking poses together. Grainne laughed out loud now and Lulu clapped.

'I'm me and I'm free cos I sit to do peepee!' she repeated, chanting like a cheerleader. 'But seriously, I can't miss not being myself, now can I? That would just be *impossibly* silly. I'm not saying I'm not silly, but *that* would be impossible,' she said. Then she sat up straight and looking round, gave a proud little wiggle of her breasts and shoulders. 'I'm a Miss under the law now! It's on my national insurance identity, and my passport, definitely Miss... Lucille Emily Farouk.

Grainne quickly recognised that the main difference between them now was that while Lulu was proud because she had become a girl, over the same period of time she herself had gone from being a girl to being a woman because she had had a child, but with no particular pride at all. Should she be sad about that? She had never been proud about anything in her life and you cannot miss what you've never had.

'So what *do* you miss?' she asked Lulu.

'I don't know. Nothing really. Nothing from the past anyway. Here and now? A man maybe, but I'm not even sure about that.' She sighed, looking around at the people on the other tables, a woman of the world, poised and elegant. Then belied the whole effect by crossing her eyes like a school kid and declaring, 'I'm not a virgin anymore, either, so I do know what it is I'm not sure about! His name was David. What about you?'

'What about me? Am I still a virgin or what do I miss?'

'Yes, that. I know you're not a virgin.'

'I miss sleeping at night. I miss having some feelings. Mere trifles like that. I even miss my family sometimes.' She paused, glad that Lulu looked a little shocked at this reply. There was no way she could pretend to be happy and fulfilled. She softened her voice. 'I've missed you too, Lu. Sometimes.'

'Me too – you,' Lulu said softly, looking into her eyes.

'So, what's he like, your boyfriend?' Grainne asked, changing the mood back to upbeat again.

'I already want to dump him. Mum says I'm a monster.'

'Why? Was he no good in bed? Don't tell me you didn't enjoy it after everything you've been through?'

'I did. It was lovely. It's just he's – he's boring.' She pursed her lips, shrugging her own incomprehension. 'I am bad, aren't I!'

But her smirk contradicted this self description. She looked very pleased with herself. Not unbearably smug, but close to it. Kind of monstrous then, thought Grainne.

'How we change!' she said, looking down at Sean stirring in his pushchair. 'I've got a baby and you –

'And I? I wish he was mine! He's so gorgeous, Grainney. I'm so jealous! Don't you just want to eat him up? I do!' Sean was still asleep so he couldn't have responded even if he were capable, to Lulu going into baby-talk mode. 'I do, I do, I do! I want to eat you all up, don't I, little baby?'

For a change, Grainne's smile was genuine. This kind of gushing over babies usually just made her feel inadequate because she couldn't feel it herself, but if anybody meant it, Lulu must, which made it acceptable. More than acceptable, welcome. And necessary. Sean needed this kind of thing – when he was awake and able to enjoy it – for his development. She knew he did. She was worried he was failing to thrive because she herself didn't have it in her. She was unable to feel much, if any, warmth for him herself, no matter how hard she tried, so it was definitely her fault he wasn't doing as well as other babies his age. Not just because of what she did to him when she was pregnant, but also, now, for not being able to be as loving as she felt towards him in the way he needed, with sensitivity and responsiveness, with her heart.

She just did not have it in her.

'All he does is howl,' she said.

They looked down at him again together. Even in his sleep he appeared to be grimacing, about to cry. He had always been like that.

'You can see who the father is just by looking at him. You probably ate *him* up a bit yourself actually, if you know what I mean.' She hadn't intended to sound bitchy, but her words hung in the air after they were spoken, persecuting both of them.

Lucille glanced at her and frowned, not getting it. Not at first. She looked down at Sean again, staring at him for a few moments. Then had the grace to blush. Immediately Grainne felt the last trace of her residual hostility towards her finally leave. This was her one-time best friend! For a few moments they sat in a close, but awkward, memory-filled silence just looking at Sean together, unspoken thoughts and feelings racing between them as they sipped their coffees.

'Why didn't you tell me, Lu? What Ron was doing to you, I mean?'

Lucille shook her head. Her cow-like eyes flashed angrily for a moment, then she looked like she was perhaps going to cry. Well, Grainne wasn't going to give her the satisfaction of that. Not yet anyway. Not till she had found out how Lulu had felt about her when she was having it off with him.

'But I suppose I already knew the answer to that question really,' she continued, determined to clear the air between them over this. 'I guessed it must have taken two to tango. You could always twist him round your little finger, anyone could see that. So, to be honest, I do think looking back on it, that I did already know in a strange kind of way. I just chose to pay no attention to it because I didn't really care. And when I read your letter I knew if you had been having it off with him it could only have been because *you* wanted to, and that your note to me had to be a lie. I know you Lulu. I used to anyway. I mean we were always talking together about men, weren't we ? You must have thought I was completely stupid, writing me that silly note. I was insulted! That's why I never got in touch. I was angry because you treated me like I was stupid. Not because you lied. Everybody lies about sex.'

Lucille shifted in her seat before looking up and away studying the décor and the walls with a fixed half-smile on her face. She looked very much like the worker in a hair salon she actually was, with her prettily styled hair and her cheap trendy clothes. If she was obviously more comfortable and relaxed in herself than she used to be, she still slapped on a bit too much make-up. Not enough to hide her discomfort though.

'I'm sorry, Grainney,' she said eventually.

Even allowing for the plastic surgery, the expression on her face did seem to be genuinely contrite.

'That's alright. I'm actually glad now. I am really! It helped me get away from him. Our relationship had been dead for months. We needed to end

131

it. But I'd like to think you wouldn't have moved in on him if there had still been something between us?'

They looked at each other with narrowed eyes. Lucille nodded her head, then shook it again, at the same time shrugging helplessly. Grainne loved her for the honesty of that.

'You can keep him,' she said, smiling.

'No, thanks. I couldn't help it Grainne. You're right it wasn't all him. But I've actually not seen him again since the day I left. Truly.'

'We were best friends Lulu! You and I, I mean. I didn't care as much about him as I cared about *you*, you know? Not by then, anyhow. So I kept on thinking how could you have done that to me? To our friendship? How could you?'

'I know. I was selfish. I didn't think. I – No, that's all it was really. I was selfish and I didn't think! I know it sounds stupid and unbelievable, but I didn't realise, I honestly didn't, that I only had one thing on my mind at that time and that was sex. And I think I just wanted to have what was yours, including your man, I suppose.' The expression on her face was somewhere between a wince and shrug.

Though she didn't say it aloud, Grainne could feel Lulu's truthfulness soothing and healing the hurt she'd felt ever since they'd gone their separate ways. But her mother was right, she was definitely a bit of a monster.

'Please forgive me,' Lucille implored. 'I owe you. I would love to be your friend again. If you'd let me. Really be your friend this time. I'd do anything.'

Lulu's intensity was a gift-horse. Grainne's mother always used to say you shouldn't look in their mouths, so she didn't. Instead, she blurted,

'Well, there *is* something you could do for me. Could you look after Sean for me sometimes? I need a break from him, Lu. He's too much, on my own all the time. Would you? You'd certainly find out a lot more about what it really means to be a woman, I can tell you! And for me it would be a little bit of heaven.'

Lucille looked wary, unsure. Was her face beginning to harden into refusal? Don't say no, Grainne begged her silently. Please don't say no.

'Please Lulu, would you? After all we shared his father !'

Whoops! Why did she always have to get so aggressive when she wanted something from someone? They looked at each other coldly for a moment. Perhaps they could never truly be friends again. Not in the same way as they had used to be. Not with that between them. But they could still pretend. They could lie to one another sweetly for old times sake. Wait and see whether, with the passage of time they did actually get to like and trust each other again.

Nevertheless, with an anger she didn't fully understand, Grainne also found herself wanting Lucille to know what it was like looking after a handicapped, permanently fractious baby. She really wanted her to know the realities involved in caring for a child who needs more from you than everything you have to give emotionally and in return gives you nothing back at all. She really wanted Lucille to know, sitting there with her lovely long legs and her manicured fingers, that there was more to life than sex and gender.

'Oh Lulu, I'm so sorry. That was cheap of me. It really was. But I meant what I said about Sean. I need all the help I can get. He's damaged, maybe autistic. He's too young at the moment to really tell. It's still too early for the doctors to say just yet what precisely is wrong, but they know he isn't normal. And so do I, believe me! And I need a break. I so very badly need a break, Lulu. And I know it would be really good for him too. It gets too much sometimes, between him and me. He is so full of need that I just switch off. His neediness *makes* me switch off, which is no good for him at all. He needs stimulation. He needs someone else he can have care and attention from and make a little bit of an attachment to, someone who'll respond to him a bit better than I do,' she finished lamely. 'It could be like he was *your* baby too for a few hours.'

'I would love to look after him. I really would. And I will, if you really want me to. I'll try anyway! But Grainne, I just want to say I am sorry too. Not just for what I did with Ron. For lying to you, treating you, as you said, like you were stupid or something, and like our friendship wasn't real. Okay?'

'Okay.'

'Are you sure you don't mind? Me looking after him, I mean, knowing what I am and everything?'

Grainne nodded so emphatically she gave herself a little headache over her left eye. 'Don't be silly,' she said, sounding, she thought, rather like a grizzly bear because she didn't want to hear such nonsense.

'He's such a lovely-looking baby. Are you still breastfeeding him?'

'What, with these shrunken things? You look like you could do a better job of that than me now! But seriously: no, he never took to it.'

They chatted for a while longer, getting up to date with the details of each others lives, all the time becoming easier and easier with one another again.

Except when Lucille tried to enquire about her weight loss. Talking about that always made Grainne tense, it didn't matter who it was with. It was so hard to make sense about something so private, and despite clearly having no intention at all of making her feel uncomfortable, Lucille's questions did make her wary. It was difficult enough telling her a little bit – enough – about what she had done to try and get rid of Sean before he was born, without telling her that emotionally all she really wanted to do now was join him, become a damaged child herself; and that not eating helped her do that. At the same time, of course, counting calories all the time and staying in control of the situation made sure that actually she was still in charge of what she did, was responsibly adult so that she could still be there for Sean however inadequate to the task of looking after him she knew herself to be.

Lucille looked confused and a little horrified as she listened to her, but in the end needed little persuasion to arrange to come round on Sunday and take Sean out for the afternoon. They agreed Grainne would pick him up again in the evening, perhaps meet Rose. Lulu said if it went alright, she would love to take him out on a regular basis. She adored babies, she said. Grainne was naturally delighted, but felt she had to warn her again that this particular baby was not so lovable at all. Then she got up and hugged Lulu, almost overcome by relief and gratitude.

They'd kissed goodbye shortly after that, but for the next week Grainne couldn't get rid of her headache. It became a migraine. It pierced her head with so much more pain than the drops of boiling water she deliberately spooned out onto her arm from the saucepan she used for sterilising Sean's bottle, in an attempt to divert herself from it. When she couldn't divert herself from it, she found that in between the stabbing photophobia and the nausea all she could feel was that she was failing. Failing personally. Whereas Lulu seemed to have found herself, she couldn't stop being concerned about how fat she was, even now when she was 'objectively' thin. And it made finding the energy to love Sean in the way he needed terribly difficult, if not impossible. It was irrational, she knew, but she wanted to punish herself for being so stupid, because however much her behaviour might belie it, she did in fact want to do what was best for her little baby son.

Amidst all this confusion and contradiction, scalding herself provided respite from the pain in her head and the noise of Sean's incessant tears. It also prevented her from dwelling too long on the vague, irrational, but persistent anxiety she felt about having invited Lulu back into her life. Whatever she felt about her now, and however much she may have forgiven her for it, Lulu had once betrayed her. A part of her knew that it wasn't very clever to renew your friendship with a betrayer. But she couldn't help it. It was what she wanted to do. Which made her head hurt.

Back in the here and now Mr Andrews seemed to be droning on forever with his litany of her sick leave.

'Then there were two days off sick at the end of February with sciatica.'

'I got up off my chair too quickly one night after I fell asleep feeding my baby. He was crying. It was two a.m. You know what it's like Mr Andrews. When you are very tired – you get up suddenly and you trap a nerve.'

She looked at her watch. Ten to five. He would want to be off soon in his big car to go back to his big home and his big wife in nerveless, trap-free suburbia. She gave him her most efficient smile, willing him to get this charade over with. She was good at her job. There was not only a national shortage of nurses, this hospital was running up astronomical agency bills. There was no way he would do anything more than merely threaten her with the sack.

'I see you are in a commendable hurry to get back to your patients, Miss O' Riordan. I think we can safely say, and I am sure you will agree with me, that the conclusion of this investigative interview must be that the high incidence of sickness sustained by yourself over the past year is regrettable, but was in fact unavoidable. Mrs Salmon will closely monitor your performance over the next year and will want to meet with you from time to time to discuss any health concerns you may have which might adversely affect your ability to work. I do not think that termination of your contract by mutual consent on the grounds of ill-health is presently advisable, but I think we would both want to urge you to try and take better care of yourself in the future.' His powerful, pseudo-benign smile in another life would have incited her to kill him. Instead, she nodded her head in abject humility as he added, 'but particularly over the course of the next year, if the three of us are not to meet up here again.' He looked at his watch. 'Er, thank you very much, Staff Nurse O'Riordan,' he said with a flat smile.

Grainne continued to nod her head from the shoulders, forcing herself to behave to the end as the ritual required. For his part, he closed his file, looked at his watch again, and ignored her. It was the cue for switching off her nods and her polite manner and leaving. The Salmon woman hardly even glanced at her as she said goodbye, too busy attending to the director's inconsequential patter about the perils and pleasures of driving home at this time of year, with that irritating, fawning falseness so many women affected for the alpha male in their working lives.

Grainne still had four and a half hours to work and it would be dark as well as wet when she had to go and wait for her bus.

She took her time returning to the Accident and Emergency dept. It was usually fairly quiet this time of day. The school age broken bones would all have been x-rayed, plastered and sent home an hour ago and the drunks usually didn't start coming in with their cuts and grazes for another hour or so.

In the event she turned out to be very busy for the rest of her shift. There had been an unusual number of road traffic accidents that evening because of the rain. She felt so tired by five to nine that she didn't even hear the next name on the treatment list being called out by the receptionist.

'Mr Siamese. Mr Roenahld Siamese, please.'

As he lumbered towards her in a tired shuffle holding his left wrist gingerly with the palm facing upwards and pain furrowing his brow, she didn't really notice him at first. She was busy directing someone else up to the medical ward and wasn't looking his way. *He* must have seen her though, because when she turned to show him into a cubicle he had a puzzled grin on his face.

'Grainney? Grainney? It is you, isn't it? You've shrunk. You look like, like a fucking stick insect! What's the matter with you, sweetheart? Are you ill? When I knew it was you, my wrist stopped hurting for a moment!' He beamed happily. Then frowned. 'I didn't like that woman calling me Siamese. I've never been called that before.'

For a moment she was stunned. Ron! And talking to her as if they had never been apart. What a surprise. And what a nuisance. Now of all times, when she could hardly stand up she was so exhausted. Ah well. Che sera, she thought. It would be handover in five minutes, then she was off.

'Ron! Hello. It's nice to see you. I suppose! But please don't call me Sweetheart. My, how you've ballooned,' she said, the shock of seeing him again making her revert to her earlier briskness. 'Swollen up like a melon since I last saw you! What a surprise to see you here. Could you come over this way please, slip your shoes off and sit down on the chair beside the bed. What have you done to your hand?'

She drew the curtain and looked from Ron to her clipboard and back again. Damn. Damn. Damn. Why couldn't someone else have been allocated to him?

'I've missed you Grainne. Ever since you left, my cancer has just spread and spread.'

She wasn't listening to him. She didn't want to. She had a viable plan of escape. She would invoke non-existent regulations. He wasn't to know.

'In view of our former non-professional relationship, hospital rules dictate that it would be unethical for me to continue to deal with you, so I am going to hand your case over to a colleague, if you don't mind. If you would like to wait here for a minute or two, I will just go and call someone over to see to you.'

She put up her hand to draw the curtain again.

'What? No! Please don't do that, Grainne. I do mind. I want *you* to be my nurse.'

'I don't think that would be at all appropriate.'

'Oh Grainney, go on! I won't do you no harm. You know that. Please. You be my nurse.'

She couldn't help softening in response to this appeal. It would only be for the briefest period anyhow if the note from the receptionist about the nature of his injury was any indication. And he was, after all, the father of her child.

'Very well. You hurt your left wrist in a fall earlier this evening it says here. So I suppose you can't take your shoes off yourself.'

She bent down to untie the laces of his trainers and to give herself some time to collect herself. What a shock! She looked at his calves. Massive. He had always been big, but now he was enormous. At least a hundred and ten kilos. It was shocking.

He had a hand on her hair and was stroking it. She shook her head away.

'Please don't do that, Ron, or I *will* get someone else to work with you straight away. Do you understand?'

He nodded.

'You're losing your hair, Grainney. It's all thin and straggly. I can see your scalp. Are you ill – being so thin and everything? Have you got cancer too?'

'I'm fine, Ron. Life has just been a bit hard since I last saw you. Alright? Now show me your wrist.'

He held it out. She examined it, asked him a few questions, said a doctor would have to see it but he needed to have an x-ray first. It would take a little while for that to be done and by the time he got back from the x-ray department she would have gone off shift. So she would say goodbye to him now.

His face fell. He was so easy to read. He always had been. It had been one of his less exciting, but more endearing qualities.

'I'll stay and chat with you for a few minutes now,' she said. 'But what's this about cancer? You've got cancer?'

He nodded.

'It affects my vision. I see things. I see how people really feel. And I see the future sometimes.'

'Tumours behind the eye can make your vision become distorted,' she replied carefully. 'But there is no way any kind of cancer can make people see the future, Ron.'

'Mine does.'

'What medicines are you on?'

'Only one. I have to take it three times everyday. It's called Olanzapine. Oh Lands of Pine. It makes me think of forests and loo cleaner. It use to be Respiridone, but I haven't done respiring, have I? Not yet. So I asked for a change.'

Grainne nodded. They were both anti-psychotics, and he was talking nonsense so it fitted. He didn't have cancer at all. He must have had a breakdown. The medication would explain the weight he had put on too.

'What makes you think you've got cancer?'

'My psychiatrist told me I have.'

'What you've got is you've gone simple in the head, you silly man. You should stop taking those drugs and get an interest in life. Oh, would you look at me now! I'm doing exactly the same thing to you now as I was when we lived together. Telling you what to do. It's hard to change the way people relate to one another, Ron. I've got no right to talk to you like that anymore.'

'I like it.'

She smiled perfunctorily. She wasn't going to give him any kind of encouragement.

'I see things which come true,' he said after a moment.

'Like what, Ronnie?' She laughed as politely as she could.

'Like you just want to get away from yourself and the more you want to, the more you can't.'

'Well, yes, me and all the other billions of people on the planet.'

'Like you never want to be a mum because your own mum let you down.'

'I'm sorry Ron, but now you have just got too personal. I think I'll tell you something for free. For auld langsyne: if you want to get a proper life you need to stop taking psychiatric drugs and smarten yourself up.'

'That's what that woman Rose told me this evening too. I think I'm really going to have to do that, aren't I? If I can. Or I'll always be a mess all me life. I can't have two people telling me that in one night and not do nothing about it, can I?'

'I'm not talking about your appearance here, Ron. Although you do look a sight! I mean your brain.'

'She did too. I think.'

'I'm not interested in what other women are telling you, Ron, although of course I am pleased there are actually other women in your life.' She stopped herself adding, 'hard though that is to believe'.

'It's not like that. She's–'

'I'm not interested Ron. All I'm saying to you, as someone who once tried to love you, is that you need to smarten up your brain; learn that you don't say horribly personal things to people, especially people you used to claim to love, and expect them not to be offended. And you haven't got cancer. You've got a psychiatric problem of some kind, that's all. You imagine things. That's what that medicine is for. To stop you imagining things. You would probably 'see' things even better if you weren't on it. And it's the medicine that's probably made you so fat, if you ask me. Now I'm sorry, but you'll have to go along to x-ray.'

'Is it, 'Fuck off, Ron.' time?'

'You could say that.'

'Can I see you again?'

'Don't be silly, Ron.'

He looked so disappointed that she relented a little.

'You can have my phone number if you like. But don't ring unless you have smartened up, because I won't speak to you. But if you ever do manage to get your act together there is something I should tell you one day. Something important. You couldn't cope with it at the moment. Anyway never mind that.' She looked at him sideways. 'I don't know why you would want to see me again,' she said, changing the subject, feeling wicked. 'I thought Lucille was the 'girl' for you now?'

It was bitchy. She didn't care. She was tired and this lug of a man had after all once cheated on her. Nevertheless she immediately regretted the way she'd spoken.

'How do you know about me and Lulu?'

'She told me all about it. We're friends again.'

'I want to be your friend again, Grainney. Anyway what d'you say it like that for? Was it cos you were jealous or something?' he asked, cunning lighting up his face.

'Don't flatter yourself! I can assure you I'm not jealous of her in the slightest. We both used to be very jealous of each other, but we're not now. I was just being a bit of a bitch that's all. For the hell of it, cos I've had a bad day and I was once angry with you both. I'm not anymore. I was just winding you up. But I can tell you're still holding a candle for her, as we say back home.'

'I'm holding one for you! Why did you leave me, Grainney? Was it cos you knew about what me and Lulu was doing?'

'That just helped me decide the time had come. I'd been thinking about it for months. We'd gone in different directions you and I. We weren't right for each other anymore, were we?'

'Yes, we were.'

He looked at her and she saw him cogging that he would go nowhere if he pursued this particular line.

'Er, I mean, no. You're probably right, I spose we couldn't have been, seeing as how you did leave me, didn't you!? It was dead weird, Grainne, you and Lulu both going within a day of each other. It shook me up it did, cos it was so sudden.'

'Well, it's all history now.'

'I wish it wasn't. I wish I hadn't done what I did, Grainney. I wish you and me was still together.'

'We have our history. Be satisfied with that, because that's all there is ever going to be, Ron.'

'I thought you said there was something you wanted to tell me one day.'

'That's different. But I've already said I am *not* telling you unless you get your act together.'

'I will. I will.'

'Until you do then.'

She wrote down her number for him and popped it in the breast pocket of his jean jacket. She pointed the way down the corridor and told him to follow the signs. Then impulsively she kissed him on the cheek and said, 'Fuck off, Ron.'

He smiled gratefully and did as he was told.

Grainne went back to the nursing office. It was time for handover. Then Sean. Then home. As she and her colleagues let the night staff team know what was happening – how the afternoon shift had gone; how long the queue of patients was now; what the most urgent cases were and what they knew of the current bed state in the medical, paediatric and elderly wards – she found herself feeling woozy again. She prayed to the God she no longer believed in, that Sean would be asleep when she arrived to take him home. She couldn't remember yet leaving work after a PM shift on a Monday night to pick him up from the minder and finding that he was. He just wouldn't seem to settle with her. Then again he couldn't settle with anyone. And it was only once a week that he had to stay with Carol, who was always very positive about how well he had coped in between the long periods of disturbance. But Grainne couldn't trust that this wasn't just a sales pitch. The woman was too slick and too confident. She was also expensive, but there it was. She didn't really have much choice.

The handover was interminable. For some reason night staff always wanted more information than they got. Always. As if they deliberately wanted to keep you from going home. When it was finally over she hurried to get up out of her chair to go to her locker for her coat and bag. As she did so she felt herself swaying, becoming dizzy and sank gratefully back down into her chair waiting for the sensation to pass. She hadn't had her mega vitamin pill or apple and banana this morning. She had told herself at the time that it was because she was in too much of a rush, what with getting Sean dressed and ready. He had been so consumed by his own screaming this morning, and so unresponsive to her admittedly feeble attempts to coax and cuddle him out of it, that she had felt something inside her snap. It wasn't that she had forgotten to eat the apple and the banana. A core part of her had simply decided that if he could scream then she could starve and then they'd both be suffering. So that would be alright. Or at least fair.

And anyway she was determined to get down to somewhere properly below size eight and back into children's sizes. She would stop there. She wouldn't allow herself to get any smaller than that, however much she might feel driven to. She didn't want people talking. And, she supposed, she did have Sean to think of. In the meantime it was such a nuisance always wearing clothes that didn't fit. But the fact was she felt almost permanently light-headed and heavy-bodied at the moment, like she was walking underwater. It had been a long shift, true. But if she just lost a little more weight and then stabilised there, perhaps she might be better able to feel a little more lighter-bodied and therefore find her hard days and disrupted nights easier to manage. Sean never slept longer than an hour at a time. Then he'd cry for two hours, his little body wracked and shaking till his throat was sore and exhaustion knocked him out again. Despite exhaustive tests, the paediatricians still couldn't find anything specifically and treatably wrong with him. They counselled patience.

She was beyond patience. She had accepted this was how he was from the beginning. It wasn't patience she needed. It was a miracle. In the meantime she had to find the best way of coping with her own guilt about what she had done to him by trying to 'spontaneously' abort him during her pregnancy. And the best way of coping with that was to feel physically lighter. Undoubtedly. It was a bit bonkers, she knew that, but she wasn't completely mad. At least she wasn't cutting herself so much anymore. The odd little scald now and again, but it was only what she deserved after what she'd done. She knew that whatever she felt to the contrary she was physically as light as she could ever remember being since she was a child. Forty kilos. She would stop when she had lost another kilo – well, perhaps two, just to be on the safe side, so that she was definitely and completely under six stone, or just maybe three – maybe – to allow for re-hydration once her weight was stabilising. But until then she wouldn't actually feel light. Afterwards, of course, it would be a different matter. She was sure she would feel as light and buoyant as air.

Then she would be able to carry Sean like the wind; through the howlings and gusts of the rest of his life, if need must be.

She got up at the second attempt. Doris, the night charge nurse, noticed how weak she was, told her in her warm Grenadian tones that she didn't mean to intrude or anything, but she was so thin she looked ill, she needed to go home and put some meat on them bones. Grainne retorted she was fine, hoping Helen, the sister in charge of her own shift, hadn't heard. She had already had a go at her last week. Adopting Grainne's own practice of saying what she thought, she had not just told her she looked ill, she had said she *was* ill and she was going to send her home at the slightest sign of her not being able to perform her work properly. Grainne had told her in equally unambiguous terms that she was perfectly well, thank you very much, perfectly well, and the officious woman had backed off. For the time being. But it was getting more and more difficult, which was such a shame. Especially as not actually eating was getting easier and easier.

Grainne went out to the toilets where her locker was. She was always so cold nowadays. She put on her coat and glancing at herself in the mirror was almost, but not quite, satisfied with how bony and hollow-cheeked her face was looking. Like her weight, her appearance was now not very far from being true to her sense of who she was. Dressed anyway. Except for her hair. It was becoming so thin and lifeless. Everyday she found more strands lying on her pillow and even on the floor beside her bed. She couldn't wash it nowadays without finding handfuls of dislodged strands curling round her fingers. So it couldn't be denied. But what was far more difficult to admit was that her freckled white body with its useless, rippling folds of sagging skin, which used to cover and contain her back in the past when she was twice her current size, was becoming hairy. Up along her arms and legs and across her back, soft fine gingery hairs had sprouted up like new grass, almost without her noticing it. A bit like an orang-utang, if the truth be told. But she knew it was related to her weight-loss, felt confident it would disappear once she was no longer actively losing weight, once she was on a maintenance diet and her periods had restarted. But in the meantime, it wasn't nice at all. She would have to buy a depilatory cream.

She dabbed on some orangey red lipstick. She had bought it just a few months ago because it went with her hair, a shade darker maybe, but no more. But now it was so much brighter that it made her look like some kind of washed out clown, or if she was honest, clown's skeleton. She wiped it off again, and made her way slowly out along the corridor to the lift which would take her up to 'ground' level. Even going up one flight of stairs was a chore nowadays.

She pressed the call button and felt herself swaying again. It was so annoying. She waited for the lift, which needless to say had to come all the way down from the top floor, and as it did so she struggled not to black out. She leaned against the wall, forcing her eyes to focus on the Magritte picture of a train coming out of a fireplace on the wall opposite. When the lift let out an electronic ping to signal its arrival, sweat was pouring off her brow and down her bony back. She decided she must have flu as she staggered into it. She pressed 'ground' and as the doors shut so did her consciousness. When the lift rose she felt herself falling and by the time it had reached the ground floor above, some five or ten seconds later, she had collapsed into a minute crumpled heap of bones, hardly noticeable beneath her uniform and over-sized woollen winter coat.

When she came to, she thought for a moment she was back at work because she was lying on a bed in one of the cubicles reserved for more serious cases. What in the name of heaven was she doing here? The SHO who had earlier looked with her at Ron's x-rays, was bending over her trying to get her attention. The dreadful Doris was hovering by his side saying she was so anorexic that she was in serious danger of catching whatever passing infection came her way and dying. Grainne pushed the SHO away and sat bolt upright. At least she tried to. She fell back again immediately. She just didn't have the strength even to sit up. But she was alert now, wide awake and thinking of Sean and Carol.

'Hi Doris,' she said cheerily. 'I heard what you were saying. You're quite wrong about me having anorexia. That's completely ridiculous. Complete-ly! But you *are* right about me being unwell. I think I must have caught a virus from a patient or something. One of the perks of the job! Smile Doris, that was a joke!

'But I'm afraid I've got to go now, thank you. I'll treat myself at home. I have to pick up my little boy or the minder will charge me double for the extra time he's been with her.'

She looked at her watch.

'Oh my God! It's already nine forty-five! I must have been asleep for twenty or twenty five minutes.'

'You weren't asleep. You were unconscious. You collapsed in the lift, going home.'

She made another, more concerted attempt to get up and leave. She didn't want to hear Doris's drivel, but as soon as she tried to raise herself from the horizontal she found she was again unable to. Not out of faintness now. Not at all. She was simply too weak to move. But it exactly reminded her of how completely helpless she used to feel when she was a little girl with Uncle Jack, which made it quietly terrifying.

She noticed her bag had been placed on the chair beside her and reached over to it for her packet of Proplus. A shot of caffeine would soon set her right.

'You are not going anywhere my darling!' said Doris. 'You couldn't make it even if you tried. Your blood pressure is dangerously erratic and you are ill. You're running a high temperature. We've asked a psychiatrist to come and see you. To see if he can get some sense into your head, young lady!'

She laughed with a good humoured heartiness as if she expected Grainne to join in or something. Stupid interfering cow.

'As to your little boy, don't you worry about a thing! You just give me the phone number of your minder and I will ring her and explain what is going on. There's no way – no way – you are going home in the state you're in. So just forget it, darlin, you hear?'

'How dare you? How dare you call a psychiatrist? There is absolutely nothing wrong with me mentally at all. I'm off duty now and I am leaving. And we both know there is nothing you can do to stop me. Thank you for looking after me,' she added with a brittle smile.

The SHO tried to make a joke about putting her clothes at the end of the bed because she was too weak to be able to even get as far as that. She told him to shut up.

'Grainne!' said Doris who was religious and didn't hold with even the hint of an expletive, 'You are being unrealistic. You are physically unable to go anywhere at the moment.'

'We'll soon see about that. Just get me a drink of water Doris, and then I'll phone the minder myself. All I need is a few minutes to perk up again. I'll be completely fine in a minute.'

Proplus and water always worked when she was feeling especially run down.

'If you want to convince the psychiatrist of that, I think the best thing you could do now would be to present him with a cooperative patient who knows how to behave in a mature and adult manner.'

'Okay Doris, I know. I know.'

'And if you can get up, which you shouldn't even try, then the first thing I want you to do is strip off down to your underwear. After that, if you've still got any energy left I would like you to step on these scales. Unless you want me do it for you.'

'No. No way.'

'Yes way! We have to organise a proper medical and nursing care plan for you. You have been admitted as a patient now, and Barry here needs to listen to your heart which you know perfectly well is stressed by how little nourishment there is in your blood. I'm not going to tell you all about it. You know perfectly well –

'Stop repeating that!'

'Repeating what, for goodness sake?' asked Doris, unable to prevent her exasperation from smothering her goodwill.

"Perfectly well', 'perfectly well'. I am perfectly well. Enough anyway.'

It was a concession. She wouldn't give her the satisfaction of making another.

'So prove it by cooperating with us then. The psychiatrist will be here in a minute.'

'You are a manipulative cow, Doris, do you know that?'

'I've heard worse from patients, Grainne, but never from a colleague in all my years of nursing.'

'Alright! Alright. I give up. Tell him to go away.' She nodded at Barry, the SHO, 'and I will do as you ask. I will show you I am now well enough to do that. All I have got is a touch of the Uncle Jack's– what did I say that for? I meant the flu. And then I'll show you! I will show you I'm well enough – perfectly well enough – to put my clothes back on again and leave to pick up my child and take him home.'

'I'll get you the phone.'

Grainne sat herself up slowly and was pleased to see she managed it without undue wooziness this time. She swung her legs over the side of the bed. They might *look* a bit bony in artificial light, but she knew they were actually still elephantine. Extremely big and extremely strong. Well-capable of taking her wherever she wanted. Anyone could see that. No-one in their right mind would think otherwise. Certainly not a psychiatrist. It would be okay. It would! It had to be.

But Doris was right about one thing. She must cooperate. Or be seen to be cooperating anyway. She would get home quicker that way, and what damage she had done to her reputation in terms of gossip amongst the other staff on the ward would be at least a little less terminal. She slowly swung her legs over the side of the bed. The feeling of faintness immediately returned and she sat still for a moment fighting it. When it receded once more, she slipped onto the floor and leaning against the side of the bed, found herself fighting it off yet again.

It involved no more willpower than cutting herself had used to do.

Holding onto the bed with one hand, she started undoing the buttons of her uniform with the other. It was difficult staying focused, but just about manageable. It had to be flu she was suffering from. It had to be. And if it wasn't, if Doris's ludicrous suggestion that she was dying was possibly true, then it was a good thing that she had written a do-it-yourself Will a couple of weeks ago to ensure that Sean didn't fall into the hands of the social care services. Well, it was only sensible. Things did happen to happen to her all the time. They always had.

Doris still hadn't got back with the phone. No matter. She would prefer to weigh herself on her own anyway. She didn't want Doris doing it. She'd tell her the result herself. She staggered over to the machine and stepped onto it. Thirty eight and a half kilos. Well under six stone. Well under. She had made it! She was finally there – here! – where she belonged. She felt a triumphant surge of achievement coursing through her, reinvigorating her, giving her the strength to deal with all the interfering Dorises the world might throw at her.

Then she realised that this was far lower than Doris or any psychiatrist would find safe enough to agree to her discharge without first asking for an ECG or whatever. In fact they would probably say she was more at risk from the flu and from infections generally just because her weight was so low, that she therefore ought to be admitted onto a medical ward for observation, until her temperature had stabilised.

Right, okay then. What could she do to get around that? Of course! She would need to fix the machine so that it would show her to be heavier than she was. That would do it.

She stepped off the scales without fainting and studied it carefully as she waited for her heart to stop racing under the strain. It was a horrible, modern digital thing. The more she looked at it, the more she could see no way of altering it to show the wrong weight. So much for plan A. Plan B was she would just have to bluff her way past Doris by exploiting her trust, conning her into believing she had completely changed her tune.

She could hear her footsteps approaching the door.

'Hi Doris! I'm so sorry about the fuss I made a few minutes ago. But I'm up! And I really am feeling fine now. You have made me change my mind. Because the more I think about it the more I think you're right.' Fishing out the most grateful smile she could find from her ancient handbag of lies, she said,

'I will see the psychiatrist of course I will.'

'Oh my goodness, Grainne, I've never seen a grown woman as thin as you, in all my years! You're just skin and bone. I'm so glad you are being sensible. So glad.'

She stood with the phone in her hands, her eyes nearly popping out, her mouth wide open, staring at Grainne who was perched back on the weighing machine again. It was time to be disingenuous.

'I've been worse you know, Doris. And you must be fibbing! With all your experience I am quite sure you have seen people thinner than me.'

'Not many, I can tell you. What is your weight?'

She made to come over and look at the reading but Grainne said,

'Could you plug the phone in for me Doris, I am feeling a lot better, but I don't think I want to risk the blood rushing to my head again by bending down.'

'Yes, yes of course.'

Doris went to the back of the bed where there was a socket for the phone line. As she plugged it in Grainne stepped off the scales.

'I'm ninety eight pounds dead on. Forty nine kilos. It is a bit low, I know. You were quite right. But I am going to make a concerted effort to get myself back over fifty again for the sake of my child.'

Over her dead body she would.

'I am so glad you are finally seeing sense, honey.'

Grainne sat down on the edge of the bed again and reached for her uniform.

'Yes I must have been overdoing my diet. Silly me. And it's stress-related, of course. My little boy is learning-disabled, handicapped if you must know.'

God preserve her from hell and damnation for using Sean as an excuse like this.

But it was doing the trick. Doris was easily being lulled back into trusting her. She quickly lifted the uniform up over her head and struggled back into it before Doris could ask her to step onto the scales again. In her rush she could feel the faintness returning. Fuck off, fuck off, fuck off, she said to it silently, doing up her buttons again. The sensation receded.

Doris picked up the clipboard with her notes on it.

'Yes, well the little darling needs you all the more then! To keep yourself fit and well. It is your duty. What did you say you were? Forty nine kilos. Oh Grainne it is so little for a woman your height. So-o little. A bird weighs more than that.'

She wrote it down on the assessment sheet.

Grainne felt elated. Perhaps it was turning out to be good day after all. She would get away with it.

She rang Carol and with her voice full of apology she explained there had been an emergency so she would be up to an hour and a half late. Miraculously Sean had fallen asleep two hours ago, Carol told her, and still hadn't woken up! Relieved, Grainne said she would see her later.

But she didn't. She collapsed at the bus stop and was returned unconscious to A and E by ambulance. Doris and Barry conferred with the psychiatrist who had seen her earlier and who now said he would have no compunction about telling her if and when she returned to consciousness that his professional opinion was she was suffering from complications connected with a clear diagnosis of anorexia nervosa. Whereas earlier he had to tell her that if she left the hospital it would be formally recorded as being against medical advice, now he was arranging for her to be admitted to a bed, re-hydrated and drip-fed with a view to transferring her to a specialist eating disorders unit once she had regained consciousness. If necessary, he said, he was quite prepared to do all this against her will, under a section of the mental health act. He was confident an approved social worker and another psychiatrist would share his opinion about her.

With a warm friendly smile Doris nodded her head in sage agreement.

PART TWO

Then there was this

(Ten Years Later)

Chapter 10.

'Mishis– I mean, Missis. That's Mrs Roje McElvey.'

'Address?'

She didn't have one anymore but she gave him her old one, as usual. If she had bothered to keep any proof on her, it would have shown she was still the legal owner of the property.

'Age?'

'Fifty. No, that's wrong. I know! Fifty three. No! Fifty four.'

'Your date of birth?'

She rattled it off. As he laboured over typing it into his machine she looked at the buttons of his uniform and remembered with some sympathy what it was like to feel self-important, to belong, to be ruled by sets of institutional rituals.

Poor little policeman.

'Occupation? No. I don't think we need bother with that. It's quite obvious you haven't got–

'Conshultant! Conshultant Family Therapist.'

'Okay, okay. Conshultant Family Therapist.'

The plump, greasy-haired arresting officer with Groucho Marx eyebrows invited her to laugh with him at his mimicry. He typed in her words with the plodding pedantry of the one-fingered, removed the paper from his printer with a facetious flourish and asked her to take a look at it. His tie was askew and he smelt of cheap aftershave and sweat. Of someone who goes through the motions.

Well, she would forgive him. Who was she to judge her fellow human beings about such matters? And it *was* a very hot night. Nobody she knew nowadays even pretended to take care of their personal hygiene. Not on the streets. And not that she actually did know anybody anyway, not in the old, non-biblical sense of the word. Young people would sometimes cling on to some semblage of style in their appearance, but they were often high on crack or heroin at the time and could briefly believe that such trifles still mattered. The more outlandish they tried to look, the more she found herself smiling at how sweetly trammelled by convention they still were. Once their drugs had worn off they reverted to being interested only in scoring again, of course, nothing else. Much as she disliked doing it, she didn't feel too bad about killing them under the circumstances. They were, in a sense, already dead, which somehow meant murdering them didn't matter so much. And if it helped prevent others from resorting to sleeping rough and treading the same sordid little mills, then, in her case anyway, the end had justified the means.

'This isn't the first charge sheet you've ever been issued, so you don't need me to tell you that it says you have been arrested for being drunk and disorderly. You are required to appear at West London Magistrates court in three days time – that's Monday morning, Rose – at 10.00 am. Again. Will you remember that?'

She glared at him. What an imbecile! He was treating her like she was an old woman, or someone with Alzheimers. It was insufferable the lack of courtesy and respect one got from officialdom nowadays.

'Will you remember that, Rose?'

'How dare you call me by my Christian name?' she growled, considering whether to scream obscenities at him.

No, not now. It wouldn't be wise at all.

She took the piece of paper, made a pretence of carefully scanning it line by line and then held out an imperious hand for a pen. She signed it with a flourish of her own, and passed it back to him with her eyes on the exit. She wouldn't gratify this lackey by even glancing at him again. She was going to get away with it. Again. And even if he did mistake her triumphant grin for a drunken smile, she still didn't want him to see it.

'If we come across you once more tonight you will be locked in a cell till then.'

'Thank you, officer,' she said with all the dignity she could muster, holding out both hands just as she had a few hours ago so that they could handcuff her. She wanted her plastic bags back. In them were her blanket and various odds and ends picked up off the streets, together with her most precious possession of all, wrapped like the prize in a Pass-the-Parcel game in page after page of newspaper tied up with string. Her picture of Lukey in its plain wooden frame. He used to like Pass-the-Parcel. At parties he would get so excited he'd lose his breath sometimes and become unable to play anymore, but she always used to make sure he got a consolation prize anyway. And all the other children too.

The policeman looked at her blankly.

'My posseshuns, Cunschtubl, if you please.' She was careful not to slur the s in 'please'. She had her pride.

'Of course, madam.'

She was not too drunk to know when someone was taking the piss out of her, but she couldn't be bothered now to raise the small matter of his insolence. Not when she hadn't yet been given her things back, and when she seemed to have just got away with murder for a second time. Anyway the problem was not that she was too drunk, it was that she wasn't drunk enough. She was feeling shaky, a little unsteady on her feet if the truth be told. Tell-tale tremors in her arms and hands and wobbliness in the soles of her feet had to be ignored. She actually needed a drink to get her bearings back. She was always better after topping up her alcohol levels. It made her feel more sober.

'Sign for them, just there please, and then you can be on your way.' He pushed another sheet of paper towards her.

'I want to see them first, check everything is still there. One cannot, indeed should not, make the mistake of trusting the integrity of the modern law enforcement officer, you know. Not nowadays, I'm afraid.'

He clearly didn't have a clue what she was on about and wouldn't have given a callous fuck if he had, thought Rose angrily, as she watched him lift the bags on to the table beside her and invite her to be his guest. She dove straight into the black bin liner and satisfied herself her picture frame and its studio photograph of Lukey was still there.

'You think I'm like one of these things, don't you?' she said, nodding at her bags.

'I'll have to ask you to examine them over there on that bench, madam please, so that I can attend to the next, um, customer.' He had no more time for her. She'd been processed.

She stared right through him and saw that his soul was now no bigger than the buttons of his jacket, poor thing.

'I am free to go now? You are dismissing me?'

'That's right.'

She manoeuvred the bin liner carefully over her left shoulder. Light as it was, it was still heavier than her carrier bags. She had inherited her father's arthritis, there was no doubt about that now, and she preferred to carry her heaviest things on the left side of her body to counterbalance the pain running down her right hip to her knee. Then she picked up the plastic shopping bags and trundled, limping slowly towards the protective glass-door exit. A young man coming in up the steps didn't bother to hold the door open for her as he swept in and past her like she wasn't there. She felt like shouting at him, telling him how much she was doing and how much she had always done for the likes of him. For those who had slid further down life's spiral. But there was no point. Just as the policeman had, she knew, he would have no more thought of her than of the old bags she was carrying. So she just stood there, waiting for a worried looking middle-aged black man with a teenager in tow, to come up the steps and push the door open. The man was too preoccupied to notice her, but the boy did and he held the door open for her. She thanked him with a grand little nod of her head, feeling like the queen, and then waddled outside into the heat of the street.

It was early evening in high summer. She had to find somewhere to settle for the night before all the pitches were taken. She fancied a park to celebrate escaping from the jowly jaws of the law just now. Rain was coming on. She could smell it in the air, hot and cloudless though it was at the moment. There would certainly be a downpour before dawn. You could hardly ever stay in a park overnight anyway because the parks police did regular sweeps every few hours. And tonight she just didn't feel her hip could take being moved on again. Not after she had settled herself down. She tended to stiffen up after a few hours of rest nowadays and sometimes took just as long again to recover her ability to move freely once more, or as freely as she was capable. She had had to do a lot of standing up in the police station which had left her feeling sore. The best thing would be to just keep on walking now until she found a likely place to lay herself down. Anyway it was probably safer to get as far away as possible from this area after what she had done last night.

She was on a mission to save the children on the streets from themselves and from their exploiters. If her quest to try and kill one whenever the opportunity arose was to have any chance of success, then it was probably better to always move on, so that when or if the killings ever did get the publicity she wanted them to have, she could continue her work somewhere else and thus also continue to bring publicity to their plight. Ultimately she considered herself to be an Angel of Mercy. The greater good of the many was her only concern, and if that meant that the suffering of a few had to be final, then unfortunately and regrettably that was just how it had to be.

It wasn't as if she wanted to kill them. Not at all. She had no choice. It had to be done for the sake of the children. Not individually of course. God forgive her, No! She hated murdering each dear one of them. But for all of them collectively. So that eventually the government would have to act to protect them. Not just take 'rough sleeper' initiatives for the media before Christmas each year, targeting grown-ups like herself. It was kids who needed to be rescued from the horrors of the street, not middle-aged or elderly drunks. Her plan was simple and it kept her going, kept on giving her a reason to live another day: If by killing a runaway child she could draw attention to their terrible plight then eventually, she hoped, something would be done.

Some of the things she had seen had been dreadful. Utterly dreadful. Children as young as fifteen or sixteen, at least that was what they always said – many of them looked much younger, sleeping on the streets like her and using prostitution to buy drugs to keep themselves going; riddled with disease, malnutrition and all the other effects of destitution, and treated by the adult world, other dossers and the rest of society alike, as if they should be blamed for their situation and given no credence as human beings whatsoever. Charles Dickens would have understood her concern. He wouldn't have approved of her solution of course, but he'd have understood. She used to enjoy Dickens before she decided to live on the streets.

And it had been a decision. At first she had just found herself deriving simple enjoyment out of getting out of the house and wandering around for hours on end locally. Then she had noticed that she began not to care where she went or how long it took for her to get home again, as long as wherever she wandered was somewhere new. London was a big city, but after a year or more of this she began to care very much indeed

154

not to wander anywhere she had ever been before. It became an obsessional need. She had known all along that it might, of course, but somehow it hadn't worried her because it was the obverse of how she had felt indoors at home. And it took her further and further afield as time went by. Away from the predictable prescribed patterns she had made herself conform to at home after Lucille had left some eight or nine years ago, away from the loneliness too. It had been a curious thing at the time, if it wasn't now, that she had very quickly felt so much more of a sense of belonging when she was out freely tramping the streets and going where she chose, than when she was alone at home, trapped in and dominated by her Book of Rules.

At home she used to think of her obsessional patterns of behaviour as The Boundless Book of Rules. It had been boundless because there had always been something else she could do to tie herself further in to a life of ritual and repetition. Every day after Lucille left she had been able to discover something else she could be doing in order to stave off loneliness and thoughts of suicide. It didn't matter how small or trivial it was, she was always able to weave a pattern of behaviour into and all around it so that she was caught up in yet another rule. From what time the post dropped in through the letter box onto her doormat in the mornings, through where precisely it landed on the mat and what direction the envelopes were splayed, she used to generate a whole range of different rituals each of which in turn circumscribed precise knock-on effects for the rest of her day. And that was assuming she had been able to get out of bed in the first place and wash and dress herself. She used to allow herself to do each of those things if and only if the consequences of each action had been consciously embraced beforehand by the successful achievement of a previous task. She could not get up in the mornings unless she had had precisely five hours of uninterrupted sleep. If there had been any interruption, then whether she got up within ten or twenty minutes of waking depended upon which side she had been facing when she woke up, whether or not she had got up in the night for a wee, things like that. The details were a long forgotten haze. All she was left with was the sense that her own home had come to feel like the last place she could in fact feel at home in. Even breathing had had to have a rhythm. She remembered that only too well: two deeps breaths followed by three short ones and then two deeps ones again. Being at home had been like being in hell.

The streets of London in contrast had become more and more welcoming to her, as long as they took her further away from her semi-detached house in Balham. In fact she had become so desperate to get away from where she lived that she used to find herself getting bad-tempered if she recognised where she was while 'out on a wander', as she used to think of it at first. Booze had helped. Instead of merely being irritated, slightly annoyed if she found herself in a street she had walked along before, the fuel of alcohol would cause her to fly into an almighty rage about it. She would also rant if someone ever had the temerity to bother her in any way. She remembered the day long ago when she had finally decided to make a permanent home of the streets. Obviously choosing to ignore her grime and stink and the half-bottle of cheap gin in her right hand, a woman of her own age, wearing expensive clothes and too much powder, had stopped her to ask the way to Nightingale Lane. Rose had had trouble making out what she was on about, past the distractingly alcoholic exoticism of the fragrance the woman was wearing. Then when she did realise what she was asking her she had wanted to say 'how should I fucking know?' Instead she had looked round carefully, riled to realise she did fucking know. With what she knew to be the ponderousness of the alcoholic she had begun to explain the way, but found herself getting tied up in knots because the woman wasn't concentrating properly on what she was saying. Rose's patience had run out and exasperation rushed in. She'd started shouting at her, and the woman backed away and then walked off hurriedly towards Tooting. Rose yelled and yelled at her as she kept on going the wrong way. All to no avail. Then she noticed for the first time that people were crossing the road to avoid her. So she started shouting at them too; that she wasn't going to do them any harm and how could they be afraid of a woman like her, weak, powerless, her sense of purpose and personal direction completely gone. She could have cried, or screamed. So she screamed, and it seemed to wash people clean away; unless they were stupid like the arrogant-looking young man coming towards her after the woman had scurried off. It took a lot of yelling to wash herself clean of him. Too preoccupied with his phone call to notice her, he didn't deviate from his path, just grinned powerfully to whoever he was talking to and kept on coming straight towards her. She couldn't believe it. She couldn't stand it either. She stared at him as if he was mad. Then she screamed again as ear-splittingly as she could and for as long as she was able. It worked. He pulled up short, his face registering the shock that it really was him her rage was directed at, then quickly crossed the street. She felt so safe and so at home after that, that she had some estate agents rent her house out exclusively to Israeli holiday-makers on a permanent basis, made a standing order out for aid to Palestinian children from the proceeds, and formally set up permanent home on the streets. If she wanted them to, everybody, but everybody crossed the road to avoid her.

From then on she used her scream all the time. It was as loud as the squealing brakes on the tube trains she sometimes managed to slip down onto in order to take herself somewhere new. She let it have complete control of her when she used it. And she used it often. It came in so useful in so many situations. At night, particularly in winter, street

156

people jockeyed for possession of shop fronts and porches with covered doorways where heating and ventilation outlets blew warmer air towards them. Pitches were jealously guarded. Rose found if she just stood where she wanted to settle and screamed at whoever was already there, they would moan and groan and tell her to fuck off, but eventually they'd move, finding that even in the vagrant life having a nutter screaming at you for hours was just not conducive to a good night's sleep. She'd been in lots of scrapes, but had been seriously assaulted only twice in eight years. On the first occasion she had simply carried on screaming at the drunken male dossers who were trying to punch her and kick her for the bottle of Bushmills they had seen her secreting into the cavernous pocket of her tattered old skirt, till eventually they left her alone with her bruises and without the whisky; and on the second she was punched so hard she was knocked unconscious and knew no more. When she came to, she had found her skirts up around her thighs and the contents of her bags strewn around her. But nothing had been taken because she hadn't had any kind of alcohol or money in them and nothing of value worth stealing. And as to her person if she was a bit sore she didn't care because she hadn't known about it while it was going on. Out of sight and out of mind meant it simply hadn't happened, as long as she could find another drink.

Now she was the one who assaulted people.

It was difficult, very difficult because to kill them she had to get close to them and when you got close to a person, especially a young person who called up all the pity in your maternal heart, it was terribly, terribly difficult to do away with them.

Two nights ago had been particularly hard. By preference she would always want to kill boys and young men but they were the last people to let themselves be befriended by an old woman who smelt of booze and dirt and sweat. The boy she had killed a couple of weeks ago had been easy only because she had watched him fall into a stupor smoking crack on his own. After checking that the coast was clear it had been a simple matter to wander over to his unconscious form and bring a brick crashing down on to his head. She had been careful to keep hold of it with both hands, having a vague memory of another brick going flying and hurting her some years ago when she had locked herself out of her house. So she held onto it and hit him over and over again till she was absolutely satisfied he must be dead. Sixteen or seventeen years old at most he was, with his downy beard and his soft womanish hands. She had hated doing it, even felt like weeping afterwards when she took the brick down to the canal and disposed of it in the dark water. But it had all been so curiously easy. The boy hadn't groaned or stirred in any way before she had been sure he was dead, and she hadn't, thank goodness, had to sit down beside him, get to know him and befriend him.

Not like with that poor young girl last night.

She had wondered whether their deaths would make it into the newspapers or TV. That was her hope and intention. There was no point otherwise. No point at all.

'Excuse me, Miss,' the girl had said, sitting down on a bench beside her in Eelbrook Common as she watched the sun going down behind the railway line beyond the houses across the park. She spoke as if Rose was some kind of school teacher or something. Her manner had immediately irritated Rose, who then realised she should be grateful because at least the girl was presenting her with another opportunity to draw public attention to the plight of homeless children. So instead of barking at her, Rose forced a smile as the girl asked her if she knew of anywhere where she might find a bed for a night. She seemed very young indeed, and although her face was grimy and her clothes looked unwashed, Rose didn't get the feeling she had been on the streets for very long. She looked a bit like Lucille had the first time they met, dark haired and pale with nervous staring eyes. And so, so young.

'There's nowhere around here, dear, so far as I know, and I have been living on the streets for some years now so I *do* know actually. You'd be best off sticking here with me for the night. Till we get moved on. But the nights are short at the moment so we may be able to stay here till dawn. You never know. Where are you from, dear, and why aren't you at home with your mother? She must be worried to death about you.'

She hoped she wasn't overdoing the 'dears'. She was using them to put the girl at her ease. She couldn't recall having ever called anyone 'dear' very much before, although it was always possible, because she couldn't actually recall anything very much anymore. Referring to the girl's mother was also deliberately intended to make the atmosphere between them more homely. She wanted her to relax, let go of her wariness.

'She isn't. She's living with a dick,' the girl replied, her angry choice of language jarring with the innocence of how she looked. 'A dick,' she said again, 'who hits her and who is always trying to get his hands on me as well, but my mum don't really mind. So I couldn't stay. She thinks I'm with friends.'

'How old are you, dear?'

'I was fifteen the beginning of last week. Monday.' She said it with pride so it might be true.

'When did you leave?'

'This week, Monday. I've never liked Mondays.'

'When was that, dear? I'm a bit out of touch with dates and things, living on the streets. You get that way, you know.'

It was important to be a bit doddery but, well, nice. That way she wouldn't feel threatening.

'Two days ago. Today is Wednesday.'

The girl was now sounding just a little bit superior. That was good too.

'Have you eaten at all?'

Nurture questions always made people feel cared for, no matter what their age.

'Not yet. I was told by someone I should go to a place called Centrepoint. Do you know where that is?'

'It will take you an hour or two at most to walk there from here. But they'll sign you in, I think, and they will want to contact your family or social services because of your age.'

Rose shook her head, frowned her concern. She wasn't sure whether this was actually true or not, but the girl had to stay with her if she was to become her Angel of Mercy, and safely dispatch her to a better place.

'Oh, no! I can't go back. I just can't. I would rather die, to be honest. I tried to convince Mum she should come too, but she wouldn't listen to me, told me not to be silly, said all men are like that, said, deal with it, like she always does about everything.'

'Have you no relatives you could stay with, dear?' Rose asked in gentle voice, continuing to lull her. She would honestly rather die, the poor, poor little darling! But how perfectly wonderful.

'Mum has got a brother up in Halifax. Up north, you know? But I have only met him once in all my life. That was when we went to my Nan's funeral. I haven't got a dad and my mum never had one neither. It runs in the family – no dads!'

The girl laughed and her laugh turned into a hacking, almost whooping cough which lasted several minutes. Rose didn't like it. It was a horrible intrusive interruption to the proceedings. It reminded her of her past too much. She could never bear the sound of anybody coughing. Eventually, just when she thought the girl would never stop, her coughing ceased.

'I think you had better stay with me for the night, my dear. I may be a bit of a grizzled old thing, but I know how to look after myself and I can keep you safe from men. I'm sure you have noticed most people who sleep rough are males.'

'I know that,' The girl said importantly. She shuddered, adding, 'But actually I haven't seen any men. I've been sensible, sleeping in people's front gardens the last two nights. Ones where they've let their hedge grow and there are lots of bushes. But I can't believe how many foxes and cats are out at night! It's a good thing I like animals. And at least it's not been cold. Think positive, that's what I say.'

Rose couldn't agree more.

'That's right,' she said. 'warm summer nights are a wonderful thing.'

Should she offer her a swig from her bottle of Jamesons? Probably not. Doing so might make her a bit wary, even if the effect did relax her, loosen her up. She was so new to life on the streets, poor thing. Not like one of the usual homeless teenagers at all. Not yet anyway. Not someone who'd take anything to get away from how they were feeling. Just as she herself would.

'What's your name dear? Don't tell me if you don't want to. It's just friendlier that's all. Mine's Rose.'

'I'm Fran. Francesca, my mother calls me, whenever she's being serious. So she always calls me Francesca actually. I prefer Fran myself.'

'How do you do, Fran?' Rose held out a grimy hand with a gentle, friendly smile. 'Where are you from?'

'Not far really. New Malden, but it's taken me all this time just to get here. We're in Fulham here, aren't we? Yes? Yes I thought so. It's taken me all this time just to get here because I haven't really known where I was going, just that I couldn't stay at home. So I wandered round streets I knew for the first few days. I wanted to stay with friends in the evenings. But I don't have that many friends, to be honest. I used to, but not now. It's terrible how people can be so bitchy. My mum's been right about that. I wanted to stay at Hannah's. She's my best friend, but her mum and dad hit her and I didn't want to get her into no trouble.'

'That was nice of you, dear. Never mind. Things change. I have often found that they do, anyway. Eventually. Just after I've given up, usually!'

They both laughed, sitting in what Rose felt was certainly a companionable silence with the roar of the New Kings road traffic rumbling behind them. They were facing the last of the sun as it finally disappeared in the west. Stars immediately began coming out. Rose pointed them out to Fran. Just a harmless old lady who could recognise the scything shape of The Plough.

'Isn't it wonderful? We don't usually see so many stars in London. It must be a special night tonight. You know what I think? I think there is a star up there for every single one of us. There's one up there for you, you know. I'm sure of it.'

The girl nodded in emphatic agreement with her. The old ones were always best when it came to uttering clichés.

'Why are you a bag lady, Rose? What happened to you?'

Before she could reply, Fran started coughing again. It would undoubtedly be an act of mercy for her to stop having to cough like that. Just as it had been for Lukey.

Rose felt herself shaking, going into a cold sweat as if she hadn't had a drink for twenty four hours or more and was beginning to suffer Delirium Tremens. Lukey. She hadn't thought about him in years. Felt him, yes. And felt his absence, always. But thought of him she had not. Not since she had left home and started walking the streets. Not once.

Now this little waif was bringing back all those old terrible feelings in a flood of love and helplessness. Every cough reminded her of him, and the girl just didn't seem to be able to stop. Instinctively she put a hand onto her bony little back and patted it to help dislodge the mucus and phlegm, just as she had used to do so long ago with Luke. And Fran only seemed to cough and splutter more painfully and uselessly, just as Luke had used to do. Without thinking Rose pulled her bottle of whisky out of the plastic bag which also had her serrated kitchen knife in it. Much as she'd counted on her scream over the last few years, she liked having the knife with her as well. Just in case. It was her bottle, and only hers, and no drunken fucking dosser was ever going to be able to take it from her without a serious fight.

The girl was coughing into her cupped hands and though her sight wasn't what it was, Rose thought she did notice little flecked globules of bright red on her palms as she reached for the bottle. Rose uncapped it for her and she tried to take a swig, but the paroxysms of coughing made it impossible.

I'll let her share the bottle and wait for her to fall into an intoxicated sleep like the one the boy a couple of weeks ago was in, thought Rose. She'll be so relieved to be out of all this, the poor little thing. Her body will be found and it will hit the headlines and there will be such a public outcry that innocents like her can suffer such short little lives and die such terrible pointless deaths. And then something will be done. She will have died so that others may live.

Rose knew it was mad. She didn't mind. It was what she *felt* was right and that was that. This wasn't about sanity or reason. It was about knowing what was right and doing what had to be done to make the world a better place. No amount of social work or government policy had ever done anything for these kids. The media and the public always responded with wholesome repugnance and righteous indignation to children being murdered. But that was all. They didn't make people think or put their money where their mouths were. Her killings wouldn't just trigger outrage. They would bring about systemic change, because they would go on and on until she was caught. Headlines would scream 'Something Must be Done' because the children should not have to suffer. And then finally, something might actually be done. Nevertheless, she thought, they ought to bring back capital punishment, if only for me.

Fran's coughing eventually subsided and she accepted a swig from the bottle. It immediately set her off again. Rose found herself patting her back once more and then massaging it in slow large circular motions, just like she had used to do with Luke. This time it seemed to work. Fran coughed a few more times and then stopped. She smiled at Rose happily.

'Thank you. My mum never done that for me. Don't get me wrong! I love her, but she never offered me a massage and a drink. But I don't think I will have anymore of that stuff just at the moment, thank you, if you don't mind.'

'Oh I really think you should, you know. Look how quickly you stopped coughing just then.'

'Ye-es, but it was the drink that set me off again. What is it?'

'It is Irish whisky. Very mild. It will keep your insides nice and warm as the night gets cooler. And you get colder.' She was actually encouraging the girl to take up alcohol. She couldn't believe the depths to which she had sunk.

Dubiously as if she was only doing it to oblige, the girl screwed up her nose like a much younger child and took another small swig. She made a face and shook her head.

'Thanks Rose. Really. I've never drunk alcohol before. Maybe I'll have some more later if I get cold and if that's okay. I don't think I will, though. It's so warm.'

'Of course it's alright, Fran. I'm just glad to be of help. I used to be quite an expert in physiotherapy and massage. Long ago, in another life.'

'Tell me! Please. Why is an old lady like you out here? Why don't you live at home?'

'I just found I was happier out here. Less troubled by painful memories. More rewarded by the experiences the present was giving me. That's all.'

Telling the truth, even in headlines, gave her more conviction, made up for the mistake of having offered the girl her whisky.

'What memories?'

'Well that's the thing you see, my dear. I've lived on the streets in order to forget them. And actually I *have* forgotten them, mostly. So I can't really tell you. Honestly I can't. But, like you, I think I had things I had to get away from. I can remember that, at least.'

If Fran could identify with her she would relax even more, become less and less wary.

'What was it like being a physiotherapist? I'd like a job like that one day,' Fran asked.

'Well, if you lean forward a little I will do the back of your neck and your shoulders and then you will know directly, and it will tell you so much more than words ever could. Anyway, as I say, I haven't really allowed myself to recall very much of my past life. I like to live in the present.'

It was time to get on with it. Any more of this and she would find herself getting too personally close to the girl to be able to do what had to be done for the sake of all the street children living in squalor and despair in all the major cities.

Fran leaned forward trustingly. Rose flexed her fingers as much as she was able and putting her thumbs on the back of the girl's neck she massaged her small bony shoulders with her fingers. The last dog owner had just left, walking away through the rapidly descending darkness

162

towards Parsons Green. There was also a woman over to their right about a hundred and fifty metres distant, but she also was walking away from them, in the opposite direction, towards Harwood road. The park was otherwise now completely empty and she could hear no punters spilling into or out of the pub behind her across the road. Conditions were perfect. The only drawback was that she was unfortunately going to have to be messy. There was no way she had the strength to struggle with this waif, tiny though she was, so strangulation was out of the question.

Rose put a little more pressure on the girl's left shoulder, which reflexively caused her to lower it, lift her right shoulder and look away from Rose into the murk. It was time. Rose reached with her right hand for her trusty kitchen knife in the bag lying on the bench beside her. Just grasping the handle always made her feel safe. She gritted her teeth.

It was all over and done with one quick slice across her carotid.

Rose had pushed her away even as she did it, so that the blood would pump over the graffiti on the back and side walls of the shelter. She immediately got up off the bench, wiped the serrated blade on the grass, her temples throbbing with anxiety, anguish and guilt, telling herself over and over again that it was all in a good cause. It was. It was. Then she whisked up her things and left without a backward glance. By the time she got as far as the World's End she had finished her bottle of whisky. Her feelings of guilt and fear had joined all the others she kept in a permanently open if long forgotten drawer, filed under confusion and shame. But it was curious how no sirens wailed.

She had to punish herself now. For the last forty eight hours or so she had been walking around the well-heeled streets of Chelsea in a haze of recrimination and doubt. It was all very well doing what she did for the greater good, but killing that girl had also felt as if it had killed what little she had left of her own soul. The boy a couple of weeks ago had been so much easier because she hadn't spoken to him. But these last two days had been like being in hell. She had taken the life of some poor mother's child. There could be nothing worse. She deserved the ultimate penalty. And yet she had just walked out of the police station scot-free. As if she was just another harmless, itinerant old woman. Capital punishment was what she deserved and she would be her own executioner in due course of time. She most certainly would. In the meantime she had to do something to punish herself now, as an initial down-payment for her terrible crimes.

How in heaven's name did she ever allow things to come to this? How could she possibly be the same person who had once tried so genuinely and for so long to be as kind and as caring as she could? Or even the same person who had once tried to kill her*self*? How could she be?

But there it was. She was.

What would the Boundless Book of Rules prescribe now? Just what she'd got, probably: protracted spirals of spurious homelessness, around and round the streets of London as a dosser. She had always told herself that eventually she would go back home and return to a normal life. It somehow kept her going to tell herself that, kept her from ever actually returning, knowing that one day she finally would. For nearly eight years now.

Not anymore. Not after this. She could never go home now.

Something had to be done in the meantime though, as some kind of personal atonement. She ruminated on what it might be as she made her way with painful slowness along Lots road and over Battersea Bridge. Although it was dark and the close stillness in the air made it feel even more likely that rain would be falling heavily before the night was out, she felt she didn't want to be under any covers tonight. Pausing to give her hip a rest she leaned against the side of the bridge and looked down at the Thames below sliding quietly out to sea. She could spend the night on the stones down there, she thought. She would like that. The discomfort would be meet and fitting. The tide was going out. She could be up and on her way before it was fully back in again. If she could already hear the sky grumbling with the occasional crackle of thunder far away to the west, it didn't matter. She had been out here winter and summer for all these years, no matter what the weather, without ever suffering any ill effects. She couldn't remember when she had last had a cough or a cold.

Life was completely incomprehensible.

Half an hour later she'd successfully negotiated her way down to the slippery stinking stones of the river bed below. And she knew what she would do now. She would destroy her most precious possession. That would be the most fitting punishment of all.

A lot of the stones were actually quite dry. She found a nice big one to sit on, plonking herself down beneath the walls of Battersea Park with the leaves of a solitary willow tree rustling gently above her. If it did rain they would afford her some protection. She leaned back against the smelly, slimy wall, placing her bags carefully beside her. It was such a hot night. The sound of distant thunder was muted, curiously quiet as lightning flickered across the night sky just a few miles away. Over Ealing and Southall, she thought. The tide was still going out and the river was down to a trickle, but she was up here rather than down there by the water because she didn't want to have to leave till the last possible moment. She hoped it wouldn't be before dawn. She didn't want a painful ungainly scramble to get away from the rising tide whilst it was still dark, especially not if the rocks and stones were already wet with rain. Apart from that, her sight wasn't what it was and her hip would be very stiff and very sorry for itself after sitting here for hours.

It was so still and so close right now, although clouds did not yet seem to be building up, so perhaps she was wrong about rain coming. Then again, what did she know?

Only what she felt. And what she felt was that she should be punished.

She felt she had to put an end to the last connection she had with her previous life. It was the only way she could live with herself as the Angel of Mercy and Death. The Boundless Book of Rules would certainly sanction what she was going to do.

She let herself doze for a couple of hours. A rat nosing its way into a carrier bag woke her up. She looked up at the sky above. It was now full of leaden cloud, reflecting the orange glow of the city back down again. Lightning flickered in trails directly above her. But it didn't thunder. It merely crackled and occasionally rumbled, was otherwise almost silent.

The Thames had begun to refill while she slept. Even though it was still some ten or fifteen metres away, she heard it gurgling as the tide came in. She got herself up off her aching bottom and stood there staring at it, rubbing her back and side, trying to encourage the blood to start circulating again. Then she started hobbling about looking for dry twigs, anything that would burn. After fifteen minutes she had gathered a little handful, sufficient for her purpose. She went down to the dark water's edge and from amongst the flotsam and detritus bobbing along the now rapidly rising river, she fished out a small plank of wood no longer than her arm, and a few minutes later, a frayed and flappy length of begrimed orange tape, the kind of thing found around road works or building sites. She walked with it back up to her carrier bags and sat herself back on her stone. The river was swollen by this time, big and black and monstrous and now only five metres away from her. She took a swig from her bottle and delved into her black plastic bag. She took out seven or eight pages of newspaper and scrunched them up.

She had to hurry. Big droplets of rain were starting to fall, hot wind beginning to gust. If she didn't act quickly it would be too late. For the moment she was alright here under her tree, but she really had to carry out her plan right now if it wasn't going to have to be aborted.

She placed the scrunched newspaper onto the plank and carefully jammed some of the twigs in amongst it. She wanted to get it right, but the rain was increasing with every minute. Hurriedly she put the rest of the twigs carefully on top of the newspaper and poured some of her whisky over it. Then she tenderly unwrapped her picture of Luke and removed the protective glass front from the frame. She threw it aside without a glance, heard it tinkle satisfyingly behind her.

The Thames wasn't so much creeping now as rushing in towards her. It was a metre away, no more. Big, black and heaving. If she didn't get on with it right now she might not be able to scramble up the old metal ladder built into the side of the wall ten metres away. Not that she minded terribly, but she had to stay alive in order to continue to do what had to be done. Laying Luke's picture on top of the newspapers and twigs, she bound it to the plank with the plastic tape so that it almost looked like a sacrificial mummy or a papoose; then she delved in one of her plastic bags, pulling out this and that and throwing it away, until she found the box of matches she knew she had had there all the time. She struck a match and lit her whisky-sozzled bundle with a panicky, irreverent haste. It took immediately with a sudden, shocking whoosh. At once the plastic tape melted and she saw Luke's perfect smiling little face begin to crinkle at the edges as flames started to consume it. Luke means light, he used to say proudly. She smiled at the memory and ignoring the pain, stood up quickly and took the flaming raft, for that was what it was meant to be, to the water.

Out from under the protection of her tree, the rain was now bucketing down. Hurrying as much as she was able, she went down on one knee, the genuflection sending waves of pain up and down her hip in huge rollers. Gritting her teeth, she launched the picture's pyre, wanting to watch it float away with all her memories – her very identity – gloriously aflame. But unfortunately, it immediately turned over in the churning water. The fire was snuffed out and her slightly singed photograph detached itself from the plank. It floated off, face down and out of reach, with all the rest of the debris being swept in by the incoming tide down towards Wandsworth and Putney.

Chapter 11.

At fifty four, Richard McElvey was a distinguished looking man. Tall, a little plump around the middle and the jowls, he had only slightly thinning, albeit completely grey hair and small elegant sideburns. He affected blue suits and striped shirts and a blundering self-effacing manner which most people found charming in such an evidently successful man, but which his wife continually found irritating because, she said, he always brought it home with him and they both knew it was a put-on. He was particularly proud of his nose which he thought of as aquiline, but which she referred to as his hook. He liked to think that though his looks were rakish, his ways were those of a gentleman.

His increasing irascibility with her wasn't very gentlemanly. He knew that. Nor was his intense jealousy or the friction it was bringing to his marriage. But at least he recognised this latter was probably due to the fact that he was more highly sexed than she was. An addict, his wife said. And that was the beginning and end of the problem as far as she was concerned. She could be such an uncompromising little bitch. If he wasn't such an addict, she said, he wouldn't be so irrationally jealous of what she might be up to with other men. That was why they were here. In their recent rows she had made it quite plain that she felt she played no part in causing their marriage to be dysfunctional at all, none whatsoever. It was just him. Her only concession was a pouted, grudging admission that it took two not to tango.

He looked at her across the waiting room sitting with her legs crossed reading a magazine. She too was wearing a blue suit as if she wanted to match him in some way. Hers was a pale turquoise colour with a skirt that stopped just above the knee and drew his attention to her thighs. He looked at her as she tapped an elegant pink suede heel, pretending to be absorbed by Harpers and Queen. He couldn't help feeling proud to be her husband, could always ignore the embarrassment of being old enough to be her father. She had an exquisite little Fuck-me-or-Fuck-off face with lovely high cheeks, big beautiful eyes and a perfect mouth. Gorgeous. The trouble was it was usually Fuck-off nowadays. She hardly ever wanted him to fuck her anymore, and old as he was, he was still as horny as a man half his age. She told him she still fancied him, insisted she wasn't having an affair, said she was just different from him and didn't feel like having sex all the time.

All the time? He was lucky if he got it once a month nowadays. But no matter how much he pressed her, she insisted there was nobody else. Every day he struggled with morbid jealousy to believe her, was always having to swallow his anxiety that she was lying to him again. That was another reason why he had agreed to come here. She told lies all the time, even when it wasn't the slightest bit necessary. She even lied to herself that she lied. So it was very difficult not to be jealous under the circumstances. Who wouldn't be? She could understand that, she'd said, but he still ought to trust her, otherwise how could *she* ever change? That she could still put him in such a bind attracted him to her almost as much as her looks. It annoyed the hell out of him as well.

They had been living together for nearly eight years, and married for five. She was his third wife. They had married and honeymooned in Toulouse, where her father and mother had met treading grapes more than thirty years before. She hadn't changed a great deal since the wedding. Her hair was a bit longer and she was a blonde now; her lips were a little fuller. Her occasional hydra-gel treatments had obviously added something to them, but so had all the pursed petulant disapproval she was forever expressing toward him. With her cute arse and perfect tits, she still had a figure he couldn't see naked without immediately desiring. He should have been pleased that she constantly required reassurance that she looked good, and that she always dressed to allure. As a man, he should have been content she was so attractive. He would have been – if it wasn't for the irony of her lack of interest in sex.

He had studied their wedding photograph on his desk at work before leaving the office to meet her here. In those days he had had a trimmer waist, a more definite jaw line and hair that had been so much darker. He looked boyishly confident, even triumphant, in the picture as if he had just won a Nobel prize, or something. And she looked happy, hanging on to his arm and staring up at him adoringly in the lacy two thousand pound wedding dress which cinched round her waist and clung to her tits in a way that had made him want to get her out of it and fuck her as soon as she tried it on in the shop. It was the dress of her dreams, she'd said at the time. They bought it off the peg in New Bond Street before leaving in a taxi for Heathrow.

Nowadays she never looked either happy or adoring.

Nevertheless, there had been compensations and distractions. He was a fairly rich man who could afford to buy fine wines for himself and designer clothes and exotic beauty treatments for his wife. He had consequently put on weight over the years and she had come to look more expensive. But their relationship had remained resolutely stuck. Any attempt at a deeper understanding of what they meant to each other or of how they affected one another, invariably resulted in failure, and an increased sense of separateness. Such attempts were therefore few.

'Dr and Mrs McElvey?'

'Yes,' they both chorused in reply to a tall thin middle-aged woman in flat sandals and a cream cheesecloth frock which looked like it had seen better days. She had a strong-boned face, lank brown hair shot with grey, and wore dark lipstick and gold half-moon reading spectacles attached to a red pince-nez. Richard thought he could recognise an aging ex-hippy when he saw one. Her nose was a bit red too. Was she a boozer? If he didn't find her very prepossessing at least she was his own age. It might make up for her natural female bias against him .

They followed her up the stairs to a consulting room with red and green flocked wall-paper and five small armchairs arranged in circular fashion in the middle. The chairs seemed to take up the whole room and he immediately felt a little claustrophobic, a little trapped. The woman invited them to sit anywhere they liked and for the sake of a bit of space he parked himself down with a chair between himself and each of the other two so that he could see them both.

The woman pushed her glasses up her nose and looked down at her notes, then she took them off again. With a rather tired, mechanical smile she exclaimed upon the stifling heat and introduced herself.

'I'm Sheila Jackson,' she proclaimed with the kind of posh nasal twang he both disliked yet felt at home with. 'I am a registered counsellor here. I understand you would like some Couple Counselling because you have been experiencing problems in your marriage recently. Perhaps it would help if you could start by summarising those problems for me, and if you don't mind I would like to take some notes. Then I want to take a brief history both of your marriage and of any relevant personal details from before the two of you met. Family background. Important life events. That kind of thing. After that we can discuss whether I might be able to help. I think that's probably all we'll be able to manage for one evening! Is that alright? Good! Who would like to start?'

He looked across at his wife and nodded. She shrugged, shaking her head not keen to go first. 'Actually, I'm afraid I really don't know where to begin,' she said, with a half-apologetic smile at the lady. 'Perhaps you had better start with my husband.'

Richard recognised this reserve was composed partly of modesty, partly of loyalty to him – angry as she was, she had never slagged him off in front of other people before – partly of shame, and partly of not wanting anything to change. For all her anger with him and his frustration with her, and despite the fact that she had been the one to suggest they seek help, there was a big part of her that wanted things to remain exactly as they were between them, he was sure of it.

'Start wherever you like,' said Sheila Walton. 'Most people find it helpful to begin with the things that currently concern them. Sometimes they come here having thought about those things and,' she smiled at them both over her half moons, 'how on earth they are going to say them on the way here. Perhaps you did something like that?'

Did the woman sound slightly tetchy? Richard wondered. Had she said these lines too many times before? Maybe she had had a long day and wanted to go home. She had big feet and long fingers which looked unwieldy and slightly bent, as if she suffered from some kind of arthritic complaint. That could make you feel a bit irritable.

'Well perhaps I should start then, love,' he said in a helpful, friendly tone of voice. 'It will give you a bit of time to gather your thoughts while I gabble.'

Neither of them offered him a grateful smile for this self-deprecating offer and feeling slightly annoyed, he decided he wasn't going to beat around the bush. They hadn't come here to fuck about umm-ing and ah-ing. If he was anything, he was a man who knew how to get straight to the point.

'We're not having enough sex. It's as simple as that as far as I am concerned. I would have no problems with her, none whatsoever, if we just consummated our marriage more often. And I am therefore afraid she might be having it off with someone else, although she denies it.'

He glanced across at his wife who suddenly stood up without looking at him so that for a moment he thought she was going to leave. But with her perfectly mascara'd eyes modestly downcast, she said the late evening sun had been streaming in onto her back, she was a little warm and just wanted to take off her jacket. She laid it carefully across the armrest of the chair beside her and sat down again. Her face nevertheless now matched the salmon pink of her silk top. She was clearly smouldering, shocked and embarrassed by his bluntness. Oh well, never mind. There was no point in being here and not coming out with the truth. He cleared his throat.

'I realise I am a great deal older than my wife and I recognise that that may be a part of the problem. She sometimes says I remind her of her father when I'm angry which makes her feel frightened. But all I can say is, she really doesn't do anything to help us function as equals. She is always moaning about this and that. Non-stop, sometimes. I try to listen to her and understand, and do what I can to help, but when it comes to giving me back something in return – I mean sex – she always complains she's too tired. Well, not always, to be absolutely fair.' He thought it wise not to burn his all bridges with hyperbole, not if this session was to have any chance of being successful. 'But far more often than not. Too often. It may be hard to believe looking at us both, I know, but it's almost as if she's the one who is nearly twice my age, rather than the other way round.'

He waited for the woman to respond but she just continued writing in her notepad. His beautiful little fridge of a wife continued to avoid eye-contact with him. Bloody Hell! He cleared his throat.

'That's it. That's it in a nutshell,' he said. 'As far as I am concerned anyway. Oh! And, of course, she lies. She can't help it. Usually I don't mind, but it can be a problem between us. That *is* all, I think. Yes, I think I have given you the flavour of it anyway.'

'Thank you Dr McElvey. Now, Mrs McElvey would you like to say what the problem or problems are that brought you here this evening? From your point of view? They may or may not be the same as your husband's.'

The ingratiating smiles they gave one another were identical. What was it about women that when they were together with him on his own like this, they often looked so knowing with one another? Even when, as with this one, they didn't actually know him from Adam?

'Well I'm not sure I would actually *like* to, thank you very much,' his wife replied with a tight smile. 'But I'm so glad you said that because I certainly don't think sex *is* a problem between us. Not really. Not for me. I just don't need it or want it as much as my husband does. I want it, but at the same time I don't want it, if you know what I mean? For me sex has always been a comfort really, a reassurance that everything's alright between us. Or, at least, it used to be. Whereas for him it is an overwhelming need. And just to make one thing perfectly clear: my husband is a jealous man. His anxieties about me lying about other men are just that, anxieties. Insulting and upsetting anxieties. There is *nobody* else in my life.' She turned to look at him with that particularly condescending combination of pity and contempt that he always found so irritating. 'I'm not lying, Richard, whatever you may think.' Turning back to the counsellor and with a fragrant furrowing of her delicately fuckable brow, she said, 'So in my opinion there is a lot more to what's gone wrong between us than just sex. Or lying. I will admit it's true that I do a lot of complaining. He *is* right about that. I know I do. But I actually think I've got good reason to, most of the time, anyway.'

'Which one of you decided it might be worth trying marital counselling?'

'Well, it was me, I suppose, who actually rang up and arranged this appointment, but I think it was both of us actually. I really don't feel there's very much wrong with our marriage, despite what my husband has just said. Not in itself. I really don't. It's the other things which are spoiling everything between us. His age has got nothing to do with it either. Not really. At least, only sometimes. I fell in love with him partly *because* he was so much older than me. I wanted – want – someone mature who can look after me, give me a bit of care and understanding. Not make immature demands upon me all the time, like an adolescent. Or like a jealous child.'

'Do you want to tell me what those 'other things' are which spoil things between you?'

'Well, it's not things, really. It's people, if you know what I mean, people I love. Family, you know. And you can't really blame your loved ones, can you? It's not nice. You can't blame people for being themselves and having needs. My mother is dying of emphysema and our little boy has ADHD and mild autism and it's – it's sometimes a bit too much. I just don't have anything left for Richard.'

She smiled, her face lighting up incongruously as tears started flowing down her cheeks. The counsellor passed her a box of tissues.

'I should have mentioned those things, of course,' said Richard. 'I do realise she is under a great deal of stress with her mother and with the boy. Naturally. It's understandable. I think it's particularly difficult because he's not really ours, if you know what I mean. And I have three step-children of my own from my previous marriage and of course that's not easy for her either. Not that we see very much of them nowadays. They're mostly grown up. But she feels I have had more experience of children than she has, and for some reason that sometimes adversely affects her confidence with the boy. That's my opinion anyway,' he added, failing to keep the certainty of the professional diagnostician out of his voice.

The woman nodded her understanding without looking at him. Her attention was still on his wife.

'Is your father still alive, Mrs McElvey? How is he coping with your mother's illness?'

'No, he died nearly ten years ago but I hadn't seen him for two or three years before that anyway. He wasn't the type of man to cope. Or not to cope. He just did what he wanted.'

'So your mother only has you? Or do you have any brothers or sisters?'

'No there's only me, and to be honest, Richard is not a blind bit of help. I struggle with Sean all day until he gets home and then I go over and see Mum for a couple of hours most evenings – she's in a nursing home, waiting to go into a hospice – and then when I get back home, Richard wants a bonk. He doesn't really want to know how I am or how my mother is or how Sean's day has been. He just wants a bonk. And if he doesn't get one, he starts ranting about who else I might be doing it with!

'And that's my life!' She continued, her voice on one whingeing note. 'I don't want it. I don't want it at all. At least, I want more than just that. The education department have promised Sean a place in a special boarding school, but unlike Richard I really think he should stay at home with us. I know he needs discipline, but what he really needs more than anything else is love. We have to wait anyway before making a final decision, visit some of the schools they have suggested around the country. They are all so far away! In the meantime, unfortunately, he bites me sometimes, screams when he doesn't get what he wants and runs riot up and down the house all day when he's not on his computer. We're lucky if he sleeps more than a few hours at a time in the night.'

She blew her nose. Richard got up out of his chair and gave her shoulders a squeeze. They were rigid, tense, unyielding beneath his hands and he felt ashamed, neglectful, insensitive and plain stupid. Putting it like this, it was glaringly obvious that she should be tired and complaining. The trouble was she wasn't usually so clear at all. She tended to put on a brave face. Normally she only talked about her mother's deterioration with a fond smile rather than tears, so he had assumed she was managing things very well. And as for the boy, she would never hear a word said against him no matter what the provocation, even though he tended to play her up the most, because she was alone with him all day, every day.

But she would continually whinge and moan about him. And about his sexual approaches in particular. That much was true. She had just done so again. At least she was owning up to it. Pleased she wasn't trying shrug him off, he began massaging her small shoulders. He felt them stiffen and then surrender beneath his fingers.

'I'm so sorry,' she said to the counsellor. 'It's just that it's all a bit of a strain, you know.'

'How old is your little boy?'

'He's ten.'

'How long has your mother had Emphysema?'

'Oh, years now, but it's only in the last few months she was told she was finally dying of it. She's got weeks, if that, before she goes. It will be a relief in some ways. For *her*.'

The counsellor clucked with sympathy before changing the subject. 'Can I ask you about your childhood? You said your father left you?'

'No, I didn't. I said I hadn't seen him. Well, that's not true. We did pass one another in the street once, but he didn't recognise me.'

'How was that?'

'Awful.'

'I meant how come he didn't recognise you?'

'Oh, I'm so sorry. I had had some corrective surgery for – for a birth defect. My parents thought I was a boy when I was born. Which I am afraid I was, physically. But as I grew up, and they saw I wasn't behaving like one at all, my mother accepted it and encouraged me to be myself, but Dad didn't. I had a gender reassignment operation just before I was twenty – eleven years ago – to put me right. I don't really like talking about it – it's, embarrassing now even thinking about it. Anyway, at the same time, as you can imagine, it was a *huge* relief for me. But Dad didn't approve. He was a Muslim. Not a practicing one, but he had very traditional values and he thought I should have been given male hormones and put in the army.' She gave a brittle, tinkling little laugh which evoked an empathic smile from the therapist. Richard bent and kissed the top of her head to show his solidarity too. Her hair smelled like the bathroom, and he suppressed the wish to be at home again having sex with her under the shower.

'When we passed each other in the street shortly after all my surgery was over, he didn't recognise me and I couldn't say hello. A few weeks later he died after falling over drunk in front of a car.'

'But you have since been able to have a baby?'

'No,' Richard interjected, continuing to massage her. As a doctor this was his domain. 'Lucille unfortunately cannot have a baby of her own, she was not intersexed. It has been a source of deep regret to both of us that we haven't been able to have a child together. As I said just now, Sean isn't really ours.'

Sheila Jackson failed to hide her confusion, which angered him. She was obviously tired. He had been perfectly straightforward.

'Let me try and understand this. You have adopted him?'

'We are his legal guardians and Lucille has been looking after him since he was a year old. Before that really. He calls her Mummy and she *is* effectively his mother. His natural mother did in fact want us to adopt him formally, but Lucille refused because she said no-one can replace your real mother. In my opinion she's proved herself quite wrong about that.'

'He is actually my best friend's child,' said Lucille, glancing up at him and acknowledging his gallantry with a tiny, grateful smile. He felt the stirrings of an erection again as she reached up and held his left hand on her shoulder for a moment. Perhaps sensing how he felt she shrugged him off, signalling she had had enough. He went and sat down again, not entirely pessimistic that he might just have begun to turn the tide of her resentment towards him. 'She used to tell him he was lucky he had two mums,' Lucille continued speaking to the woman. 'I tried to stop her saying things like that, but she insisted it was true; and then she got ill and couldn't cope and asked me to have him for a while. And 'a while' has turned out to be ever since. She was so ill she nearly died, so I couldn't refuse, for her sake or for Sean's. When she got better she didn't want him back. She said he needed someone who could be interested in him and love him whole-heartedly. And I did love him, with all my heart. And as she still wasn't very well at all, I happily signed the papers for her, without really looking at them. Happily! I mean I was so young, it wasn't really about papers, it was about doing a friend a favour and caring for a little boy I adored. In himself he is the sweetest little boy you could imagine. It's just his behaviour that's been so impossible, not him. Grainne – that's his mother – still sends money to help, even though we have a five bedroom house in Oxshott and my husband is medical director as well as consultant at his hospital. Money isn't a problem for us. And, before you ask, I don't work myself - I couldn't work and still manage Sean. I once wanted to train as a nursery nurse. I have always loved children, but it just wasn't to be. I am actually doing a foundation course now for a degree with the Open University when I get the time. But I just don't get much time at all, I'm afraid. I think Richard thinks I'm a bit thick, don't you sweetie?'

'Not at all. I just don't think it's very sensible looking after him all by yourself.' He turned to the counsellor. 'We have tried having au pairs, but they all leave. Lucille says nobody could look after him who didn't love him. Well, I spend a lot of time with him at weekends and I can't honestly say I love him, not in the same way as she does, but he responds to me quite well. I tell Lucille the trick is to be firmer with him, but to be perfectly frank, she isn't at all. He is becoming a big boy, I suppose, and therefore more of a handful, but even so –

'He responds to you because you are a man, Richard. And like a father to him. And to be fair to him, Richard is very good with him, Miss, er, Mrs ?'

'Sheila. Please. Sheila Jackson.'

'I'm Lucille. My husband is brilliant with Sean he really is. Strong and firm. Sean really respects him. But also, perhaps because he is a man, Richard doesn't understand what it's like for me, when I have spent a whole day struggling with Sean and he hasn't responded well to me at all, just given me endless hassle all day. He loves me. I know he does. He can be very affectionate when he wants to be. But respect and good behaviour he reserves for Richard, and for Richard alone. I get none.'

Sheila Jackson nodded her understanding and Richard's head sunk into his hand and he sighed aloud. The gender card was being played again. It always stumped him. You couldn't argue with it because inescapably childcare and everything else for that matter was altogether different for women. Even transgendered women whose chromosomes were essentially no different from his own. Perhaps it was all a matter of hormones.

'Lucille, in order for me to understand your difficulties better I have to ask you both a few more difficult questions. First about your sex life. Do you want a sexual relationship with your husband?'

Why was she bloody concentrating on Lucille all the time, Richard wondered, although he too was interested in the answer to that question. Is it because I am a doctor? I have to be ignored, treated as if I was a second class citizen? But it was a very good question. He noticed Lucille was flushing again, and almost glaring at Sheila Jackson.

'Of course I do. It's just – well, the difference between us is that I think we've got one, he doesn't. He can be an attentive lover sometimes and I do still fancy him. I really do.'

She has to be lying, thought Richard. She shows no sign of fancying me whatsoever anymore. Again he sighed loudly, and shifted in his seat. Lucille ignored him.

'But he somehow makes me feel I am not good enough,' she said, 'which does put me right off having sex with him, it's true. When you've got a history like mine your sexual confidence is very easily dented, do you know what I mean? Especially if you are always so tired anyway. I start feeling I'm unattractive, which is just not a sexy feeling at all.'

'If I may explain,' said Richard. 'She used to be passionate and imaginative in bed, but as time has gone by, I don't know, I don't know whether it is a reaction to the shame she feels about having spent her childhood and adolescence in the wrong gender, but she has developed an antipathy to any kind of contact between us that doesn't involve the missionary position. I enjoy fellatio for example, but she will only do it with the greatest reluctance.'

Lucille's sharp intake of breath was almost a yelp. There was no other word for it. He felt mildly gratified in a vengeful sort of way. She sounded like a fucking poodle. There was a resounding silence as his words and her yelp hung in the air. He grimaced, hearing how angry and unpleasant he sounded. Oh, well, – fuck it. He was angry and he wasn't used to this kind of thing. He didn't know how to behave here. Did she expect him to pussyfoot elliptically around the reasons why they'd come? What good would that do? He felt confused, uncertain. Like a patient. As a consultant he had always relied on being the competent and charming man of knowledge and power. He grimaced at how coarse and brutal he was in fact now being. Never mind, at least he was being honest, even if it did mean the counsellor was getting a distorted picture of him. He wondered whether he was overcompensating for Lucille's phoniness by being so boorish.

'You are insulting me, Richard, and it's also not true. I do like it. Sometimes. I just prefer, you know, the missionary position as you call it. It's just your appetite for sex of whatever kind is so much greater than mine. That's all. The real problem Sheila, since you ask and as he is being so charmingly blunt about it, I will be too; the real problem is that he is like a bull in a china shop when it comes to sex. And I suppose that makes me feel kind of, I don't know, like I'm some kind of Ming vase, for goodness sake! You know, precious and easily broken, which I'm not really. Truly I'm not. It's just he doesn't realise it takes me far longer than him to get in the mood for sex and feel relaxed and ready for it. Because more than anything I need comfort and care and love to feel properly interested in it. He's always up for it. Always. I can see he's all leering and horny before I've even got undressed! I mean I just can't keep up with that. I really can't. It makes me feel inadequate. I wouldn't mind if he just wanted to, well you know, get on with it and bonk me. But he expects me to be immediately all interested and involved myself when he wants it. When all I'm actually feeling, most of the time anyway, is shattered!' She turned back to face him again. 'You simply don't seem to understand that, Richard. I really do get exhausted.'

'Every night?'

'Yes every night, sometimes. Oh dear. I'm crying again. I really hate this. It's awful. Just awful.'

Again she smiled brightly at the counsellor through her tears.

'It may be of no consolation to either of you,' said Sheila Jackson, 'but it is never easy for any of the couples who come here to talk about such things. But I am sure you will both agree it is best if all the cards are on the table from the outset.'

'Well this is the last thing I want to say on the subject of our sex life. It's so embarrassing talking about such intimate, private things. I just want him to show me some respect and recognise that there are some things I feel uncomfortable about. I love it when he just treats me like a woman. That's all I need. And all I want. A little consideration about how I'm feeling, would really, really help. Put me in the mood, perhaps make me feel like I used to when we first met.'

'Which was how?' asked the counsellor.

'Wonderful! There's no other word for it. He was the man of my dreams. Tall, handsome, mature, intelligent. And interested in me! I couldn't believe how lucky I was. He would want to know what I was feeling all the time in those days. All the time! And what I was thinking and if I was alright. Whereas now I find myself grateful if he shows any interest in my feelings at all! And even when he does I am never sure anymore whether he really wants to know, or whether it's actually only because what he really wants to know is whether he'll be able to get his end away or not. I am sorry to be so crude. But that's how it is.'

'That's really not fair, Luce.'

'It's what I feel, Richard. You know – feel.' She spelt it out for him. 'F.E.E.L'

'And what about you, Richard?' Sheila Jackson asked.

'What about me?'

He was feeling hurt, morose and miserable. He always tried his best to be honourable. He never cheated on Lucille. He might flirt with junior medical staff and nurses sometimes, in the mildest way, but really Lucille was the only person in his life he cared for. She knew that. So it hurt to effectively be told that his only interest in her was sexual.

'I mean what do you feel about what your wife has just said?'

'I am a man. As such the foundation of my interest in all women is sexual, of course it is. But I love Lucille and regardless of my sexual desire, I am actually interested in her as a person as well. I'd have never actually married someone nearly a quarter of a century younger than myself if I hadn't been, for God's sake. And I still am. That's why I'm here. What she hasn't told you is that when I do enquire after her feelings she invariably gets very nervous, as if telling me will somehow make them worse. So out of deference to her propensity to become too anxious, and out of a wish to avoid upsetting her, I always try not to talk about emotional things with her too much at all. I do it out of love.' He looked at Lucille and spelt it out for her. 'L.O.V.E.'

'It seems to me that you two have actually got a lot you need to say to each other,' Sheila Jackson interjected. She has a talent for stating the obvious, thought Richard. Perhaps it was an essential part of her job description. He stared at his humiliation by locking his eyes onto the now orange evening sky out the window. 'In fact if there was any one thing I would want to say to you both so far, it is this,' the counsellor continued. 'I am surprised by how two such intelligent people can have such a naïve – and please don't get me wrong I use the word 'naïve' in a non-pejorative sense – can have such a naïve understanding of how relationships actually work and of how feelings can affect them. I am almost tempted to suggest that it would be helpful for you to have some psycho-educational input. Not from me. I am a therapist. But there are short training programmes which might help you to learn something about how human beings grow and develop emotionally.' She must have noticed his scowl at this ridiculous suggestion because she cleared her throat and changed direction. 'But we can perhaps save that thought for a subsequent session assuming you both decide you want to come back again. You may feel dragging things out in the open like this and talking about them actually does more harm than good. That is something you will have to discuss together. But in the meantime we still have twenty minutes left. I think it would help now if you told me how you first met, when you were married and so on.'

Richard kept his exasperated eyes on a gannet wheeling high up in the sky as Sheila Jackson kept hers on Lucille.

'We met in Balham ten years ago,' Lucille replied. 'I was living with his ex-wife, his first ex-wife who had looked after me and actually paid for the corrective surgery I needed – purely out of generosity and the goodness of her own heart because we were friends. It was amazing of her really and I still don't properly understand why she was so sweet and generous towards me. She said it was a mother's gift. But of course she wasn't my mother, so it was unbelievably kind of her. I dread to think what would have happened to me otherwise. But she did let me pay rent – I had a job as a stylist in a hair salon in those days – and she said I could pay her back if I really wanted to, if I was ever in a position to do so. I did send her a cheque after Richard and I were married. But she never cashed it. She'd actually stopped speaking to me a couple of years before that,' Lucille added in a quiet, hurt tone. 'After I moved out from her place and moved in with him. She wasn't horrible or anything. It wasn't like she suddenly refused to ever see me again. There was no, what do you call it, animosity between us. She was very nice really. But I suppose he was *her* husband before he ever was mine, and he never would have been mine if it hadn't been for her. So I did understand why she decided it was best to have no more to do with me. It's all ever so complicated!'

She laughed as if that was funny. The counsellor smiled politely. Richard didn't bother.

'What I never could quite understand, though,' Lucille went on. He knew what was coming. He had heard it countless times before. 'Was how two such lovely people could ever have split up from one another in the first place. But Richard will tell you about that, I'm sure. If he wants to.'

I don't think I will, thought Richard, his attention held by the gannet leaving its thermal with a single flap of wings and gliding off in the general direction of the setting sun.

'When I first got to know him,' Lucille went on. 'I thought he was the handsomest, kindest and sexiest man I had ever met. And so good with children and animals. I used to take Sean out for walks on Wandsworth Common and he told me that he sometimes walked his dogs there. And I knew it was true because the second time I met him – at Rose's – he apologised about his dogs having chewed up Sean's bottle of Ribena in the park. Months before, it was, and I hadn't even known about it, but he produced a brand new one he bought specially!'

'They weren't my dogs!' Richard growled. 'My second wife and I bought them for her children,' he explained to the woman, wondering why he felt he had to be defensive.

'Then accidentally on purpose somehow, after I met him properly at Rose's', Lucille went on. 'because – honestly! – we didn't deliberately arrange it, not at first anyway, we started to meet regularly in the park. It was summer. The weather was wonderful, the evenings were long and one thing led to another, you know. I mean I knew he was married and everything, and when he first kissed me I knew I shouldn't have let him. But I couldn't help it, I wanted him to. And if I'm honest, I'd lost touch with reality. I was still on a bit of a high, you see. For a year after my surgery I was, well, free. And I became a bit too free, if you know what I mean. It was so wonderful to be out of the prison I'd been in all my life. I'm a bit embarrassed about that period of my life now. But I can't really regret it.'

'You're saying you were promiscuous?' Sheila Jackson asked, looking at her with what Richard felt was far too much compassion from above her half-moons. Lucille, of course, was in her element. She loved talking about herself. She nodded her head at the woman with a solemn shrug.

'I was. But even then it wasn't because I wanted to be. It was because of the effect it had on my confidence. Every time a man showed interest in me as a woman it helped me feel a little bit more sure of myself, you know? But the truth is, by the time I met Richard I really didn't need that anymore. And I would never have let him touch me if he hadn't told me his marriage to Mary was over. Never! Not just, you know, because it's wrong, but also because it was finally getting through to me that I'd had

179

enough by then; quite enough, both of men letching, and of myself for wanting them to. But Richard was different. He was so much mature than the boys I had been going out with. He still looked at me like a man, but he didn't, you know, immediately try to get inside my knickers. I know it's a cliché, but he was the first man and so far the only man in my whole life to ever buy me flowers. Which is a bit sad, isn't it? But I loved that. Boys my own age either didn't want to get close at all – not to me – or they wanted to get *too* close. As I watched him getting Sean's attention and actually playing with him one afternoon in the park, I realised what I had always known really. I wanted a man to take care of me, and get close to. Not a boy.

'And I still do. But I don't think he really wants to get close to me anymore. He's only interested in sex now, like a boy, not a man. Just sex. Nothing else. Certainly not in who I am anymore. Well, it doesn't do anything for me.' Her voice rose an octave and she gave him a baleful glare. 'It doesn't turn me on one little bit.'

Richard noticed he was gawping. At least half of all this had to be lies because it was completely new to him. Why hadn't she ever told him before? Admittedly he hadn't asked, but still, how come she had never before told him how promiscuous she used to be? She had to be lying. She always lied when it was important not to. One of her favourite songs was an old Simon and Garfunkel number from his youth. It had come out long before she was even born. The Boxer. Lie-la-lie.Lie-la-lie-lie-lie-lie.Lie.

'Richard, do you want to respond to what your wife has just said or would you prefer to leave that for another time and tell me some of the relevant highlights of your life?'

'I think Lucille wants to be wanted but she doesn't want to be had. I call that prick-teasing myself. She's telling you about the past, but I am concerned about the present. Our marriage is nearly on the rocks. This is my third one. I don't want it to fail too.'

'Do you want an emotional relationship with Lucille?'

'Of course I do. But I cannot separate having an emotional relationship from having a sexual one as well. Not if we are to have a marriage. Plenty of men take their sexuality off elsewhere – pornography, prostitutes, that kind of thing – and consequently don't have a proper marriage at all. In my opinion, anyway. I admit I do need to show Lucille more interest, but if looks could kill I would be dead in the water every time I even glanced at her with any desire nowadays. At the same time she always makes sure she looks so completely fucking desirable –

'Richard! Please.'

'Completely desirable' he said, looking her up and down in a frankly sexual manner till she averted her eyes, shaking her head. 'Which is difficult for me. I'm a man.'

'Tell me a bit about your past,' said Sheila Walton.

'There is nothing much to tell. A conventional middle class upbringing. Grammar school. Cambridge. I've always liked women. Never been gay at all. So I was bit – no, I was *very* – shocked when I found out about Lucille's past. As a heterosexual man, and knowing nothing about her background or history at all, I'd actually fallen for her as a female. There was nothing remotely masculine about her. Not a thing. But after Rose let slip the truth, the fact of her transsexual status remained and I had to deal with it one way or another. I told myself it should matter, that my desire for her should be undermined somehow. In a way I actually wanted it to be, but it wasn't. The truth was I found didn't care. She was still who she was and I still wanted her.' He paused, took a deep breath knowing what he was about to say would upset Lucille, but needing her to know what he felt.

'I still do want her. It's not my problem. It's Lucille's. And it's what is getting in the way of our marriage. As far I am concerned, she's all woman. I've never known her any different, and that's that. No. The problem is with her. She never, ever, even mentions, let alone talks about her childhood or adolescence. It's as if she believes she can't be who she really is – now in the present – because of her past. When, of course, the very opposite is the case. She wouldn't be who she is now without having been the person she was before. So she was once a boy? So what? Accept it and let it go. Sometimes it makes me wonder whether, after all she's done, she may not actually like being a woman very much, after all. She clearly enjoys all the trappings of femininity. You know – the lifestyle, the interests, the clothes, the friends, the feelings, all that kind of thing. The gender role. But not, if what she says about there being no other man in her life is true, the actual sex role of a woman, just taking a man inside her and being fucked.'

Shit. He was being too coarse again. His anger with her would keep on slipping out. He'd blow it if he wasn't careful. He raised his hand in acknowledgement. 'Sorry.'

'Richard, how could you say such a thing! You know that's not true.'

'I don't think you enjoy sex, Lucie. Not any more. Not with me, anyway.'

'I do,' she almost screamed. 'I would. If you just gave me more time.'

'We will have been living together for eight years in October, Luce. I think you have had enough time. You used to enjoy it. Unless you were pretending. But I think something has happened. Either your past has caught up with you in some strange way, like I said, because you can't let it go, or else you were lying just now when you said you still fancied me. Then again, maybe there is somebody else.'

'I've told you, Richard. There isn't anybody. Please don't start that nonsense up again. No-one! Oh god, this is too much! I *wish* I hadn't come. I feel completely torn apart. I have to go.'

She stood up, hurriedly hoisting her bag over her shoulder and picking up her jacket. She started for the door, angrily stifling sobs and wiping loose strands of tear-damp hair from her mouth. It was a melodrama Richard could do without.

'Lucille, please! Could you wait just a moment,' Sheila Walton interjected, sounding slightly flustered. 'Of course we have only just met, but it seems to me that perhaps these and many other issues between you both need further elaborating and understanding.'

What a pompous old windbag the woman was.

'In the meantime, if I may say so, Dr McElvey, you have said a lot of things to your wife without actually letting *her* say very much to you. Perhaps as a way of balancing things up it might be helpful for Lucille to have her say now. Then, I think,' she looked at her watch, smiled at them each in turn, 'we really must stop.'

'I've said all I want to say, thank you very much, Sheila,' Lucille said from the doorway. 'I don't think he heard me and if I was to say it again he still wouldn't. But you have insulted and hurt me, Richard, and whatever may or may not happen between us in the future I will say for the record, for Sheila, that I enjoy being a woman in every way. In *every* way. I would just like a man who could accept me and love me for who I am, not for who he would like me to be. That's all.'

The session ended with tears streaming down Lucille's face. The perfect, doll-like creature who had met him here fifty minutes ago was now just another red-nosed, blotchy-cheeked woman with a marriage problem. She glanced at herself in the small round mirror by the door, looked horrified and said she was going to the loo and would see him downstairs. Giving Sheila Jackson a curt nod she swept out. Richard felt like a bastard. He also felt he wasn't going to come back here again despite setting another appointment with the Jackson woman for the same time next week and giving her a cheque. They were definitely leaving the session feeling worse than when they had come in, and what was the good of that? Why pay good money only to feel even more fucked up?

'How do I make you feel you're not good enough?' He asked when she eventually joined him outside the building, her appearance restored.

'I couldn't believe you said that,' she replied, eventually as they looked out for a taxi.

He saw the hurt set of her mouth, realised he should be taking a different tack.

'And I can't believe I make you feel unattractive when as far as I'm concerned you have got the cutest arse and the finest legs in London.'

182

He put a hand on her backside with a big friendly smile and tried to squeeze her bum. She pulled away from him, the disdain in her eyes was absolute, which made him feel angry and eroticised at one and the same time. He had only been trying to show her she was attractive and cheer her up.

'Richard! Please. Not now. Not out here. Not when I am so upset. You're the one who's unbelievable. How can a man as intelligent and experienced as you, be so completely – and grossly – insensitive and stupid? I just don't understand it!'

'Lucille I –

'Just don't speak to me Richard. Don't say another word. And don't try to grope me again, please.'

'We don't understand each other at all sometimes, do we?' He tried to rationalise, as if what was going on between them was not out of the ordinary. 'Still, all relationships have their ups and downs I suppose. As long as we still fancy each other, that's the important thing.' It was another attempt to be light, jocular. He was certain he didn't sound as sarcastic as he felt. He reached out to give her a final, friendly pat on the bum.

'Richard! Please! Not now!'

The hysteria in her voice was over the top. If she didn't want his attentions, she didn't have to be such a drama queen about it. She was almost shouting at him again, for God's sake. Out here on the street. He couldn't help smiling, though. No-one had done that to him since he was fourteen or fifteen and his mother had slapped him, just once, across the face outside Sainsburys. He couldn't remember why. Oh, yes. He had seen a woman packing shopping into her car and he had happened to mention he would like to shag her. Mother had put down the bags she was carrying and slapped him. Fancy remembering that after all this time.

Lucille now looked at him with visible loathing, contempt and disgust written all across her face.

He wasn't so stupid that he didn't realise that this was an occasion when he had better do as he was told. He looked up the street for a taxi, trying to suppress the erection which her anger, unfortunately, so often seemed to arouse in him nowadays. She wasn't much more than half his age, yet so often she made him feel like a little boy.

183

Chapter 12.

The flight to Northern Ireland had been bumpy, the weather back in Manchester drizzly and grey. But as Grainne sat in the back of the bus heading towards Belfast city centre from the airport, the sun was streaming down out of a cloudless blue sky, lighting the serrated roof tops of the smoky, grey and dirty terracotta lines of terraced houses. They almost seemed pretty, certainly familiar and homely which felt bizarre after all this time.

Grainne was coming home after a gap of sixteen years. She had decided it was time. Her mother would be turning sixty tomorrow and was having a combined retirement and birthday party. Over a hundred and fifty people were expected, family, friends and a few work colleagues, and nobody she wouldn't want to see, her mother had written begging her to come. She was desperate to see Grainne again and promised only to be delighted if she would, nothing more and nothing less, because she loved her and missed her so much. Grainne had allowed a flood of warmth and longing to come over her as she read that, decided to suspend her memories for a few days and risk it. After all, she wasn't a girl anymore. She was thirty five years old.

Anyway, there would be little time for any awkward intimacy, she hoped as the bus pulled into the terminal. What with all the preparations for the party to be made, deep emotional contact could hopefully be avoided. If there was one thing she had learned about herself whilst living in England it was that minimising emotional input and output was much the best way of keeping her equilibrium. It prevented all kinds of messy feelings slopping about. The best way of reducing emotionality was to distract herself by concentrating on other things. Work, calorie counting, exercise, anything which could prevent close personal contact with other people. That's why she did the work she did. It was odd, sure, but close physical contact with her clients precluded genuine personal closeness with them. Thank goodness! The fact that she got paid also helped her to distance herself from them. Some of them genuinely came for massage rather than the extra services she offered, but those were usually female clients, whom she tended to like better anyway. Their physical needs were less messy. She still worked on a bank basis as a nurse to supplement her income; but as a masseuse offering special services she made so much more money so much more quickly than she ever could in the health service. She lived off the money she made from her sex work and massage, and always sent her child benefit, plus whatever she made from nursing, to Lucille each week for Sean. She insisted upon it. Some years ago when Lucille had tried to argue over the phone about it with her, saying it was completely unnecessary as she and Richard had more money than they knew what to do with, she had angrily replied that if

184

Lucille wouldn't accept her money than she would have Sean taken into care instead. She was Sean's mother and she wanted to pay for the painful and humiliating fact that she wasn't emotionally equipped to care for him properly and didn't want to see him again. It was a matter of pride.

She had learned a lot about pride ten years ago when she only just managed to avoid being compulsorily admitted into hospital under the Mental Health Act. She had ended up staying in the awful eating disorders unit for what turned out to be the best part of a year. She'd reluctantly agreed to being admitted 'voluntarily' as an in-patient. The sense of having been coerced into something she didn't actually want to do had re-awoken all her old childhood demons and it had taken her six months before she could begin to own the voluntary nature of her admission into hospital and sometimes genuinely co-operate with the treatment programme. Pride had had to be swallowed like food for those first six months until she could feel she was doing what she wanted to do, rather than pretending. But even then it had only been up to a point: the truth was, she'd only decided to eat in order to be discharged, not because she wanted to eat like other people at all. No way.

The fact was that anorexia had become so bound up in her sense of who she was that it was now an essential part of her, because it was an aspect of her personality that was authentically hers and hers alone. Others might see it as an illness, and she could understand that now, but for her it was as much a part of who she was as her hands or her feet. She had, however, learned to keep it in check, to stay just within acceptable limits so that she would never again suffer the indignity of unwanted hospital admission, and so that people didn't stare too much. But it was still hard. It still required all her concentration to force food into her mouth and make herself chew it, then, more difficult, swallow it and then, more difficult still, keep it down knowing it could be ejected at will.

Would her mother recognise her? Probably. She never dressed like a whore or a mental patient. She made a point of always looking healthy and sportive nowadays. She was wearing an expensive green and white track suit over a clean white T-shirt and tennis shoes. She had had her hair done yesterday in a short spiky style which she was quite pleased with. She felt she didn't look much different from the eighteen year old girl who had left for England full of hope and excitement to train as a nurse all those years ago. Thinner, of course, much less lumpen; like someone who had grown up and who didn't depend on food or its absence for comfort anymore, yet still recognisably herself.

As she walked along the old familiar streets, rolling her neat little wheeled suitcase behind her, she felt nervous rather than frightened. She was doing what she wanted to do. It was a definite choice. When she had been walking in the opposite direction sixteen years ago she had been terrified and despite her optimism felt like she had no choice whatsoever.

She'd just had to get away. Ridiculous as it seemed now, the prospect of not only training to be a nurse in England, but in the glamour of London at that, had seemed a wonderful opportunity.

She turned the corner into her street, was immediately struck by how small it was and how little it had changed. It looked cleaner now, less grimy. More double-glazed windows and identikit front doors and a plethora of big shiny cars parked both in the driveways and on the street. It was otherwise still terribly familiar. As if she had never been away. She wondered if Ma and Da still kept the front door on the latch like they always used to when they were in, so that anyone who knew them also knew they could just walk right in. She hoped not. She didn't want to walk right in as if she had never been away. She didn't know them at all anymore. She would bang on the front door knocker and wait for her Ma or Da to come to the door. The knocker was small and black, shaped like a lady's elegant hand tapping on a ball. She could remember her mother paying twenty pounds for it when she was a little girl, a huge amount in those days. It had been Ma's pride and joy. She'd been so excited scolding and praising Da as he screwed it into the door, making sure he did it in the right place without damaging it.

But when she got to the house the door was a plasticised, panelled mock-Georgian affair with no knocker at all and a huge wisteria clung to the front wall. She felt a ridiculous resentment towards it for being there. She stopped and stared at her childhood home, trying to take it in. In contrast to all the other semis in the Close, it did look completely different from the place she had left without a backward glance. Then it had been a white-painted, pebble-dashed eyesore. Now it was an anonymous modernised building just like the rest. She pressed the door bell which created a bland sonorous ding-dong somewhere inside. Sixteen years ago there had been no bell. Through the frosted plastic in the door panelling a wide figure lumbered slowly up the hallway towards her. Ma.

The door opened.

'Ma! Hello. It's me.'

'Oh Grainne, Grainne my darling. It's so wonderful to see you. My, how you've changed! I can hardly believe it! A grown woman! No, no. Of course, you are! Of course, you are. Come in my darling, come in. Come and let me look at you. Don't you worry, I'm not going to cry.'

She followed her in and shut the door behind her. Her first impression was that nothing had changed inside at all. Not even Ma. She was a little fatter it was true, and had joined those ladies of a certain age for whom a blue rinse is a good solution, but that was all. In fact Grainne was sure she had seen her before in just that same pastelly pink, pleated dress with the Forget-me-not print.

'You look wonderful, Ma. You haven't changed at all. I can't believe you're going to be sixty the day after tomorrow.'

'Oh get along with you! And look at you – you've lost all your puppy fat somewhere along the years, haven't you?' She put her hands on Grainne's hips, gave her a little squeeze. 'There's not a spare ounce on you anywhere. And I just seem to put more and more weight on. Here now, hang your jacket up on the hook there, and give me a big, long hug. That's right. Oh Grainne. You are so thin. Are you sure you're alright?'

'Of course I am, Ma. I just keep myself fit. That's all. I have to. Where's Da?'

'He's in the garden fast asleep. Go and wake him up. I'll put the kettle on.'

Grainne went through the tiny lounge she had grown up in. It was still magnolia coloured and her father's tacky little collection of snooker trophies still adorned the fireplace. Memories came flooding back. All of them warm. None of them bad. She went out through the French windows into the garden. Sure enough there was Da lying in a deck chair with a straw hat pulled down over his face. She went up to him and knelt down.

'Da,'she whispered quietly. 'Da, it's me. Grainne.'

He snored, then twitched violently awake, his sun hat falling down into his lap.

'Grainne! Come here, darlin, let me hold you. How long is it? Too long that's for sure. Where has all your beautiful ginger hair gone? You've had it cut. Oh, it's good to see you again after all this time. So good. And what a beautiful woman you have become! Moira,' he shouted. 'Our little Grainne looks just like you.' He put his hat back on his head, gave her a knowing wink. Grainne remembered his tomfoolery. 'No man in tow, is there, inside, talking to your Ma? No? Well, there should be, my darlin.' He shook his head 'Why did you have nothing to do with us for so long?

It was rhetorical, he wasn't looking for an answer just now, but Grainne was nonetheless relieved to be saved from answering by her mother.

'Now, Paul, don't you be starting on her as soon as she's arrived,' said Ma, wobbling a little as she came out carrying a tray of biscuits and a pot of tea. 'She had her reasons I'm sure. Now I'll just go in and get the mugs and we can drink your health, Grainne. I've brought you some biscuits. You were always such a lovely plump little thing and now look at you – so slender we can hardly get a hold of you. You be careful, Paul, you don't break her, holding her hand like that.'

'Don't be silly, Moira.'

'I'm very strong Ma. I do weight training.'

Grainne couldn't help lapping up all this fussing over her, even as it irritated her a little. When she had lived here as a child, as the eldest she'd been expected to help make a fuss over her younger twin sisters -

she couldn't remember her parents ever making a fuss over her. Not like this anyway. She decided not to be churlish, to let it be as comforting now as a rare drink of hot milk at bedtime had been when she was a little girl.

'How are Aislinn and Siobhan?' she asked.

'Oh, you'll never believe it! Aislinn has just announced she is pregnant again and Siobhan is flying in with Mark from Boston on Sunday morning. Mark is her er, partner I think you call it. And as far as I know they are both fine,' said Ma, also determined to be full of good cheer.

They drank tea in the sunshine, her father and mother both being careful to keep the conversation light and easy. It was the right thing to do and Grainne felt a rare warm glow growing inside her which she knew to be illusory but which she wanted to enjoy all the same.

When she finished her tea, Grainne insisted on going upstairs to her room on her own with her suitcase. It hadn't changed very much at all. Newish wall paper, that was all. And a certain unlived-in quality. Still the same books in her little bookshelf though, which was a surprise. Dianna Wynne-Jones, E.E. Nesbitt, Louisa M Alcott. Many long hours had been whiled away with them in the dim and distant past. She must have been reading them when she was about nine or ten or maybe even younger, certainly twenty years ago at least. Remembering, like it was yesterday, the feeling of lying on her bed with the late evening sunshine streaming in through her window loving to read, she flicked through her once treasured copy of the Ossianic Tales. There was a pressed clover inside it which she couldn't remember putting there, of course, but it felt a part of the book and the book felt a part of her. She closed it and inhaled the intervening years since she last opened it. She had done the right thing. Her home had been a safer place since she had been gone. Her books had stayed put. She recalled once telling her mother that she wanted to keep them all, if her little sisters didn't destroy them, and had written her full name inside each and every one in her best childhood handwriting. It had been one of those things she said to Ma which she must have heard and for a moment the sweet consideration of this made her question the memories that had driven her away from here all those years ago.

She delighted in the odd combination of familiarity and strangeness that the old books with their dated covers evoked in her, removing one after another and immersing herself in the unexpectedness of discovering good feelings and cosy memories from her childhood. Here of all places. Life was so complicated. It was a miracle Aislinn and Siobhan hadn't destroyed them or walked off with them. Specially Aislinn, now she had children of her own.

She put the books back and lifted her suitcase onto her bed to unpack. She took out the simple, long-sleeved lilac dress she'd brought with her for the party on Sunday. Normally, and whatever the occasion, she always wore trousers. Buying this obviously had something to do with

188

coming home. Ma always used to make her wear a skirt or a dress for church on Sundays. Some residual, forgotten memory of this must have prompted her to go into Hennes yesterday and buy this outfit. There was even something slightly frumpy and churchy about it, now she looked at it. It had seemed to trendily cheerful when she'd tried it on. She smiled. It didn't matter, she'd only wear it the once. She hung it up in the empty cupboard thinking she might even go to church with Ma too. For old times' sake, to please her and to thank her for keeping her childhood books for her.

Wallowing in the strange, unexpectedly pleasant sensation of nostalgia and memory impacting with the here and now, she freshened herself up and went back downstairs.

Over the next twenty four hours she was thrilled to rediscover the fact that she still loved and was loved by her Ma and her Da. She had somehow completely forgotten this in all the intervening years over in England. Made herself forget it perhaps, because forgetting it was what had enabled her to have so little contact with them for such a long time. What a stranger she was to herself and how little she knew her own feelings that she had been so full of trepidation on the way over here.

Well, she knew why of course, had perfectly good reasons for it. There was the little matter of Sean, and of guilt, and of horrible memories which she didn't want to think about right now, but which had all too often been the only thing she had been able to think about at all, for far too long.

All of which had nothing to do with her parents. That was the sad thing. Ma and Da had never really done her any harm at all. It had been all her own doing that she had kept herself away from them for so long. Almost as if she had wanted to protect them from both the facts of what had happened to her, but more than that, from her inexplicable, inexcusable rage with them about it.

But now she was here she wasn't angry with them and it was alright. It was really quite alright. And that's how it stayed.

Till Saturday evening.

She and Ma were washing up the dishes. Da was in the next room in front of the television. Grainne had forgotten that washing-up had often been an opportunity for some truth and plain speaking between them when she had been a teenager. Not the whole truth – some truths were unspeakable and had never been talked about – but they used to feel close over the dishes, or at least they would try to. A team. Grainne had that feeling now as Ma brought her up to date about relatives and friends she had not seen nor heard about for sixteen years. It seemed that those who hadn't died would all be coming to the party tomorrow.

She was at the sink washing the plates and Ma was drying them up. Everything was going along swimmingly as they talked about all the things they would have to remember to do to make sure the party went like clockwork, until her mother caught sight of the dull-red bracelet of fishhead-shaped scars just above her left wrist where she used to burn herself with the point of a knife which had been pre-heated over a gas ring. She hadn't done any such thing for some years now, and having lived on her own for so long, had got used to washing up without having to conceal herself. She'd been so happy here, felt so relaxed being back at home that her guard had slipped and without thinking she had automatically pulled her sleeves half way up her forearms when they got damp in the bubbles of washing up liquid.

She was immediately aware of her mother's shocked and quizzical expression when she passed her the first plate, but ignored it and hoped Ma would follow her example and ignore it too. For a while she did. But when the dishes were nearly done, and perhaps because her hands had been in the water for some time, the scarring became more prominent, at once livid yet also pallid across her orangey freckled skin. As she passed her the last glass, Ma looked from her face to her wrist and back again and raised an eyebrow. Grainne cursed herself for not having worn rubber gloves, but said nothing, pulled the plug from the sink and took a tea towel to dry her hands off with. She pulled her sleeves down, looked at Ma and shrugged.

Okay, time for some truth. It couldn't be avoided. Not the whole truth, just no lies either. That was their old unwritten, kitchen sink rule. But she would have to obey it only if Ma pressed her.

Ma did. She draped her own damp tea towel across the edge of the sink and took hold of Grainne's wrist to look more closely at the scarring.

'What is this? It was never an accident?'

Despite her intentions, Grainne felt an overwhelming urge to tell her mother everything. Just like when she was a little girl and hadn't been allowed to say anything on pain of death to the whole family if she did.

Ma pulled the sleeve up higher and saw the old mish-mash of white griddled cutting scars overlaid with the more irregular-shaped patches where she used to scald herself. Grainne pulled her arm away as gently as she could. Ma always used to be such an anxious, nervy person, but she seemed very calm now. She looked directly into her eyes with such compassion that Grainne just wanted to melt into her arms. Why, oh, why hadn't she realised when she was a little girl that Ma was so much stronger than her hesitant, timid manner suggested? She must have been too young at the time to realise, or too frightened and ashamed. And of course there had always been far more to Ma than saccharine. She had often gone around with a shrill, scary disapproval on her features, belying her hesitancy and timidity and making it difficult for the little girl Grainne was then to know if or when she could confide in her.

Well she wasn't too young now to recognise her mother's strength, despite what she felt. And she wasn't too old to be embraced by her either. They held each other for what seemed like minutes. As they did so Grainne could feel a huge longing for relief welling up inside her. She could not remember when she had last cried, but the sense of comfort now was so intense that she felt near to doing so. She found herself smiling as her mother patted her back and held her tight against her. It felt like something she had been waiting for all her life.

Eventually they let each other go.

'I want you to tell me everything, Grainne. All you have told me about so far is your work and your friends; but you haven't said anything, not a blessed thing, about your feelings or any of the more difficult things that have happened to you in your life. And if you would want to tell me, Grain, I would want to know. I'm not pressing you, but don't hold anything back now please.'

They both laughed at this. It would be alright to tell her some things, and then the relief she suddenly found herself longing for, might finally come.

'Please. For my sake,' said Ma. 'If not for yours! If I end my life not understanding or really knowing my first born child, then my whole life will have been a waste. I want to know. And I want you to know that I love you no matter what has happened or what you have done. Or what I have done to you. No, don't pay any attention to my tears. They're just tears, that's all. You don't need to shield me from the truth because of my tears.'

Ever practical, she bustled over to the kettle and gave a purposeful flick to the switch before tearing off a couple of squares of kitchen tissue from the roll on the wall and loudly blowing her nose. She passed Grainne the other one. Grainne panicked. How could she tell Ma about her own brother? How could she tell her anything? She could not speak the unspeakable. That was not actually physically possible. Oh, God.

'I wouldn't know what to tell you. I wouldn't know where to begin. But you haven't done anything. How could you have? Don't be silly, Ma.'

'Do you mind me asking you some questions then, my darling? I only want the truth, mind. Or nothing. You're a grown woman and you don't have to tell me anything you don't want to, of course, but you know how I have always hated lies.'

Grainne didn't say, 'that's why I had to leave, Ma'. She said,

'The truth can hurt. Sometimes lies are better. Less hurtful, anyway.'

'Nothing can hurt me more than the fact that I have had neither sight nor sound of my eldest daughter for sixteen years. Nothing. Do you know, I couldn't wait for your Christmas cards each year. Even though I hated them once they had arrived because you said nothing in them about how you were or what you were doing or where you were living after you moved away from Tooting. Wherever *that* was! Your father was so distressed he wanted to hire a private detective to find you. You were always his favourite, you know. The twins never meant the same to him at all.'

'What do you want to know?'

'What made you leave us Grainne? Why did you go having to do your nurse training in England? Why couldn't you have done it here in Belfast?'

'I had to get away Ma. That's all.'

'Grainne, please don't take me for stupid. I know you had to get away. My question was why?'

'Because – well, because your brother, Uncle Jack had been bullying me and I was ashamed and I wanted to get away. Get away from my shame.'

There! She'd said it. If Ma couldn't read between the lines then she could not read at all.

'Bullying you? What do you mean Jack had been bullying you? How?'

'Ma, please, I don't want to talk about it.'

'What did Jack do to you, Grainne? I want to know. Is that why your arms are like that? Is that what you're telling me? What did he do to you, Grainne?'

'I can't tell you Ma. That's the truth: I cannot tell you. I don't know how to put it into words. It's too difficult. Just accept it's the truth Ma. And then forget it. Please. I have.'

'Don't be ridiculous, girl! How can I forget it? You clearly didn't forget it, if the scars on your arm are anything to go by. Is the other one in the same state?'

'It's not as bad. And actually Ma I haven't really harmed myself for, I don't know, ten years.

'Oh my poor girl. My poor, poor girl.'

'Stop it, Ma. I'm okay, and I am not a girl anymore. I'm grown up now and I can cope.'

'I want to know what he did to you. Was it sexual?'

'It was– yes. Yes, it was sexual. There, I've told you.'

And telling her after all these years made her feel curiously detached from her past rather than connected with it. Light headed. Not really relieved at all, though.

Her mother stifled a small choking sound and sat down suddenly on a kitchen chair, staring at Grainne as if she were a ghost.

'Oh my God. Jack! Oh my God.'

She blew her nose again and Grainne knew, after all, that she had been right not to have told this to her before. She would have never coped with it.

'He's coming to my party at the clubhouse tomorrow. I don't want to see him. I don't want to see him or speak to him ever again.'

'Ma, it stopped more than twenty years ago. By the time I was fourteen I realised he was full of bullshit and I told him I would tell the police if he ever tried it on ever again. And he didn't. I had to leave four years later because of my shame and because I had never told you.'

'Why not Grainne? Why didn't you ever tell me? I would surely – surely – have sorted him out, I can tell you.'

'I was ashamed, Ma. And I didn't want to upset you or spoil things between you and Jack. And you had enough on your plate with Aislinn and Siobhan.'

'I did not. I did not! You should have told me.'

'You did. They were in the 'terrible twos' when he started. I was six years old, but I still remember you saying 'my terrible two are in the terrible twos and it's all too terribly much' all the time. We all used to laugh about it, and copy you. But I knew you meant it.'

'You were six when he started on you? Oh my God! How could I have not known?'

'He told me he was in the IRA and that he would blow us all up if I even gave a hint of what was going on. I believed him, Ma. Children can be so gullible. Anyway, I was! I believed him.' She felt guilty about *that* now, though she knew it to be ridiculous, as if she had let her mother down.

'Did he, you know, did he do everything?'

Grainne nodded. Somehow now she was actually telling her mother about it, she didn't feel as acutely ashamed or tongue-tied as she had always feared she would if or when this moment ever arrived. She was just describing facts. Facts she knew she hadn't been responsible for, even if she had always *felt* as if she had been. Always had and always would.

'We should tell the police. He could have done it to someone else.'

'I know. That's what's been troubling me most ever since, but I did tell him I would go straight to them if I thought anyone else was at risk. And I told him Father Brady knew; that I had told him in confession and given him permission to tell the police if there was even a suspicion of him being in contact with any children again.'

'Well, Father Brady has been dead five years, but Jack has been paralysed for ten so it's probably alright. To think I felt so sorry for him and Bobbie. I still visit them every Wednesday afternoon. Poor Bobbie. She can't possibly know.'

'What happened to him? I mean, how did he get paralysed?'

Grainne didn't really want to know, but at the same time his fate held a morbid fascination for her.

'A swimming accident in a hotel pool down south. Drunk, I believe. He dived straight into the shallow end at night and broke his neck. I never dreamed I would ever say 'good thing', but it is a good thing, a very good thing.'

'I don't think Auntie Bobbie needs to know, Ma. The truth would only hurt her.'

'I think you're right. Maybe there are times when the truth doesn't need to be told.'

They were silent for a few moments as some kind of mother/daughter connection re-established itself between them. Now that her mother could understand how their connection had been broken, Grainne felt a forgiveness for herself and for her mother which was almost religious, except that it felt more real than the intangible, conceptual forgiveness religion had ever had to offer,

'So I still don't understand what you were ever doing that to yourself for,' said Moira O'Riordan, nodding at her daughter's arms.

'Nor do I. And as I said I've stopped now. Haven't done it for years.'

'What have you done then, over the last few years? I want to know everything.'

'There's not much worth knowing I *can* tell you.' It wasn't a lie. 'I've taken charge of my own life, is all. Grown up a little bit.'

'Grainne, come on now. As I wrote on that invitation I will only love you. I will not judge you. I am your mother. I felt so privileged just to be given your address last month. What made you decide to get back in touch? At least tell me that.'

'I missed you, Ma, that's all. And Da. I felt it was time to try and make up for all the missing years before I lost you both.'

'Oh, we are still a bit too young to be going just yet, I can tell you. I'm only going to be sixty, you know, not a hundred and sixty! And your father is still only sixty three. I think we've both definitely got a good few years yet in which to make up for all that lost time. Yes! Yes, we must all make the most of what time we have left, whatever age we are! Now, tell me more. Is there a 'partner'?' She furrowed her powdery brows at her use of this word, moved it on into a frown of concentration as she studied Grainne's face and saw that there wasn't a partner. 'Or children? Oh, Grainne, your face tells such a story. It is so hard to believe I never picked up anything was wrong when you were a little girl. So I'm a grandmother again? Well, that's grand, so it is. 'Grand' is just the right word for it.'

Grainne nodded. What else could she do? Sean was a fact.

'What is the child like? Why didn't you bring – him? Her? – Him! Why didn't you bring him with you? No! That was a very silly question and you don't have to answer it, my darling. Tell me about him.'

'His name is Sean. Sean Lucien. He'll be eleven in a couple of months. He doesn't live with me. A friend of mine looks after him. I made her his legal guardian.'

'For heaven's sake! Why?'

'I wasn't up to it, Ma. I couldn't do it. I don't know why exactly. I think there was too much on my mind and I wasn't giving him the love and attention he needed.'

'My poor girl. Why ever not?'

Oh well, perhaps the worst question of all. The worst answer anyway.

'I didn't want him, Ma. When I found I was pregnant I just didn't want him and I – I don't want to tell you this, Ma, so perhaps I won't. Some things *are* better left unsaid. I should live with my shame without sharing it. Anyway ten months after he was born I gave him away to someone who was and is able to give him what he needs. It was my own choice which I made freely after carefully considering what would be best for him, because – I'm sorry, Ma, to hurt your feelings – but I just didn't have wanting him anywhere inside me. I looked, believe me, and all I could find was that what I wanted for him was what was best for him and I felt that what was best for him was that someone else should look after him. Someone I knew would do a better job.'

Her mother was shaking her head.

'You are right to be angry with me, Ma.'

'Oh Grainne, Grainne. I'm not angry. I'm sad. And not just about what you have told me. There are things *I* have not told you. Oh dear, oh dear. How little we know of the patterns which repeat themselves. Down through the generations.' She shook her head from side to side, a curious combination of wonder and sadness on her face. 'How little we know. And if only I *had* known. I could have looked after him. I would have happily looked after him.'

Her mother was crying; she could see that she had failed to look after Grainne properly and keep her safe when she was a child, and so it would have been quite impossible for Grainne to have let her have Sean.

'I mean I would have tried to,' said Moira O Riordan. 'I will not lie to you.'

'What do you mean 'patterns which repeat themselves'?' Grainne asked. 'What patterns?'

'I mean that I gave *you* away after you were born! Although I had you back after nine months, but when you were born, I went mad. No really! There's no other word for it. Well, there is, actually. What was it the doctor said? I can't remember.'

'PND – post natal depression? No? Post puerperal psychosis?'

'Yes that's right. Psychosis. That's what they called it. I was depressed *and* confused, but at least I was sensible enough to know I had to let the nuns look after you until I got better. I knew that much. For my sins. And, you see, I thought that that was my own carefully considered choice too. I really believed it was. Your father couldn't look after you. Not full time. He was driving trucks all over Ireland, and even Europe sometimes, for

O'Keefe's Transport. And we couldn't do without the money. He did visit you though. Every time he had a day off. So the nuns looked after you for most of the first year of your life while I – I tried to regain my sanity. But, sure, that's not all, you see.' She lowered her voice to a fearful whisper and again spoke as if in wonder. 'The pattern affected your grandma too. You're Grandma gave *me* away when I was a child! Who knows if her mother, your great grandmother, gave *her* away too? I wouldn't be surprised now if she did, I really wouldn't.'

'Why, Ma? Why did Grandma give you away?'

'If I never told you it was not because it was a secret. I just never felt I could talk about it.' She shrugged. 'I felt like you felt just now: I cannot put it into words. I have never told anybody and it's all so long ago – more than half a century ago. And anyway it doesn't matter now.'

'What happened, Ma? Tell me, please. Be fair. It matters to *me*.'

'I don't really remember. Well, not everything. I was four or five years old. Goodness knows where your grandfather was at the time. Out drinking with friends? I don't know. He wasn't in that night anyway. The four of us lived in my grandma's fine stone house in Armagh. My grandfather – your great grandfather – had died some years before, but the house wasn't too big, even though it had three bedrooms, one for my Grandma, one for me and one for my ma and da. I – I had a little straw doll which my grandmother had put on the mantelpiece above the fireplace. I asked her for it one evening when I felt too cold to go to sleep. Winters *were* cold in those days. I had been sitting on my grandmother's lap in front of the fire trying to get warm. It was late. We were all in our nightdresses. My mother had gone out the room. I don't know why. To make some tea or a hot water bottle for my bed I think. And I asked Grandma to pass me my dolly. So she put me down from her lap and went to the fire place to get it. Her – her nightdress was set alight by a spark from the fire as she bent forward to reach for it, and I watched her go up in flames in front of me. The terrible thing was, she'd managed to get my dolly and had dropped it on the floor. It was fine, not burned at all.

'She didn't die immediately. It took a few days. Screaming the whole time. Her pain was unbearable. And it was all my fault. There was no ambulance service in those days and we had no phone of course – so she didn't get any relief from it. I would fill jugs of cold water for my mother to wash her with but she couldn't stand being touched. By anything. Most of her skin was burned in huge black-red blisters and weeping wheals. I still see them in my dreams. My ma made me watch as she bathed them. So I would learn, she said. I think the burns must have become infected. Or maybe she hurt so much that the stress and shock was just too much to bear. I don't know. But she died in her bed a few days later still whimpering and groaning with the pain and the agony of it. I won't ever forget her cries. Piteous. Absolutely piteous. And all because of me. My mother never forgave me. I think she loved me. I think she did. And I think it was *because* she loved me that she sent me away to live with my Auntie Caitlin, my father's older sister, long dead now of course, so that I wouldn't be exposed to her anger with me. She knew it was unfair to blame me, I think, but blame me she did and she felt it would be best for both of us if I went away. I can still remember so vividly – like it was yesterday, Grainne – my father putting me into our pony and trap with my suitcase and that awful doll, driving me to the next village and leaving me with Auntie Caitlin. I ended up staying there for three years. So you see, your little boy is at least the third generation in our family whose mother couldn't cope with him. There, now.'

Looking at her mother staring back into her past, Grainne shuddered and said,

'Oh, Ma! What a terrible thing to have carried around with you all these years.' She reached for her mother's plump be-ringed hand. She felt so sorry for her. Yet glad too. Glad to have in common with her the burden of carrying a guilty secret all her life.

'What happened to the doll?'

'I sewed a heavy stone into its belly with a darning needle and drowned her in the Boyne, just before grandfather prevailed upon my ma to have me home again,' replied her mother the murderess.

'At least we all – I mean you and Grandma and me – we all tried to do the right thing. We all recognised our deficiencies didn't we, Ma? At least that can be said in our favour.'

The silence between them was so stressful that Grainne found herself desperate to cheer her mother up. She fell into platitudes.

'We knew our weaknesses. We tried to make sure our babies wouldn't be too damaged by them. By giving them away. Not *too* damaged. At least we can say that.' She tried to pull her sleeves further down over her hands 'I am not damaged, Ma. Whatever I have told you. Truly I'm not.' She nodded her head repeatedly, making her face fierce with the demand that her mother should agree with her.

Moira O'Riordan understood this, blinked away her tears and nodded her head over and over again too. With her other hand she patted Grainne's which still lay on top of hers.

It *was* chilling that their shared pattern of being separated as children from their mothers and then in turn separating themselves from their children when they become mothers, seemed so much bigger than their good intentions. They both felt helpless together now, tiny cogs in the process of this awful pattern unfolding across the generations, but at least they didn't have to feel so alone anymore. Being joined with Ma as a victim of this pattern made it feel so inescapable that Grainne could feel the shared weight of all her ancestors and all her descendants each burdened by their own part in the same theme. It was chilling. She felt like running back into the bosom of the church and crying out for help to escape. But it was too late now. She'd given Sean away ten years ago, and stopped going to church with any faith when she stopped Jack from doing what he had to her ten years or more before that. She'd kept up appearances every Sunday for four years until she left for England, but she would never go back again. A brief visit for the sake of appearances tomorrow for Ma was one thing. She could manage that. But belief in a benign divine providence was quite another. What kind of a God could allow so much horror to happen to little children and their mothers?

Her poor mother. How terrible all her life to feel she killed her grandmother.

'Perhaps your little Sean, by being a boy will break the pattern. Perhaps he will be different from us when he is grown up. Perhaps he will keep his children.'

'I hardly know what he looks like. Lucille – that's my friend who looks after him – says he finds it almost impossible to relate with anybody except her husband and herself. And even then it's difficult. He's got a developmental problem, you see. He was born not quite right. It was my fault. I wanted to get rid of him. That's what I didn't want to tell you just now. He's quite clever, but he doesn't cope with anything very well, especially changes or unpredictable things. Or so I understand. I haven't actually seen him since he was a baby. I just prefer not to, but I think I understand a little better now *why* I don't. Lucille used to send me videos she made of him each Christmas, but after a few years I stopped her. It upset me too much.'

'So that's why you don't feed yourself properly,' said her mother, her powdered face now sunken like a soufflé. She was visibly trying to stop herself shaking her head from side to side and could not take her eyes off Grainne.

'What do you mean? And stop looking at me like that, please Ma. It's too much.'

'You feel so bad about not wanting your baby that you don't even want to feed yourself! And you were such a lovely plump girl when you were younger.'

'You've said that enough now, Ma. I heard you the first time. I had the symptoms of what they call an eating disorder long before I ever was pregnant with Sean. That's the diagnostic term. You had your post puerperal problems - I've had an eating disorder. Having a disorder doesn't necessarily mean that you are ill, just that you are not quite right and you can get ill with it sometimes. It's not serious unless you let it get out of control. And I don't. I can manage it very well by now. It's not a problem anymore at all.'

'It's my fault. I should have protected you from Jack. I should have realised there was something wrong. I don't know how I didn't. It's like I was blind to you. Oh Grainne, I have let you down so much. So very, very much. It's no wonder you could never come back to see us.'

'That's just a feeling, Ma. The fact is you never let me down. You did your best to look after all three of us girls, and Da, and you couldn't help what you didn't know, could you? You did fine. I am certainly alright myself and I'm sure Aislinn and Siobhan are too! Aren't they?'

'They're alright. Yes. As far as I know.'

'There you are then!'

'Sean is such a nice name. Why did you keep him for ten months only to give him away just when, well, you know Grainne, when babies start walking and trying to talk? Was your little Sean's development very delayed?'

'That wasn't the problem at all, Ma. There just wasn't anyone I felt I could let look after him till then. My friend Lucille had cared for him regularly for some months, but I only properly realised he was more likely to thrive with her, when it dawned on me how much better she was getting on with him than I was. Consistently.'

Her mother wouldn't stop shaking her head.

'Then I dropped him,' Grainne said, with a deliberately cold edge to her voice.

'You dropped him? Oh my good God, you poor girl! Was he badly hurt?'

'I don't think so, no. I was giving him a bath and he was all soapy and slippery. I lifted him out of the water. You know, so that I could refill it with fresh water and rinse him off. He slipped out of my hands and banged his head on the side. I picked him up immediately and he was alright, I knew he was, but I felt terrible about it. He hardly even cried and there was no bump or bruising or anything, but I felt so useless as a mother that I just didn't feel he was safe with me anymore. I knew it in my bones, you know? I was no good for him. In fact I was bad for him. When I told Lucille, she said that a bad mother wouldn't have bothered to pick him up at all. She didn't realise that it was purely instinctive, that there was nothing good about it at all. Anyone would have done it. But when she said that, I realised that she herself was such a positive person, a person who picks people up when they have fallen. In fact that's how we first met eleven or twelve years ago after I'd literally had a fall – slipped – in the park. It was Lucile who came to help me up on to a bench. She's a warm, friendly person. Not the world's brightest button, but really, really nice. So I thought and thought, and decided she was perfect for him, he would be far better off with her than with me. In fact I knew he would.

'I hadn't just dropped him because he was slippery, you see. I wasn't very strong physically at the time cos of my eating disorder. Not like I am now! I'd dropped him because he was too heavy and too wriggly for me. I just didn't have the strength to cope with a child. I wasn't eating at all, really at that time. To tell you the truth, Ma, I could hardly climb the stairs on my own, let alone with a baby. So I *knew* I was doing the best thing arranging for her to have him. And events have subsequently proved me right, I'm glad to say.'

'What about the father?'

'Hopeless. Actually after I had finished with him, he and Lucille were an item for a while. But that didn't last long either. He developed schizophrenic-type symptoms. Not a great genetic inheritance is it, when both your parents are mentally ill? Like me, Ron could hardly look after himself properly, let alone a baby. So I decided not to tell him he was a father. I felt it would be easier for both of them if he didn't know.'

'Grainne, this is such a sad story. I had so many dreams for you when you were a little girl. So many.'

'I know you did. That's why there was so much I couldn't tell you cos of what it would have done to them. But my life is sorted out now, Ma. I enjoy nursing. I *know* I made the right decision for my son. And there is absolutely no secret about it, so it's not as if he'll never know me. If he ever begins to consistently express a wish to see me, Lucille says she will be in touch straightaway and tell me. And then we'll meet, and that'll be fine. She tells him all about me whenever he asks. I send him a Christmas and birthday present each year. But so far he hasn't been curious about me at all, which is just how I want it to be. According to Lucille he's quite okay about it all, accepts things as they are, as natural, which for him, I suppose, they are. You don't miss what you don't know. Or who you don't know. Do you, now? So it's not actually so sad at all!'

'I realise now I never really knew you at all,' said her mother. 'But Grainne, I missed you terribly once you were gone, worse than if I had lost a part of myself. So I think you are actually wrong about that. I didn't know you, but I did miss you terribly.'

They looked at each other feeling their closeness and their distance like a sea between them.

Chapter 13.

Two weeks later Ronald Symes, Ph.D, was busy rearranging chairs for his afternoon session in the low-ceilinged hall he had hired at the hotel in Great Portland Street. His audience of professional and lay people had to be let back into the hall in five minutes time after the break for lunch. It was hot and the air-conditioning seemed to be only working on an intermittent basis. He would ask for some of the fee back for that. Bunching the chairs up more informally, he tried to move in a smooth unhurried way so that no signs of perspiration should make themselves visible on his shirt. He never sweated like he used to do when he was overweight and on medication. In public he was always as cool as a cucumber.

Some eighty people had signed up for the day at an exorbitant fee. But he did have his overheads. The morning session had gone well. His training seminars usually did. He was a psychologist and therefore well aware that when people parted with a substantial amount of money for a training course in advance, it meant they had an expectation and an investment in the subsequent experience being a satisfying one. He would aim to confirm their expectations. Of course there'd be the odd trouble-maker for whom nothing was good enough. But he was used to that by now too. It didn't matter. He had become adept at managing large groups of people and moving them in exactly the way he wanted .

The afternoon session involved a demonstration exercise with self-selected members of the audience in a small group, with everybody else observing and commenting. It usually went well because the voluntary nature of the role-playing ensured that there was high energy and enthusiasm amongst the participants, creating a spectacle which under his direction usually proved to be highly engaging for the audience.

Psycho-Educative Experiential Training, or PET as it was increasingly coming to be known thanks to his expert marketing skills, had proved gratifyingly popular since he had first started presenting one-day workshops and weekend residential seminars on the subject some fifteen months ago. Using his personal and professional contacts to access data bases belonging to various health, counselling and psychotherapy organisations, had reaped immediate dividends. A combination of carefully placed adverts in both professional and selected women's magazines, press releases, targeted mail-shots, leafleting, and e-mails had proved of great long term benefit for generating on-going publicity and interest, even though they had initially cost a lot of time and money. By setting himself up as a limited company, which he called PET Consultancy, and stressing in his publicity the relevance of psycho-educative experiential training both to the general public and to the helping professions, he ensured that it appealed to the widest range of people. The odd stupid enquiry from cat or dog lovers was an occupational hazard, but their nuisance-value was more than off-set by the positive connotations most people made of both the surface and subliminal meanings of the term 'PET'. Each event he put on nowadays was invariably sold out well in advance. He never put his own name on the adverts or workshops titles, always emphasising the corporate logo of PET Consultancy and its ability to attract world renowned presenters.

It was rubbish of course. There was only him, but as he did occasionally make derisory offers they could only refuse to famous therapists to come and speak, he felt able to namedrop them if necessary as previously invited speakers. Anyway, the punters still seemed to sign up and pay their money. If they didn't come flooding in neither were they a trickle. All in all it was very manageable and nicely lucrative. In due course he would begin putting some of the money he earned into actually inviting one or two guest speakers. It would give PET Consultancy more legitimacy.

Every workshop was conducted in much the same way. Didactic, bullet-pointed information-sharing until lunch-time followed by an afternoon of active audience involvement which provided an experiential basis for the ideas he had expounded in the morning. He called them his Key Ideas. There was nothing original about them. He would happily refer to great clinicians, thinkers, writers and artists of past and present as originators of these key ideas, and cast them as supporters of his completely derivative Master Key Idea: that taking a developmental perspective enables greater understanding of self and others, which in turn empowers everyone both to be and to do what they want more effectively.

He would intone sonorously about finding and clearing away emotional blockages as if he was a mental plumber or proctologist. He always laid great emphasis on personal pronouns so that members of his audiences felt they were being spoken to as individuals and emphasised the importance of personal experience in developing emotional intelligence.

'It's not difficult. It's not rocket science. Like most therapists, I always begin and end with the attachment relationship between mother and child. It's where we all began our experience of this world. So it's the best, indeed the only, starting-off point for psycho-educative understanding. If you leave here at the end of the day with only one thing, then leave with the fact of the *continuing* importance of that first neuropsychological bond you made with your mother at the very beginning of your life. Now some of us never made such a bond. Some of us, like myself, may have been abandoned at birth and put up for adoption, perhaps experienced multiple carers during those earliest formative years. Some of us bonded very poorly, if at all. Perhaps your mother was a prescription drug addict being treated for sleeplessness or depression and therefore unable to make a proper bond with you. Perhaps she died. But for all of us, an understanding of how it actually felt to be helpless, vulnerable and dependent – an infant in relation to a mother or indeed to a mother-absence – is vital if we are to understand *why* it is that we find ourselves again looking for those things, or their opposites, in our relationships now.'

Sotto voce, so that the audience had to keen their ears forward to hear him, he repeated, 'Right now. We look for what we got or did not get from our mothers and fathers in our current relationships with our lovers, our partners, our husbands, our wives, our colleagues, our friends and... our enemies. Everyone in fact.'

As he had done in all his previous talks he continued speaking in this clichéd repetitive manner, imparting basic, stereotyped information about the relationship between experience and human development, until he was sure every member of the audience understood exactly what he was going on about. People liked understanding. By talking about the importance they should give to trying to understand themselves, Ron gratified their self-regard before they had even heard half of what he had to say. They also liked a good personal story. So he would tell them that the relationship between his own early development and his here and now experience had itself been a life-long problem. He would tell them he fell victim to a schizophrenic-like illness in his late twenties which involved him believing that his thoughts and feelings had more universal importance than they did in fact have and which made him feel he had superhuman powers and could 'read' peoples minds and 'know' what they were thinking.

'Emotionally I was a simpleton,' he told them. 'Because during my earliest formative years I never had a proper experience of the complex growth-enabling interactions that occur between a baby and his mother. So that nearly thirty years later I thought I had a special cancer. A mental cancer. A cancer of the mind.'

Some members of the audience helpfully laughed. Others looked at them disapprovingly.

'I know. But my genuinely held belief, which I can assure you was almost psychotic in its intensity, was that this 'cancer' caused me to read too much meaning into things. I genuinely believed I was suffering from such an illness. Delusions of grandeur and ideas of reference were the least of my problems! Now you may ask yourselves how could a psycho-educative experiential training have helped me with that very serious problem? Well, I'll tell you. It helped me realise I was thinking like a small child who believed in magic and in his own magical powers; in a persecutory world of demons and monsters in human form. But ten years after my breakdown, here I am, with a Ph.d in Clinical Psychology, talking to you coherently – I hope – and free from any symptoms of mental illness whatsoever. And emotionally I am no longer as dim as I once was, at least I don't think I am!'

He put an exaggerated interrogative expression on his face, exposing a quasi-vulnerability which modestly invited members of the audience to gainsay him if they so wished. No-one did. He nodded his head gratefully, as if each one of them had contributed to the miracle of his new-found emotional intelligence.

'Now I'm not trying to brag or sell you a miracle cure. I am simply saying that PET is learning about human development and the effect that experience can have on it, and then seeing how that relates to your own particular circumstances. Adopting a PET approach can therefore have life-transforming effects on your sense of who you are. Thank you very much.'

The audience clapped enthusiastically. He smiled, nodded his gratitude for their attention, making sure he made eye-contact with as many people as possible as he did so. But it was the almost hypnotic effect of repetition in his talks that he found tended to most involve and enthuse the punters who came to listen to him. By deliberately picking up on the most important word in each preceding sentence and repeating it in the next, he found that audiences would get hooked into even the most complex material. It was a technique he had known about academically for years because, of course, the most charismatic politicians tended to do it in their speeches all the time. He first found out for himself just how powerful it was when, in trying to escape the rain one night, he accidentally stumbled in upon an African-American preacher using it at an evangelical tub-thumping session at the old Hackney Empire. It had been a revelation to experience in the flesh just how easy it was to manipulate a large group of people into agreeing with you. He had hurried home and then spent the whole of the next month breaking his Ph.D thesis into its constituent parts and repackaging it for popular consumption in a simplified, repetitive format. Then he had set up PET Consultancy and since then had never looked back.

He might even get onto satellite television one day.

He opened the doors to allow people to re-enter the hall for this afternoon's session. He always thought of the first hour after lunch as the snooze session. Particularly on really hot days like this one. Full stomachs and warm sunshine guaranteed that at least half the audience would be struggling to stay awake – those who had bothered to come back in from the sun. Today he expected at least three quarters of them to return, maybe more. The morning had gone well enough. He'd spent the second half of it showing them the research statistics supporting his approach in brightly coloured columns, continually sugaring and spicing the dryness of his material with case vignettes, tales of personal tragedies averted, confidences regained and relationships restored to their former glories. To engage your audience you had to appeal to both hemispheres of the brain. He felt he had succeeded in that this morning. His presentation had generated plenty of discussion and a final spontaneous round of applause when it finished just before lunch.

When the room had filled up again he began by reviewing what he had done in the morning.

'Before lunch we were looking at how psycho-educative experiential training enables more effective being and doing. This afternoon you will demonstrate it for yourselves. I need some volunteers who are interested in bringing a problem, or as I termed it this morning, a blockage which they don't mind sharing with us and to which we can apply some PET perspectives, either a current one, or one from the past. It really doesn't matter.'

Hands went up. He chose two men and four women at random and asked them to join him on the raised area at the front.

The first one up decided to be clever. A soft chinless man in his late forties with rimless spectacles and thinning hair which seemed to stand up on end, he clearly wanted an audience himself. Well, he would get one. Ron never let himself be burdened by chips on shoulders, whether his own or anyone else's.

'Excuse me, Dr. Symes, but aren't you just re-jigging some of the old insights of psychoanalysis – I'm thinking about Freud amongst others – for the twenty first century? All this talk about blockages, anality in the psychoanalytic jargon, and the need to look at one's own past experience suggests as much anyway'

'Indeed I am. And yes, you are absolutely right.'

One of his rules for public engagements like this was to always disarm pompous pricks like this one with Oppositional Defiance Disorder – ODD – by agreeing with them.

'Absolutely,' he repeated. 'Thank you for pointing that out. As I said this morning, there is nothing intrinsically new in PET. Other key ideas derive, for example, from attachment theory and neuropsychology. Indeed any discipline which helps us learn more about ourselves. So you are absolutely right. At least in some ways. The main difference between PET and a psychoanalytic approach, for example, is that I believe that patients and therapists can be much more focused and purposive in what they do together. I would argue that rather than waiting, as the psychoanalysts do, for the material to arise naturally and in its own time out of the relationship between their patients and themselves, we need to get straight to the point and fast-track the development of the sine qua non of effective and successful change, namely the Relationship itself. Capital R.'

He turned to the main audience on the floor and spoke to them directly. It was important not to lose them.

'As many of you know, ladies and gentlemen, most if not all schools of therapy believe that the relationship between therapist and client is without doubt the single most important agent of therapeutic change. But sadly, whether we like it or not, time is money. We therefore have to cut the cra– I mean, we have to hurry up and get on with the process of building the relationship, by actively deciding what we are going to work on.

'But enough of these arcane distinctions. I don't want people yawning and glazing over. What I do want, this afternoon, is to bring some of what we've been talking about alive by way of demonstrations of PET in action. The first demonstration will show how groups make decisions and more particularly how a PET approach can actually facilitate a group's decision-making processes. The second will focus on an individual.'

He asked his six volunteers to sit in a semi-circle facing the audience and told them their task was to decide together which one of them, and it could only be one, would remain for the second half of the afternoon so that his or her and only his or her particular problem could be worked with.

'What I am asking you to do is to choose amongst you who is the most deserving of an exclusive personalised PET approach later on. None of you know each other, do you? No? Good. Some of you may not actually want to be the one who is selected either. In which case I suggest you leave and go back to your seat right now so that I can invite someone else to come up and take your place.'

Nobody moved. Good. You could hear a pin drop. For the moment anyway he had both the audience and the volunteers where he wanted them.

'What I would like you to do is simply discuss it together. Whenever any one of you decides they don't want the personal session later on, or decides they would prefer someone else to have it, please feel free to get up and go back to your seat in the main part of the hall. I will occasionally interrupt the discussion, ask you to freeze, and share a few observations from a psycho-educative experiential training perspective. Is that clear? Any questions? No? Alright. Please introduce yourselves by name and, if you wish, by professional background and then begin your discussion together. Thank you.'

He picked up a chair with deliberate ostentation and moved it well away from his six volunteers who looked politely at one another, seemingly at a loss, waiting for someone to go first. At the side, Ron stood up again.

'And so, right at the outset I have to make my first interruption. Psycho-educatively it is as if none of those present has resolved the delicate balance between assertiveness on the one hand and respect for, or deference to others on the other. Developmentally this suggests that as a group you have decided, so far anyway, to remain still. It is a group regression to the definitively static, helpless infantile developmental stage at which it is not yet possible to walk. At the same time however, there is considerable awareness, rather than ignorance, of what is going on in the world around you. Between six and twelve months old, approximately. So you could perhaps experiment with crawling!'

He gave the six participants a warm ingratiating smile. Light laughter rippled across the audience, and the six volunteers smiled back at them, good sports each one of them. Then they looked at each other sheepishly. All except the man with the sticky-up hair who was clearly a bit of a goat.

'Meaning no offence, I think that's an easy thing to say. I suspect few us of would disagree with it, but I don't really see how it takes us any further.'

'With equal respect,' replied Ron evenly, knowing that 'no offence' was always used offensively, 'I again have to say that I absolutely agree with you, and would merely want to point out that you yourself have now kindly taken things further by speaking up and asserting yourself. I believe it takes courage and skill to do that, and would therefore hazard a guess that experientially helping others out is something you have often done before. It may or may not be a block for you personally, I don't know. Thank you anyway, very much indeed.'

Acknowledging the accuracy of this hypothesis and unsure whether to be flattered or flustered, the man introduced himself as Aidan, a social worker from Lambeth. He looked to the others to introduce themselves. The other male waited on the women to go first. They identified themselves as Anne, Geraldine, Yvette and Lucille, a community nurse, a charge nurse on a psychiatric ward, a GP, and a student respectively. As they did so, Ron scanned the watching audience for drooping heads. None so far. The other man in the group then declared himself to be George, a voluntary sector worker.

Affirmed in his role as leader, Aidan looked to Ron for approval which he got in the form of a benign nod and an agapaeic smile. 'Yes, please do, get the ball rolling, Aidan. Thank you.'

'Well, this is very difficult. We are being asked to be both generous and selfish at one and the same time,' he began.

'I don't know about that,' said George. 'I think we are simply being asked as a group to find a way of identifying the person who would benefit most from a focussed PET session. That's all.'

The community nurse and the GP nodded their agreement with this view.

'Well, I just don't think it is simple,' said Aidan, reddening slightly.

'Neither do I' said Geraldine, the overweight, over-heated ward sister whose dyed blonde hair was sticking to her sweat-beaded, red forehead.

'Perhaps we should each spend a minute or so stating what the problem is we would like a PET session for and then we could decide whose need we felt was the most urgent or the most deserving,' said Yvette, the middle-aged GP. She had a Yorkshire accent and was wearing a crumpled brown linen trouser suit and flat sandals. She was fanning herself with her information pack, and looked keen if not impatient to get on with it.

'Yes,' said the student, Lucille, with some enthusiasm. 'Then we could take a vote on who it should be. That might be fairest, don't you think?'

Ron thought he had heard that cheerily inconsequential voice before somewhere. He looked at her intently trying to place her. A pretty enough woman in her late twenties or early thirties. And then he recognised her. My god, it is. It's my former flat mate, my little transsexual ex-lodger. What a turn up. After all these years. Had she recognised him? Yes, of course she had. He could tell by the way she wasn't looking at him as she spoke. Well, well. What a surprise. He remembered his disappointment all those years ago when he'd gone to collect his dog from that woman Lulu used to live with, and she had told him Lulu had deliberately gone out for the afternoon, refusing to see him because of how he had tricked her the year before into believing the dog was dead. And now here she was, after all this time. And of course she had recognised him. She had probably noticed his name on an information leaflet or a poster. Interesting.

He watched her face colour and fall as Aidan gave an unashamedly sneering response to her suggestion.

'I don't think that would be fair at all, actually,' he said. 'I mean if you look at it, that would all depend on who was the best one-minute-storyteller, rather than on who could really benefit most from an individualised PET consultation.'

'It's as good a criterion as any other I would have thought,' said Yvette, looking at Lucille with a smile.

'Perhaps we should put it to the audience to decide for us,' said the tall, wiry George from behind his beard and heavy-framed spectacles.

'I think Dr Symes said we had to come to a decision ourselves,' Aidan replied loftily, looking to Ron for confirmation.

'Which could, of course, include a decision to confer with the audience,' said Yvette, not concealing her impatience with the social worker.

'Well I've come to a decision myself,' announced the community nurse, getting up off her chair. 'I have changed my mind. I would prefer to observe.'

She nodded curtly at the other five with a small smile and made her way back to her seat in the audience without making eye contact with Ron. He smiled, stood up and asked them to freeze.

'A PET analysis of Anne's decision to leave the group might be that experientially Anne has a low tolerance of dithering, that she perhaps received too many mixed messages as a child which resulted, in adulthood, in her still feeling impatient with confusion in others. At the same time she has herself reflected the kind of upbringing she received – we cannot get away from our pasts – by sending out mixed messages herself, the evidence for which is in her coming and going, changing her mind about a PET consultation. But of course without knowing you, Anne, that's one hell of an assumption to make on my part and I must assure you that I am being completely hypothetical here. Your reasons for going back to your seat are of course completely your own and are just as likely to have nothing whatsoever to do with what I've just said.'

He gave her his least smug, most self-effacing smile as she sat down in her chair five or six rows back in the middle, nodding her head all the while in apparent complete agreement with what he was saying. It was important to pre-empt any hostile reaction to his words by getting her retaliation in first himself, accusing himself of what she might otherwise have accused him of. She stood up again.

'Actually, you may well be right, as a matter of fact, consistency and commitment have never been my strong points,' she bellowed across the heads in front of her. 'But I actually felt far too hot up there even though the windows are open. And as I am a little hard of hearing and the sound of the traffic outside was very loud from there, making it difficult for me to get hold of the discussion properly I thought it best to leave you all to it.'

'Thank you, Anne,' said Ron looking out at the audience as a whole. 'A PET analysis of Aidan and Yvette's different views, suggests that developmentally the group discussion has rapidly moved from infancy to adolescence. The tension between trying to come to their own decisions and/or leaving it to the adults – you, the audience – to set the boundaries, is a quintessentially adolescent one. Now I cannot over-emphasise that my continual reliance upon a developmental analysis should not be understood in any way as implying any kind of insult at all, none whatsoever. That is the mistake so many people make when developmental observations are deployed. They think you are accusing them of being like babies or children or adolescents, that you are patronising them, when really all you are doing is simply pointing out behaviours which are developmentally characteristic of that particular stage in our growth and maturation. Stages which all of us – every adult human being on this planet – has been through, and can therefore return to behaviourally or feel blocked at emotionally at any time. So it is vital not to feel personally insulted by a PET perspective.'

He turned to the group of five on the stage, nodded at them to continue and sat down again.

'Alright we seem to be agreed on what we're going to do. A few brief words from each of us in turn about why we want a PET consultation and then we'll take it from there,' said George. 'Would it help if I started? Okay? Right. My problem is work-related.' He droned on about being under-funded and understaffed and being expected to provide a service for the whole range of learning disabled people in his London borough with only three other staff. When he'd finished he glanced around at the other four. He got a lot of sympathetic noises from them and from people in the audience. He looked gratified and asked, 'Who'll go next?'

'I will,' said Yvette, the GP. 'My problem is also work-related. I am quite simply overloaded. I work in a busy Halifax surgery and we have an excellent practice manager who devotes herself to finding new ways of cutting down the volume of work and still meeting patient needs. I am considering going part-time because if I don't, the workload is going to cause me to have, well, a nervous breakdown – not to put too fine a point on it. My husband left me ten years ago and my daughter has finished university and found a job locally, so it is not as if I need to be earning as much as I was. I would like a PET consultation to help me decide what it would be best to do at this point in time. That's all.'

She looked expectantly at the three who hadn't spoken yet. They continued to be silent, until Geraldine, the plump peroxided nurse came to the rescue.

'Mine's a personal problem, I'm afraid. Is that alright?' She looked across at Ron, whose nod signified 'of course'. 'I'm worried my boyfriend, who I love, I really do, is beginning to, you know, like, play away. He complains I'm like his mother because I always nag him, which is a bit of an insult to his mother if you ask me!' There was a warm Welsh lilt to her accent and she elicited a few kind laughs from the audience. 'Besides not being strictly true. I don't *always* nag him. So I'd like a PET consultation to help give me some ideas about how I can control my tongue; so I don't lose him altogether.' She wiped her nose with the back of her hand, sniffed and said, 'When he does come in, I can't help it, I find myself *at* him, you know, asking where he's been and what he has been up to. Well, he says nowhere and nothing. He always says that. What can I do? That's what I want to know. And what should I do?'

She flushed with what looked like simultaneous embarrassment and pride. She had said what she had wanted to say. Some members of the audience started briefly clapping. Ron never ceased to be amazed at the extent to which some people would expose themselves.

There was just Aidan and Lucille left to speak.

'After you,' he said to her.

'Okay. Thank you. Well I have this little boy, Sean, you see. He's eleven. He suffers from Attention Deficit and Hyper-activity Disorder. ADHD. I won't have him medicated because I'm sure that with love and time he'll grow out of it. But a psychiatrist has diagnosed him with a kind of autistic problem as well. Aspergers Syndrome, she said, 'maybe'. Labels are all very interesting, they really are, I do read up about them on the internet and I'm fascinated – really! – but they don't actually help very much in coping with the day to day problem of caring for him. I don't really believe anything can, to be honest. He only sleeps a couple of hours at a time at night, and sometimes he kicks me and bites me. I don't know what to do. I can't send him away to a boarding school. I love him. And anyway he is always so much worse when he is away from me. But I can't go on for much longer with things as they are!' She shrugged appealingly. 'I want it both ways, I suppose.'

She dipped her head as she finished speaking and reached down for her handbag on the floor beside her for a tissue. Ron had been watching her closely and found himself wondering whether he had got it wrong. It couldn't be, could it? A husband and a son? Yet he got no sense of her lying. Perhaps the name was a coincidence. After all, it was ten or eleven years since he had last seen Lulu. She could have gone blonde, he supposed. That was quite possible. A husband too, maybe. But children were not. No, he must have got it wrong. It must be someone else. Except that that sing-song voice couldn't be anybody else's. Could it? Of course it was her. It had to be

It was Aidan's turn. Ron watched Lucille look at Aidan expectantly, then shoot a sudden glance through the group at him. Seeing that he was gazing directly back at her she immediately looked down again, popping her tissue back into her bag before returning her attention to the social worker who, with a self-important clearing of the throat, said,

'I would like a PET consultation to help me with an elderly client who for obvious reasons of confidentiality I cannot go into too much detail about. Suffice to say she is in her early sixties and suffering from fairly advanced dementia. She is always living in the past. Multiple blockages – to use your word Dr Symes – which cause her to relive, and believe she is actually in, incidents from her past. I always ask her how old she is every time I visit her and she looks at me like I'm stupid and says she's five, or fifteen, or fifty, or whatever it is. I'd like to help her to find a way of remaining in the present and letting go of the past. Although I'm not sure how kind that would be. I have to say that most of her relived/re-experienced memories are painful and unhappy ones, and that she is still able to live at home. I am concerned that if she deteriorates further she soon won't be.'

They all sat for a moment in silence digesting what each had had to say

'So how are we going to decide who it will be?' George eventually asked. 'I'd like to suggest that perhaps we decide whether it should be someone with a personal problem like Lucille or Geraldine, or whether it would be better to keep it professional and go with Aidan or me. I think Yvette's might be the one I'd choose myself, because her stress-at-work issue is both professional and personal.'

'Well, that's very kind of you,' said Yvette, 'but I feel Lucille or Geraldine's problems are much more serious than mine, as is Aidan's but I fear, Aidan that yours is insoluble. I think I will bow out myself now.'

She got up smiling and brooking no argument returned to her seat.

'From a PET perspective,' said Ron, standing up and holding up his hands at the remaining group of four to freeze, 'the ability to consider and to care for others is very much a mature adult position to take. Yvette has demonstrated this by leaving you, but so to has George by focussing on it as a group issue. Developmentally speaking, the group itself is thus becoming more mature.'

He sat down again.

'I don't mean to be rude but personally I feel a bit manipulated into behaving in a more 'mature and adult' manner by Dr Symes.' said Aidan. 'At the same time, of course, I do actually want to behave in a mature and adult manner, so I'm in a bit of a bind really because my natural inclination is to rebel like, like a teenager. If I may be so bold as to provide my own PET analysis!'

Well please do, you pompous little arsehole thought Ron, smiling benignly at him.

'I do feel your old lady is a really deserving case,' said Lucille, 'so I think I should go back to my seat now as well, if you don't mind.'

'No, please don't. Your problem is far more worthy of attention than mine,' said Geraldine, demonstrating a generosity of spirit as ample as her figure, and lifting herself heavily from her seat. 'I need an agony aunt rather than PET. And like Anne I feel it's too hot up here. But I think you should stay, Lucille, I really do.'

She left to the sound of one or two claps from the audience as she did so. Aidan, George and Lucille were left.

'What are we going to do?' George asked the other two. 'Draw lots? Toss a coin?'

'Yours I think is an organisational problem, and mine is perhaps only temporarily soluble as my client's brain cells continue to die off. I think we should let Lucille have it,' said Aidan.

'Yes, I agree,' said George.

The two men got up and both of them wished Lucille well, nodded at Ron and went along the moral high ground back to their seats. Ron stood up.

'Well, ladies and gentlemen, what you have seen this afternoon is a group of people working in an extraordinarily collaborative way – And with the minimum of conflict! – to come up with a solution to the conundrum I gave them. Psycho-educatively, I think one can safely say that rather than there being any blockage, what we had was a fully developed, mature and civilised discussion which allowed the members of the group to act in the best interests both of the group itself and of the person they in the end decided was their most deserving member on this particular occasion. On another day it might have been someone else. In terms of PET, the group rapidly developed, grew up and generously responded in a kind and adult manner to a request that was itself both kindly meant and adult in its intention to provide you with a learning experience. Do as you would be done by! The experience of being treated in a dignified and respectful manner was mirrored by a dignified and respectful group process. The psycho-educative experience of being treated as adults enabled the group to respond as adults. It's simple and it is obvious. Everything about PET is obvious. The problem is, of course, it is easy to overlook the obvious, so that we cannot see what's right in front of our faces!'

He paused to let his words sink in.

'Now I think we will adjourn for the mid-afternoon tea and coffee break, reconvening in half an hour's time. In the meantime, I'll try to find out what has happened to the air conditioning in here.'

The audience applauded enthusiastically. Then chairs shuffled, bags were picked up, and the murmur of multiple conversations quickly filled the hall as people bunched up by the doors, heading for the tea trolleys and the loos in the corridor outside.

'Perhaps I could ask you,' said Ron, turning to Lucille with a warm professional smile, 'to wait with me a while so that I can fill you in a little about what to expect from the second half of the afternoon session.'

He pulled up a chair beside Lucille and politely held out a hand to her before sitting down. He couldn't remember physical details after all this time, but the size and feel of her hand in his, the softness of her skin and the bone structure of her face were unmistakably that of a genuine female. Nevertheless she knew him. The expression on her face made that quite clear. So it had to be. There could be no doubt.

'You have the same name and indeed look remarkably like someone I knew over a decade ago,' he said, offering her the opportunity to deny it. 'I just wondered –

'It's me, Ron. Lulu.'

'I knew it! Actually I wasn't altogether sure it was you, especially when you mentioned marriage and children. I have to admit that confused me. Still does. But this is amazing. How are you?'

He held onto her hand, patted it. She was smiling at him in an almost inane manner, he thought, making no attempt to remove her hand from his. She seemed grateful to have been chosen by the group and delighted he had recognised her; as if she wouldn't have approached him or identified herself to him if he hadn't taken a lead. He warned himself not to be conned for a moment by her charms even if they were no longer so spurious, remembering with a small hollow pang of residual anger that ten years ago she had been the one to lead, knew precisely where she wanted to take him, and the upshot was his life with Grainne, even his sanity had been destroyed. Despite these feelings he couldn't help responding to her transparent pleasure at seeing him again. It was nice to see her again too, kind of.

'I hope the problem you mentioned with your son is the only serious one you've currently got on your plate, because by the sound of what you were saying just now, it's quite enough!' He looked deeply into her eyes with his customary combination of the suave and the empathic. 'Quite enough. But it's wonderful to see you again after all these years. You look very well and er, very good Lulu,' he added, giving her a once-over with the frank ballsiness he reserved for girlfriends and ex-girlfriends. He was gratified to observe her smiling and glancing down at the floor with the usual mix of modesty and pleasure so many women affected when he flattered them. When she looked back up at him again he caught her gaze and held it, giving her his warmest smile. Her face lit up.

'So do you, Dr Symes,' she said breathlessly, continuing to grin stupidly at him. '*Doctor* Symes! It's amazing! I didn't recognise you at first. Then I just couldn't believe it! You've lost a lot of weight since I last saw you. And you used to have a beard. But even so, I should have realised it was you! But it took me nearly half an hour of convincing myself I wasn't imagining things. I didn't even recognise your name on the poster – Dr Ronald Symes. Wow!'

'Perhaps you'll meet up with me afterwards and we can catch up a little on what's been happening to each of us over the years? I mean you're married!?'

'I got married in France. They've always been much more civilised over there. Five years ago. But I'm on the verge of divorce now. My husband has changed. People do, don't they? But not always for the worst,' she added, her mouth dropping open as she stared at him for a moment before she closed it again with a self-conscious abruptness which amused him. Again he recalled the shamelessness with which she had seduced him all those years ago. Perhaps there were some things in a person that just don't change at all. Well he had changed and he wasn't so easily manipulated anymore.

'I have really enjoyed today so much. You speak so clearly. And,' she furrowed her brow as if searching for the right word, then broke into another smile, 'so lucidly. And Lulu likes lucid,' she said with an inane grin. 'Very much.'

He couldn't help grinning back, but felt something close to embarrassment at being flattered this obviously. Didn't she realise how obvious she was being? He could hardly believe that he used to feel thick in her company.

Perhaps she also had a leucotomy when they cut off her *cojones*. Two operations for the price of one or something. Or maybe there had been complications and the general anaesthetic had caused a little brain damage. But she was pretty. There was no denying that.

'Everything feels so much easier somehow. Or it did while I was actually listening to you anyway,' she said. She must have noticed the slightly sceptical eyebrow he was trying to hold down because she nodded her head, added, 'I know. But it really did!' She widened her eyes in an obvious and inept attempt to emphasise she was telling the truth. 'I need to be more grown up with Sean. I really know that now.'

Many women came to his workshops simpering and gushing in this kind of way without actually wanting anything from him at all. Nevertheless the stereotyped nature of her display now both attracted and annoyed him. They used to know each other, for fuck's sake. He didn't need her playing the dumb blonde for him. Ten years ago it might just have been acceptable but she didn't have to pretend to be something she wasn't anymore. Perhaps she couldn't help it, but it simply served to remind him she was a genitally restructured, hormonally altered fake. Even if she did radiate psychological and anatomical harmony as she gazed at him with the kind of undisguised adoration he had only ever had from women. And then only in recent years. Never mind. How she behaved was her business and he certainly knew how to exploit this kind of fawning to the hilt.

He looked her up and down. Nice legs, good figure, pretty face. He deliberately let his appreciation show again until she had the grace to blush and look away down the empty hall towards the open doors at the other end. The animated murmur of voices and the clinking of cups and spoons were redolent of a successful day's work. He would let Lulu's presence here in front of him give it an unexpected extra spice, allow it to pleasantly remind him of how much he himself had moved on since he had last seen her, even if she hadn't. Not in terms of her personality anyway.

Thinking about the good old bad old days, it was quite clear she had to have told Grainne about their dalliance. There could be no other explanation. Well, he thought, who knows? Perhaps he'd like a little revenge for the distress she caused him back then.

'Will you stay on afterwards?' he said. 'We could find somewhere for a drink, maybe a bite to eat?'

'Well that's very nice and I'd love to, I really would, Ron, but I have to get back for Sean. He's spending the day with a friend of mine who's got a little boy just a bit older than he is. Not that they get on very well together really. He wasn't happy about it at all this morning. In fact he was so angry with me that Richard, my husband, ended up having to lift him physically into the car kicking and screaming. I felt so awful about it, I nearly decided not to come here today. But I'm so glad I did. Anyway, when I spoke to Richard later on the phone, he said Sean did actually settle down by the time they got round there. I rang up during your coffee break this morning to see if he was alright and he'd been surprisingly well behaved. I promised to pick him up by six thirty or seven this evening. I could ring Julia, I suppose, and ask her whether she wouldn't mind if I was a bit later. I don't know.'

She looked at him sideways, probably angling for him to show some interest. Not a problem.

'Yes do! It would be great to catch up.'

'It would, wouldn't it! But I don't know how Sean will take my being late for him.'

She was definitely regarding him more deeply than was necessary. Perhaps she too was remembering what they used to do together. Fine. It would be an easy matter to seduce her, he could feel it in his bones. If he wanted to. Whatever, it was a pleasure to feel able to turn the tables. Even after all these years. He would ring Sophy when he got a moment and tell her he couldn't go out with her tonight.

'I do hope you will. But we can talk about that later. Now about this session,' he said. 'I am simply going to interview you about your son and–

'He's not really *my* son, of course. You are one of the very few people who know that that's actually not possible, Ron. But he's *like* my son. He really is. And I have been like a mother to him since he was a tiny baby. He calls me Mum and I am his legal guardian, but actually he's not mine. He's–

Her face went white and her mouth fell open.

'He's what, Lulu?' he asked intrigued. 'Are you alright? You look as white as a sheet.'

'Oh, dear! I'm so sorry, Ron. I'm so dumb. It's only just registered. He's yours! I'm sorry, but he's yours. Oh, dear!'

'I'm sorry?'

He found himself pushing his chair backwards a little and suddenly feeling a cold sweat. Perhaps her bizarre life had driven her over the edge, poor thing. Well, he could still remember what that was like. But he was disconcerted and he didn't understand.

'Mine? I'm sorry?'

He must stay cool, not get rattled. He leaned forward again. This time she took his hand in both of hers, widening her eyes again in that synthetic way that had irritated him a few moments ago and furrowed her brows in apology and concern. There was something so inauthentic about her that she was almost a picture of herself. And just as she had ten years ago, she was upsetting him. He would seduce her and leave her. It would

216

be a nice turnaround. But he was the father of her child? That was impossible. She was obviously confused.

'I am too,' she said. 'Sorry, I mean. I shouldn't have just come out with it like that. I should have told you later. But I didn't know I was going to blurt it out. I really didn't. I'm so stupid sometimes. I am sorry, Ronnie. It must be an awful shock. He looks a lot like you, actually. The same brows and cheeks and nose, but he's got his mother's eyes and mouth. And her colouring. He's ginger like she is. Oh, dear,' she said to herself again, clearly stifling a giggle. 'Oh, dear. This is getting worse and worse.'

He wanted to make sense of what she was saying, but this wasn't the right time. He had to remind himself that although he didn't know much about them, transsexuals were notoriously borderline. That much he did know. He would have to question her carefully over the next few minutes, make sure she was actually a suitable subject for a public demonstration. It could cause incalculable damage to all the hard work he'd put into building up PET Consultancy if she turned out to be a screaming berserker. Or even a blackmailer. That was unlikely, but possible, he supposed, the cold sweat becoming freezing.

Not feeling so confident at all, his nether regions tightened. An ancient feeling of deep uncertainty and danger, which always used to be accompanied by delusions of meaning and grandeur, flitted across the bottom of his belly towards his bum. He immediately dismissed it. The feeling itself was a delusion. He clenched his buttocks.

'I'm not sure what you mean. I'm sorry, but I'm afraid this is all a bit beyond me just at the moment, although I would be very interested to know what you're talking about later. I really would. But I think we should concentrate on the task in hand right now, if you don't mind. We can talk about your little boy afterwards.'

She still had a hold of his hand. She squeezed it repeatedly as she spoke.

'She didn't tell you, did she? No of course she didn't. I remember her saying to me she wasn't ever going to because she felt you weren't up to being a father. Not unless hell freezes over, she said, or at the very least a miracle occurs. Well I think it might have. It has to have! Because she'll be so angry at me for blurting it out unless we sort it out properly.' She gave him an apologetic appealing look which said we're in this together now which didn't really appeal to him at all. Not under the circumstances. 'So thank you, I will,' she said.

He looked at her blankly. What was she talking about?

'I will meet with you afterwards, Ron. I must! I'll call Richard, explain to him what's going on and then we can take as long as we like and I'll tell you all about Sean. But now, yes please, do tell me what you want me to say or do. I'm a bit shy. You know! I have never done this kind of thing before. I think I'm in shock. I feel numb. Cold.'

She trembled, half shivering, half shuddering. He found it incongruous in the broiling heat of the afternoon, but was attracted to the vulnerability. Feeling not too dissimilar himself, he found himself wanting to warm her.

Ridiculous.

'Yes,' he said reassuringly. 'We'll talk about it all afterwards. Of course we will. Now then, all I want you to do for the purposes of my workshop is simply respond as honestly as you can to a series of questions that I will ask you about your little boy.'

She nodded repeatedly at his every other word but he could see she was not really concentrating on what he was saying at all.

'As I said Ron, he's your little boy.' She spoke very softly, full of understanding, like she was trying to soothe him, and if he didn't know how lucky he was. Fuck that.

Anyway, he didn't have time to feel patronised. People were already beginning to come back into the hall. He gathered himself together and gently but firmly disengaged his hand from hers.

'About er, Sean, you said his name was? The questions will take a developmental focus both on Sean himself and on the attachment relationship between the two of you. Does he call your husband 'Dad'?'

'No, all he knows is that he doesn't know his own mother or father, but that he could see his mother if he really wanted to.'

'Okay, we'll stay with that. I'll keep questions to do with his biological origins to a minimum. But I will be asking the audience for questions for you about his care and development. I'll field any questions you find difficult or don't want to answer, if you look across at me for help. Just give me a glance. After that I will work with the audience to formulate some suggestions in answer to *your* stated reason for coming up onto the platform, namely what are you to do to enable yourself to feel less emotionally stretched when looking after him. Does that feel alright?'

'Perfectly,' she said, thankfully seeming to pick up on his need at the moment to keep up a professional impression. 'Are *you* alright?'

'Fine,' he replied, coolly. 'We'll talk afterwards. Definitely.'

He felt angry. All his years of hard work, from his early elocution lessons and foundation courses whilst still on anti-psychotic medication, through his mastery of the grammar of social interaction, to his Ph.D, had brought him a respectable position of authority. He was now the one who disarmed people and solicitously asked them whether they were alright. Not the other way round. Suddenly in a matter of moments it felt as if the tables were in danger of being turned again by her solicitousness. They weren't of course. But he didn't like being on the receiving end of anyone's concern. It made him feel uncomfortable, as if he was mentally struggling again after all these years. Well, he certainly wasn't about to let that happen. He would reassert his power and control.

'Sometimes individual members of the audience can seem a little too enthusiastic or pushy. But don't worry, if there is anybody like that I will deal with them. Just leave everything to me. Er, I think for the purposes of the demonstration it would be better if we didn't reveal our previous knowledge of one another, don't you?'

He put this last point as blandly as possible, not letting his eyes narrow as he spoke.

'Oh absolutely! Yes. I mean, no! Of course not. I mean, we actually are complete strangers now aren't we? Well, like complete strangers! I certainly won't let on about our previous... friendship. Certainly not. I'm a respectable married woman now. And I never ever think about the past.'

Her lips pursed attractively and she shook her head. Despite the heat she again seemed to shudder slightly. From gazing intently into his face all this time she now cast her eyes down again. Was she looking at his genitals? He recalled the audible sighs of satisfaction she used to make when she'd finished fellating him all those years ago and stared across at her shapely little knees and the barely visible tops of her breasts as she sat there in her white cotton frock. She was doing such a good impression of prim and proper he would have been completely prepared to believe it if he hadn't known better.

He got out of his chair and started to shift the other chairs back off the raised stage area and onto the floor. Lulu excused herself saying she needed to go the ladies loo before they restarted. He nodded, smiled and watched her go.

But he was disconcerted. There was no doubt about that. And this baby business was bizarre. And worrying. He didn't want a paternity suit filed against him. Was she talking about Grainne? She must be. Grainne was the only ginger girl he had ever had sex with, and the only one of his past girlfriends he had actually lived with for any significant period of time. And of course she was also the only one Lulu would have known. Nevertheless he couldn't have his past catching up with him. Not in this way. He had to be in control of his history. Serendipity or happenstance could not be allowed to interfere. He didn't mind being open about his schizophrenic diagnosis, or misdiagnosis as he now recognised it to be. That was fine, that leant credibility to his status as an authority on psychological success. He wasn't a member of the Madpride group only because he actually had to trade on his history of mental illness. It gave him a vitality others lacked when it came to presenting his material, which would certainly be lost if he stopped owning up to having once been mad. But things from the past he had no control over, like transsexual girlfriends, or unknown children, could not be allowed to disconcert him and interfere with his current plans. He deliberately inhaled serenity and exhaled anxiety using Vedic techniques of rhythmic breathing.

After a few minutes he'd regained his composure and the room had filled up again. Some people had left early, perhaps wanting to spend the late afternoon in the sunshine, but there was now no-one milling about in the corridor outside. One of the hotel staff officiously and quietly shut the doors. The hall became silent with expectation.

But there was no sign of Lulu. He smiled calm reassurance at the audience and said he was sure she would be back in a minute.

A minute passed. Fucking hell, he thought, where is she?

Another minute passed. Some members of the audience started to get restless and others started quietly talking to one another again.

Yet another minute passed. He stepped down off the dais and quietly asked a nice, matronly-looking woman if she wouldn't mind just going to the Ladies for him and making sure Lucille was alright.

The hall was humming with conversation again. An interminable while later the woman was back, holding out her hands and shaking her head.

It was quite clear Lulu was gone. He might have fucking guessed.

Never mind. He was good at thinking on his feet. He asked Yvette, the GP, if she wouldn't mind standing in for her. She was happy to do so, and almost mechanically Ron asked her questions about her earliest remembered experiences of stress and her earliest memories of being asked to do more than she could manage, and traced a developmental history of such experiences. Then he invited the audience to comment or question her in terms of these experiences. An hour later she decided that she didn't want to continue to suffer such stresses anymore and that henceforth she would go part-time. The audience clapped and cheered their approval when she made this announcement. Then everyone left with a happily personalised experience of a successful PET session. They took all of his information leaflets and handouts. He was confident none of them had a clue about how disturbed he was beneath his confident façade.

When he finally left the hotel himself at six o clock, he allowed himself to think about Lulu with a mixture of anger and regret. He should have handled her differently, but there it was.

And there she was, simultaneously incognito and unmissable in dark sunglasses. Perched on her white high-heeled sandals, she was walking distractedly in little steps backwards and forwards on the other side of the street talking on her mobile phone. She hadn't seen him, but he felt certain she was waiting for him. And sure enough. as soon as she did notice him crossing the road towards her, she waved excitedly, said goodbye to whoever it was she was talking to and ran towards him. She removed her sunglasses, put them in her bag, and with a pleased smile took hold of his arm.

'I put these on so that the people coming out wouldn't recognise me. I'm so ashamed and so sorry I had to leave you in the lurch like that, Ronnie. But I just couldn't face it. I *couldn't* talk about Sean in public. Not with you of all people. So I had to let you down.'

Nobody had called him Ronnie for years. It undermined his hunky gravitas. He smiled through gritted teeth.

'I wasn't let down at all really. It actually went very well.'

'Even if it hadn't been you, I still would have chickened out. It's too personal and too painful, Ronnie. You know?'

'I should have realised that, after you had declared your reason for wanting a consultation. Of course I should. The heat must have been getting to me too.'

'Do you still want to talk? I mean I can go home if you want me to. But I've rung Richard and he understands. Surprisingly! He's going to pick up Sean for me. So if you still want to take me for that drink...?' She still hadn't let go of his arm, and looking down at her guileless trusting smile, he again felt catapulted into an intimacy he was by no means completely averse to. Not yet anyway. He had to find out more about this child.

He steered them round a corner to a pub with one or two little tables outside. One of them was just being vacated by another couple. Lulu sat down at it and asked for an orange juice. He stood at the bar waiting while his Guinness was pulled and wondered if he would still find her there when he got out again.

But there she was, fanning herself with a beer mat, the evening sun streaming down onto her slim attractive legs, looking chic and self-contained. He sat down with a smile, took some long slow sips of his beer and looked at her freely without having to keep his professional persona up anymore. She was clearly not someone who was unaware of the effect she had on men. That also was consistent with the person he had known ten or eleven years ago. He was aware of her watching him as he eyed her up. She grinned knowingly when he reached her eyes.

'It's so wonderful to see you again, Ron, after all this time. And so successful too. Quite the man of power and influence you– 'she paused. 'you never seemed likely to become, back when we were lovers! I hope you'll tell me how you did it before we say goodbye. I'm so stuck myself. I'm desperate for change in my life. Absolutely desperate.'

'You don't look it exactly,' he said. 'Desperate I mean. You,' he paused deliberately, a professional technique he often deployed, watching her face wait in expectation for him to finish. 'You look great,' he said.

Her face relaxed, pleased to be having the right effect on him, no doubt. If he did decide he wanted her, he was confident he could have her. It would be easy.

'I've always been good at false pretences Ron, haven't I? That hasn't changed.'

'So tell me what you have been doing all these years. And when you have told me that, you can tell me about this child.'

'This child as you call him, is yours, Ron. And Grainne's. I'm just the – the foster mother. I've been looking after him since he was a tiny baby. Like I said, he calls me Mum, but he knows *she* is his real mother. Although he's never actually seen her since she left him with me when she went into hospital for her anorexia. When he was still a baby, that was, not even toddling. She still won't have anything to do with him. Not directly. For his own good, she says. She always has a reason why it would be bad for him. It's sad really. But you know what Grainne's like.'

'I don't think I do actually. Certainly not anymore. Anyway, as you rightly said earlier, people change. I haven't seen or heard from her since she left me, a day after you did, all those years ago. I knew why you left. I never really did get to understand what made her leave though. I guess you must have told her something. About us I mean?'

'I do do silly things like that. I wish I could think before I speak, but I just can't, Ronnie. Too often I can't anyway. And I couldn't then. I didn't tell her directly. Honestly I didn't. Not as such. Well, not to her face anyway. Oh dear, I'm trying to lie again. The truth is I left her a note.' She gave him a lame winsome frown. 'I'm sorry, Ron, I really am.'

Another stab of ancient anger pierced him in the chest, but he didn't let it show, decided instead to gauge what she wanted from him and then not give it to her.

'Oh, don't worry. It's all history now. Or it would be if you weren't telling me I had a son.'

'You do, Ron, he's lovely. Looks just like you. He does really.'

'We'll talk about him in a while. I need time to digest the information. It's all a bit sudden. Put it in context for me,' he said, leaning forward with his most seductive, tried and tested combination of strength, vulnerability, and perceptiveness. 'Tell me about yourself first.'

Chapter 14.

Her husband was waiting for her in the Volvo outside Oxshott station four hours later. When she got in beside him Richard bent to kiss her on her lips, but Lucille offered him her cheek instead and in a no-nonsense, but not unfriendly mood asked him how his day had been. She didn't want to be horrible. After all, he'd picked up Sean from Julia's, but her own day had been so full of surprises that she just wasn't in the frame of mind to submit herself to his predictable attentions without first feeling that they had shared at least some words together. Sean was sitting in the back playing a computer game. She greeted him in a warmer manner, but he ignored her. At some point she would have to tell him she had met his father, but she would have to do it carefully, find the right moment. Confer first with Grainne and Richard. She might even tell him that they used to be lovers, but at the right time. When he was ready to listen. Everything must be done properly.

Richard started the car, switched the headlamps on and pulled out of the station. It was a five minute drive back home to Burylands. They gave each a desultory run down of the headlines of their days, but looking out into the darkness of the trees beside the road Lucille couldn't get Ron out of her mind. For the first time in over ten years she was reminded of her pre-operational past without immediately wanting to wipe the memory away. Nowadays her identity was just a fact. But in those days as she swept the floors at work and washed the old ladies' hair, or put their curlers in, she couldn't bear how slowly each day would pass. Clients and staff alike patronised her as if she was their own personal little nancy boy. She would smile sweetly, enjoying their company often enough, but always sour with envy of the femaleness they'd been able to take for granted all their lives. 'I'm not a nancy boy. I'm a girl too,' she would tell them silently, and sometimes aloud if they were interested, as the hours dragged by until she could finally rush home and freely look and behave like one. Back in those bad old days a simple thing like a man's desire – Ron's desire – had made her life both more bearable and more difficult. She used to sashay around in front of him every evening, delighting in the evidence of his obvious excitement. He was only attracted to girls and women, so her confidence in her femininity would soar as she awoke his sexuality simply by walking, talking and looking like the person she knew she really was. After rewarding him with a blow job she would usually take Milly out for her evening walk in the woods, she remembered, positively glowing with pleasure, often playing make-believe – daydreaming – she was pregnant. Some of her happiest moments in those dreadful days had involved tottering along behind Milly in her tatty charity shop skirts and cheap high heels enraptured by the feeling that his seed was inside her, holding her tummy triumphantly with a smug little smile on her face, searching her lips and tongue for the still lingering taste of him.

Pathetic really. She wasn't like that at all anymore, thank goodness! But in those desperate days she had had to be grateful for small mercies. Her euphoria had always only lasted a little while anyway before the cold reality of what she actually was would come back to her and spoil everything again. No vagina, no baby, no breasts, no self, nothing.

That's what she had really hated back then. That, and cheating on Grainne. Not Ron himself. Ron had been really rather alright. Certainly everything she had wanted at the time. And she had liked to think even then, that in his simple compliant way he had always treated her like a lady. Certainly his attitude towards her gender solution – she had refused from the beginning ever to think of it as a problem – had always been alright. The occasional bit of banter of course, but he was a man after all.

He hadn't seemed even the least bit troubled about keeping Grainne in the dark about what they were doing together while she was out at work, Lucille recalled. But then neither had she. Not bothered enough anyhow, because she'd wanted him so much, despite his beard, his belly and his stink. She used to love the fact there were secret parts of him, which she didn't really understand and which even then had made a man of mystery out of him. And for her, the mysteriousness of men had always been the most desirable thing about them, not their looks.

Nevertheless he *was* so much better-looking now. It was simply amazing. How could this even be the same man? He seemed so perfect now. When he put a finger to her cheek and briefly held it there, touching her as they said goodbye at Waterloo an hour ago, she had leaned her face into it and found herself longing for him to kiss her and hold her, every part of her body aching for him. And he hadn't even given her a hug, wretched man!

She had also felt curiously proprietorial towards him. After all, he was the first man she had ever been intimate with sexually. It made him special to her somehow and therefore legitimately desirable. She had never actually cheated on Richard before with anyone. Not in all the time they had been together. But after that session with the Relate counsellor a couple of weeks ago she no longer felt any reason to be loyal to him any more whatsoever. Her desire for him was gone. Not so much because of what he had said, or the way he looked – he was still an attractive man – but because of how humiliated he so often made her feel. It was strange the way things had turned out. She had been hoping that the counselling would bring them closer together. But in fact they were further apart than ever, going through the motions of being a normal married couple when actually she felt little or nothing for him now beyond the comfort of familiarity. He was like an old slipper.

She wanted a man not a slipper. She wanted Ron. The taste of bleach and fired almonds abruptly made her want to swallow, flooding her mouth with the sensation of her first sexual encounter with him. She almost sighed out loud. She wanted him with a desire she hadn't experienced since she first fell for Richard. It was overwhelming. She would do anything to have him. Anything. So perhaps there was after all something about Ron which hadn't changed: he still left her feeling that she wanted to be a slut with him. He was the first and so far the only man she had ever cheated with as well. *And* he was the father of her child!

She looked back over her shoulder at Sean buried in his computer game. Well? He *was* her child really. Not biologically, but to all other intents and purposes. She had certainly been a mother to him all his life. It would be so appropriate if his father wanted to have sex with her again, proper heterosexual intercourse. So right.

'Lucille!' Richard repeated interrupting this pleasant reverie. 'I said, how was your day?' Did that old friend of yours find it easy to come to terms with his new-found paternity, or was he upset, or what?'

'Richard! Not now! We can't talk about that now. You know we can't.' She glanced at Sean on the back seat again. His resemblance to Ron was striking. How on earth had she not noticed it before? He was such a lovely little boy when he was engrossed in his games.

Richard glanced at her and seeing her smile took his hand off the gear stick, put it on the inside of her knee and caressed her. Although she felt relaxed and for the first time in weeks actually in the mood for physical intimacy, she had never allowed him to do this kind of thing in front of Sean, even in the better days of their marriage. She delicately took his hand away and held it on her lap. As an afterthought she cursorily caressed his knuckles once or twice. She didn't want him to feel rejected. Not yet. In fact she might even let him have sex with her tonight if he wanted to, imagine he was Ron.

When they got in, she took Sean upstairs and tidied his room while he got into his pyjamas and cleaned his teeth. He seemed remarkably docile this evening. Perhaps it was the lateness of the hour.

'What have you been doing, Mum?'

'I was having dinner with a very nice man. You'll meet him one day. He – he's a long lost relative of yours, so you'll actually have to meet him one day, poppet. It wouldn't be fair if you didn't. He was a friend of mine – and Mummy-Grainne's – long before I ever met Richard.'

'I don't want to.'

She tucked him into bed, knowing he would be up in a couple of hours. Hopefully he wouldn't disturb her, but usually he did. She was used to it though. In fact she would probably wake herself up at night if he didn't, now she had become so accustomed to it. Richard, of course, always slept through everything. She placed a little kiss on Sean's forehead. He reached up and put his arms around her head. They held each other for a few moments. Then she disengaged and switching out the light went to her own bedroom and got undressed.

Briefly she studied herself in the mirror. She looked alright. Her tits still looked good. Her bum was nice and round, her tummy trim. She put a lot of work into her figure. Most men would find her desirable, she told herself. She slipped on her dressing gown, fastening it tightly around her. But she was anxious. As she cleaned her face off, she couldn't stop worrying whether Ron still found her attractive. He had given her one or two signals, it was true, but that could have just been his polished masculine politeness. After all, he knew her history. And as a psychologist he'd also know that because of it she was very likely to be susceptible to even the slightest show of attention from a man.

She fell back on the old empty consolation that it wasn't her fault she'd been born different from other women, incapable of remaining genuinely neutral in the presence of a man and just being herself. That was actually only possible with females, and in particular with her mum. In the presence of a man she was still as insecure as ever about her lack of ovaries or a womb. Mum once said she was monster and as the years had gone by her attitude towards men had sometimes felt monstrous when it didn't feel pathetic and silly. Not because of what she did with them, not anymore, but because of how she was with them – permanently fluttering around them and flattering them like an old spinster, or fawning and flirting with them like a teenager who'd just won an evening out with the leader of a boy band. It was really hard just to be herself.

So, in a way, she could understand why Richard was so jealous, even though she had never given him any real reason to be. In reality she had simply got on with the everyday business of trying to be a wife, a mother, and a daughter. Richard had been a good enough husband until recently, but even with him she always seemed compelled to slip into stereotyped role playing. The Tired or Nagging Wife in response to his Insatiable Male Appetite for Sex was now one of her starring roles, however much she hated playing it, and however much it left her feeling miserable and utterly undesirable.

She couldn't stop herself thinking about Ron. He would be able to have any woman he wanted now, let alone one like her. But he had fancied her a little bit. Surely he had? Examining her face neurotically in her dressing table mirror she slapped on too much moisturiser, trying to find her confidence. Even without make-up most men would still find her pretty, wouldn't they? Even though she was going to be thirty one this year? Would the touch of tightness in the corners of her eyes start to develop into lines soon? She suppressed the panic that thought induced. What if it did?   It wouldn't matter. She'd simply do whatever was necessary to get rid of them. There was no way she'd be fanciable if she had crows feet, not when she didn't even have a uterus or cervix. She began brushing and rebrushing her hair and then, even as she ridiculed herself for it, touching up her lipstick despite the fact she was getting ready for bed. The fear always gnawed that because there was something missing she couldn't be truly desirable. That hadn't actually been her experience at all, but it was what she felt. And she was nothing if she was not what she felt.

Meeting Ron had made her feel horribly young again; that dreadful, *gauche* combination of anxiety, insecurity and overwhelming desire. She needed to talk about it. It was too late to ring Mum whom she talked to about everything now she didn't have much longer to live. Neither of them were prepared anymore to rely on silent intuition together, because they both knew her days were numbered. Life was too short and time too precious. So they would talk and talk together nowadays, in so far as Mum was able to, in just the same kind of way they once used to share silences together, companionably, intimately, like they were one person with two heads. When she went round to see her in the morning, as she did almost every morning if she could, she would tell her about Ron. And Mum would help! She would know what to do!

She put on the kettle for a cup of tea.

As she reached for a mug from the cupboard above her head, Richard came up behind her and put his arms around her, cupping her breasts and breathily remarking on how attractive she was. She rolled her eyes heavenwards. Couldn't he just for once come out with something new? But then again, no! Hadn't she just been feeling that under the agitated circumstances, and even though she resented herself for needing it, her confidence in her own attractiveness would benefit from male interest; even if it was only Richard's, it would be still be evidence of her womanly pulling power. She was so stupid sometimes, so mixed up; usually, in fact, if the truth be told. She sighed and relaxed against him, turning her face up towards his and allowing him to kiss her. Immediately she felt his penis harden against her. Her usual response lately to his horniness was to immediately pull away from him, but now she let herself feel reassured by it and with a smug smile she pressed herself against him before saying,

'I want a cup of tea first.'

But he didn't want to let her. Shrugging, she surrendered herself to his ardour. It wasn't often nowadays that she was ever in the mood, but he was her husband after all. She put her arms around his neck. He put both his large hands under her dressing gown squeezing her bum before picking her up, placing her on the kitchen table, and spreading her legs as he kissed her. But nice as his hunger for her was, when he stepped back to unzip his fly, she drew the line at actually having sex on the kitchen table with him. What if Sean came down and found them in *flagrante*? She pushed him off, shifting forwards and slipping to the ground. He made a grab for her. With her best, if rather rusty look of sexual come-on she pushed his arms away, gave the large bulge in his trousers a fond pat and insisted on going upstairs.

Richard was like a dog, so beside himself that she was prepared to have him at all, that he nodded his enthusiastic agreement. She turned out the light and he followed her up grunting with excitement and muttering something about the desirability of her rear. She wiggled it amateurishly for him. Yes, tonight it really might be rather nice to be bonked. She couldn't remember when they had last had sex. Most of the time she just wasn't in the mood, that was all. But never mind that, she told herself, just think positive. Behind her on the stairs his hands were on her bum again. She stopped, pushing back against them for a moment, then broke forward running up the last few steps and into the bedroom. She draped herself against her pillows in the kind of whorish pose she knew he liked as he followed her in puffing and blowing and nearly falling over in his struggle to get his underpants off over his upstanding penis. It was almost comical. What was it about men that when they were at their most powerful they were also at their most vulnerable? For a moment she thought he wouldn't manage it and couldn't help smiling. Then they were at his feet. He was still a fine figure of man, if just a bit too old for her now; but still attractive – tall, heavily built and unambiguously male. Just like Ron in that respect, but Ron probably wouldn't have those tell-tale little love handles, nor those grey hairs on his chest. He grinned at her as she looked at him and she lifted her arms in invitation and sure enough, as one thing followed another, she found it was Ron she was thinking of with her eyes closed as Richard entered her. She kept on trying to pull him in deeper as he bonked her, and found herself coming to a climax with him. It was the first time in over a year, and as someone too long used to being in detached sexual limbo she was grateful to find it was still even possible.

It had been a good day. All things considered. A very good day.

* * *

In the morning when she got to the nursing home her mother remarked on how fresh and well she looked. She glowed. She always tried to look her best for her mother.

'You do look lovely dear,' croaked Emily Farouk from beneath the diminishment and pallor of her dying. Her colourless eyes were sparkling. 'You look ever so nice in white,' she wheezed. 'I don't think I've seen that skirt before, have I? I do love a few pleats. I really do. You see them so rarely nowadays.' She took almost as long pausing for breath between sentences as she did speaking them. Lucille stopped herself from biting her lower lip. Mum's eyesight was still as good as ever and she hated

228

Lucille to be at all upset about her. 'But all that ironing, or dry cleaning, or what not! They're just not practical, are they? Let me look at you, my love. Give me a twirl. Yes, very pretty. You've been such a lucky girl to have a husband who can afford you! It's more than I ever had.' She rasped with a feeble bubbling paroxysm of coughs, which she required that they both ignore. Her drowning lungs were a part of who she was by now. She put her oxygen mask to her nose and mouth for a minute until her chest had calmed down again. 'You suit white so well with your lovely golden skin.'

'It's all the work I put in on the sun bed,' joked Lucille although they both knew her colour was one thing about her that was natural.

'I could never wear white myself,' said Emily Farouk, not really listening. 'I do have one white dress in the back of my wardrobe somewhere, a crinoline designer thing with huge buttons on it going all the way down the back. Impossible to sit down in comfortably, it was. Must have been designed by a man! Did you come across it dear, when you went through my things last week? It was very eighties, with huge shoulder pads. Very strange. I felt like a sailing boat in it. Your father persuaded me to buy it for some christening we were going to just after he received that redundancy package from the railway. He thought it looked nice on me, you did too, but actually it just made me look pasty-faced and I only ever wore it the once. But you would probably look wonderful in it with your skin. You must wear it to my funeral if you find it. I want you to.'

Lucille smiled as she tidied up the bedside locker, rearranging things a little so that her mother could reach her spectacles and her glass of water without being in danger of knocking over the bunch of fresias she had brought her yesterday. She was used to her mother's black humour. But more than that, this kind of conversation, talking about appearances, was what had first joined them ever since Lucille had been a small child. Neither of them were going to stop it now despite their sadness, and however hollow it might sound. It was how they touched base with one another.

Lucille went over and sat down on the chair on the other side of the bed. In the requisite matter-of-fact tone she asked Mum for a bulletin on how she really was, declaring she would give her a manicure. The reply was noncommittal, uncertain.

'How should I know darling? I'm only the patient.'

Slowly, feebly, but with strength and elegance, Emily Farouk managed to move a hand out onto Lucille's lap. They were silent together for a while, sharing the feeling of quiet contented togetherness that had always joined them best.

'So what are you looking so radiant about?' Mum eventually asked in her squeaky, sore voice.

'It's just a front, Mum. Mostly I am feeling nervous. But happy too, I suppose.'

'What's happened?'

'I've been very silly. I need your advice, Mum. I met an old boyfriend. My first boyfriend. The only one I ever had from before I, you know, got fixed. I've told you about him loads of times. I used to tell you about him anyway. Ron! Remember? Sean's father. The thing is he didn't know he was a father, and what did I go and do when I met him again yesterday? I just went and blurted it out and told him, that's all. I couldn't help it. I was just too excited, I think, seeing him again after all this time. So I got confused and forgot to be sensible. Now he wants to see him.' She looked at her mother with a sombre, blank face. 'I'm terrified.'

'Oh Lucille, how could you, you silly girl! He's a lunatic isn't he? I hope you didn't tell him where you live?' She broke into another burst of coughing which seemed to last forever. Lucille put her glass of water to her lips.

'He's changed, Mum. Almost as much as I have. More. I was always who I was really, wasn't I? Whereas Ron is unrecognisable! He's a doctor now. Not one like Richard. A Ph.D. In Psychology! I can hardly believe it. He used to be so thick the sports pages of the Sun or the Star or whatever it was, were more than he could manage.'

Lucille stood up again with a vacant smile, carefully smoothed her skirt under her bottom so that the pleats wouldn't crumple, and sat down again. She always attended to her appearance when she felt stupid and unsure of herself. It helped her feel better, gave her something to do. She returned to her mother's nails. While the first hand dried she sat back in her chair. She was the thick one nowadays, she realised, not Ron, because she could not for the life of her understand how he could have changed so much.

She held up Mum's hand, crossed her legs, and put it down on her lap again. Out of the corner of her eye she could tell by the way she was looking at her that Mum knew how disturbed she was.

'Things like that, fundamental things like who you are, Lucille, don't change. You know that.'

'Well I'm quite sure he didn't use to pretend to be thick, whatever you say! But maybe he was ill. I don't know. It was endearing really. At times anyway – the way you could get him to do whatever you wanted cos he was so stupid.'

Her mother glanced at her, reading her like a book. Lucille shrugged, covering up the flush she felt coming into her face by saying,

'He's just not like that at all now. And you'd never believe he was once a big fat slob! I know! I don't know why I fancied him. But in those days I suppose I just had to take what I could get! But I do know why I fancy him now. He's so different Mum, you just wouldn't believe it. How could someone like him end up with a PhD and his own consultancy business?

But he has. And he's so good-looking now too. He could have swept me off my feet at *any* time yesterday. At any time. He didn't though. Sadly.'

'Where is Sean?'

'He's in the car.' Mum clearly wasn't interested. Even so, Lucille didn't mean to retaliate or hurt her when she added, 'he refused to come up and see you, said it was boring sitting there just listening to us two talking together. I said come up and see your granny, and he said in his usual blunt way that you're not his granny. I don't know what I'm going to do, Mum. Grainne's disappeared and isn't replying to any of my e-mails or texts, so I can't ask her.'

'What are you going to tell Sean? I mean, presumably Ron has a right to see his child?'

'Yes, of course he does. I suppose.' Her laugh was a nervous one. 'I don't really know the legal position. I don't know what else I *can* do, but first of all, tell Sean the truth. That's the first and most important thing. The problem is how. And when. I want to know, I mean I *need* to know, that if he is going to reveal himself as his father, Ron won't just disappear out of his life again straight away afterwards. Sean couldn't bear that. And neither could I. It would be so hurtful. I told him that last night and he said he understood. But I'm worried now he didn't really let me know whether he actually *agreed* to my making that a condition of seeing him. He just said he understood. But I didn't want to, you know, alienate him. So I said I would speak to Grainne first and then I would have a look in my diary. Yes, I know, Mum! What diary? – And give him a ring today to make a date for the two of them to meet.'

'A date, dear? Why did you delay it? There's no point now is there? In delaying it, I mean. Not under the circumstances. Not now you've told him.'

'I was just being sensible, Mum.'

'No you weren't. That's why you're now trembling like some poor lamb in a slaughter house queuing up to have her throat cut,' Emily Farouk replied slowly. 'The first thing is to tell Sean the truth. You're right about that, of course you are. But that means telling him the *whole* truth, and trying to find a way of doing so which doesn't hurt him. Or you! Or anybody. And that can't wait. You surely don't want the poor mite to have to wait to hear who his father is from you until you're actually with him, a stranger, or two strangers if his mother now decides she wants to become involved too! Which, in the circumstances is very likely. Make no mistake, my darling, that's what his mother and father are to him. Strangers. He hasn't seen Grainne since he was a babe in arms, of course, and he's never seen his father. So if you wait till you're with either or both of them before you tell him who his father is, you will always regret it. Always.'

'I know you're right. I thought that myself really. I really did. Then I thought I'd be being selfish if I did that, but you've reassured me, Mum.

231

Thank you. I am *not* going to tell him all about me, though. He doesn't need to know *everything*. I will tell him all about himself. I'm just so distracted — there's too much to think about — that I can't even think straight.'

Mum's nails were dry now. She reached for her other hand.

'Wouldn't that be a bit unfair?'

'What?'

'Telling him all about himself, but not all about yourself?'

'He doesn't need to know *all* about me. It would just confuse him on top of everything else.'

'It's certainly going to confuse him to suddenly find out so much more about his own life, that's true. But, maybe, sharing some more about yours would help him experience it — and you, sweetheart — more, I don't know, more completely, and because of that more genuinely if you know what I mean, dear.'

'Genuinely? No, I don't. What*ever* do you mean? He knows me perfectly well. He's known me all his life.'

'I mean I think it would help your relationship with him. That's all.'

'How?'

'I don't know, Lucille. Stop being so deliberately obtuse! All I know is what you tell me now I'm stuck in this place waiting to die. He loves you. You share the most tender moments together and — and yet he hates you! That's what you're always telling me.'

'It's not *me* he hates. Not me personally. I know it's not.'

'Of course it's not personal. He behaves badly at you because he doesn't *understand*. We both know that.'

'He just gets cross with me because he's frustrated about that, poor little poppet. *I'd* be angry if I couldn't understand. Anybody would. The trouble is I never seem to help no matter how hard I try. Not in all these years.'

She shook her head sadly.

'You are lying again, Lucille. At least be truthful with me for goodness sake. You can be so irritating sometimes! Now then, you've often said how much he hates not understanding things. That's true enough, I'm sure. Feeling and understanding have always been difficult for him, even though he's clever. But actually things are about to get much more complicated and difficult, and if there is one thing I'm sure of, it is that he needs to know that you can cope with that. With difficult things, I mean. He doesn't know it at the moment. Not really. And not yet. So he's not secure in himself. And it's no wonder, is it? What with one thing and another. But as a mother, I am absolutely certain that he wants to secure himself in you. In your love. And in your personality. His bad behaviour with you is just done to test you out. Until he can feel secure with you. That's what I think. He wants to know if you can cope with difficult things just because *he* is himself a difficult thing. And he knows it! His life is a difficult thing. Can you cope with him? That's what he still needs to know. Even after all this time. If you can't, then he can't. And until you can, he won't!'

She was so exhausted after this speech that she visibly dwindled, her chest caving in on itself beneath her peach nightie, and her head falling forward as if she hadn't the strength to hold it up anymore after all that talking. Lucille reached for her oxygen mask and held it over her nose and mouth for a minute or two. Eventually Emily Farouk lifted up a hand to hold it herself a moment longer before returning it to rest on the counterpane on the bed beside her. It was only then that Lucille said,

'But I can't! I can't. I can't cope with difficult things at all. He knows that. So do you.'

'He needs to know you can. And stop talking such nonsense. I wish you'd stop trying to pull the wool over my eyes all the time. I'm your mother, darling. Stop pretending to be what you're not. With me, at any rate. You can do what you like with other people. You may look like a – yes, a bimbo – and naturally it can be useful sometimes, but *not* with me. We both know that you are not actually the helpless type at all.' Her voice was a gruff whisper.

'I am with Sean, Mum.'

'Nonsense, chick,' her mother said with more kindness, a smile lighting up her face again. 'I'll never forget that sweltering afternoon six or seven years ago when the swarm of bees came down the chimney into Sean's playpen. Do you remember? Of course you do. How old was he at that time?'

'I don't know. Two, maybe just three. Yes, three. The balloons from his birthday party were still tied to the end of his cot. But what's all that got to do with anything?'

Her mother had stopped listening, was wandering down memory lane.

'We'd just gone downstairs to make a cup of tea. You were wonderful. I was so proud. No-one could have coped as well as you did then. First you sensed something was wrong. Intuitively. There was no obvious reason to think so at all. He didn't cry out, did he? No, don't argue with me, Lucille. I haven't got the energy. You *knew* something wasn't right.'

Emily Farouk's smile became more dreamy as she went further into her reverie, proud to be the mother of someone brave and clever. Lucille began smiling too. She liked Mum to be pleased with her. She always had.

'So you rushed upstairs.' Her voice was so faint, Lucille could hardly hear her above the bubbling of her breath. 'And I followed you and you came out of his room holding him in your arms, and he was already quite a big boy by then, surrounded by all those bees that had come in through the chimney breast in the heat. I still can't believe how many there were. Were you frightened and unable to cope? Not a bit of it!' She tailed off, seemed to fall asleep for a second of two, then snapped herself back into full consciousness. 'Of course you weren't. As I clearly recall. So don't try and make black white! The whole swarm followed you downstairs in a horrible buzzing bundle all around your head. I'll never forget it. As if *you* were their queen too! You put Sean carefully down at the bottom of the stairs and walked slowly out of the back door and then the bees swept off and away. And not one of us was stung. It was like a miracle. It *was* a miracle, which you, young lady, were responsible for.

'That afternoon I saw quite clearly that you can cope with anything, especially when you have to, when there is no choice. And you've got to now. Otherwise I fear that out of his childish loyalty to you he will make sure that contact with his father and everything else you try to do for him... will fail.'

'Oh Mum! I didn't cope at all. I was petrified. You know I was. I nearly fainted.' She gave a shrill little laugh and told her mother to wiggle her fingers.

'That was afterwards. Shock. Anyone would have.'

'It was during too. I should know,' she said. 'Hold still now, Mum, please.'

'Oh forget about my nails for a moment. Stop insulting my intelligence with your sham helplessness. What I am saying is important.'

Lucille continued painting them, shaking her head and smiling.

With that, Emily Farouk very deliberately removed her small, mottled hand from Lucille's and turning it over, wiped her shining wet nails across Lucille's pleated lap leaving a diagonal triple slash of pearlescent burgundy emblazoned across the front of her white skirt.

'Mum!' Lucille heard herself shrieking. 'What are you *doing*?'

'That's to help you remember what I said when you get back to the car and Sean asks you what happened. Tell him Granny did it and tell him Granny said you must tell him everything. And tell him Granny said you can cope. And that he can too.'

She sighed, sunk her chin into her shoulder in what this time was a very deliberate manner, brought the oxygen mask back to her mouth and closed her eyes.

Lucille was seething. She felt just like that bundle of bees right now, buzzing with anger. But there was nothing she could do. She screwed the cap back down into the varnish bottle and popped it into her open bag on the floor beside her. If she quickly applied varnish remover it would lift some of the intensity of the colour off, but it might equally well spread the stain. She felt white with shock and rage. But she couldn't just leave it there. It would never come off if she did that. She dabbed at it with the varnish remover as best she could till she was left with a diffuse red-flecked stain in the middle of an unmissably huge damp patch, the pungent aroma of which was making her feel light-headed.

She reached for her mother's hand again, almost snatching it back, but was gentle about wiping off what was left of the varnish from her old porcelain-grey fingers. Emily Farouk continued to be too exhausted to open her eyes or acknowledge her. So Lucille carefully repainted her nails anyway and then packed her things and left. As she closed the door behind her she heard her mother's now minute voice say cheerily, 'See you tomorrow, my love.'

The walk back to the car was negotiated by putting on her sunglasses and holding her bag in front of her skirt to cover the stain. The stench of the varnish remover kept on wafting up her nose. She ignored it, walked purposefully out of the front door and back to the car, reassured by the sound of her strappy heels clickety-clacketing normality again across the asphalt drive. She had to regain her composure. It would never do to be in this state with Sean. She took a few deep breaths and then got into the car.

Sean was sitting in the front passenger seat with the seat belt on.

'Get in the back please, Sean. You know I can't let you sit in the front. You're too young.' She sat back in her seat making it plain that she wasn't going to start the car up till he moved.

'You've had a period,' he said, looking at the damp patch on the front of her skirt.

Between them her mother and Sean couldn't have made it any easier to tell him the truth now, but she wasn't sure she wanted to just yet. She felt manipulated.

'How do you know about periods?' He more often responded to her seriously when she matched his directness with a blunt directness of her own. It had become something of a habit to respond to him in kind.

'Richard told me. Ladies bleed once a month and they sometimes get a bit cross just before it happens.'

'Well, I don't have periods. I spilt some nail varnish, that's all. I was born – I was born with a condition like a hysterectomy. It's why I can't have babies. No womb.' She gave him a clipped smile. 'So, no periods. Now get in the back, please Sean. *Please.*'

'What's a hiss-trek tummy?' he asked, touching the stain on her skirt and then smelling his fingers.

'Get off!'

'What's a hiss-trek tummy?'

'Hys-ter-ectomy. It's an operation some women have to have.'

'What kind of operation?'

'I just told you, Sean. It's when a lady has to have the part of her inside her tummy which babies grow in – where her periods happen – taken out because something is wrong with it and she might die if a doctor doesn't operate on her and take it away. It's very upsetting.'

'I want to be a hysterectomy doctor when I grow up and take bad babies out and save ladies lives. That would be cool.'

'Good darling. I'm glad. Now will you *please* climb into the back.'

'Why were you born with a hysterectomy?'

'I – I don't know. I don't know. I just was. Now get in the back. Please.'

'I will in a minute.'

He must be in a good mood. That was a relief. Because she wasn't. And he was usually so stubborn if he didn't want to do something.

'Alright, in a minute then. But we shan't be leaving till you do.'

She turned on the car radio and retrieved her tissues and varnish remover from her bag again to have another go at her skirt. The sun streamed down through her opened window. The stain wasn't actually too bad. Her skirt might not be ruined after all. She would send it to the dry cleaners, see what they could do with it.

'Was I hysterectomised out of Mummy Grainne?'

'No I didn't mean that there is something wrong with the baby. I meant with the mother. Although it can be with the baby too. What you are thinking of anyway, is called an abortion. But if a baby is aborted then it doesn't get to live at all. No, Mummy Grainne brought you into the world normally and I have brought you up in it.'

'With Richard.'

'Yes, with Richard. Of course. But I'm the one who loves you, aren't I?'

'You're my mum. But Richard's not my dad, but he still loves me too.'

'I'm your sort-of mum. People call women like me 'foster-mums', whereas Grainne is your 'birth mum' – your real mum.'

He had never been interested in this kind of thing before. Whenever she had tried to talk to him about it he had found a way of shutting her up or leaving.

'Is Richard my foster-dad?'

'Well, it's all very complicated. He's my husband and he is like a father to you, so in a way you could say he was. But I don't think he loves you like I do. No, he couldn't because I love you completely, poppet. But he's very fond of you.'

'I like men better than women.'

'That's because you are still a little boy,' she replied primly. 'Just. Most eleven year old boys think women are a bit yucky. I remember when I was your age at school we used to think the boys were all silly the way they'd do anything to shy away from girls. Most of them. Except for their own mums, of course!' And then just a few years later they'd do anything to go out with one.' She laughed lightly and patted his knee. 'One day when you are grown up, when you are a man yourself, I'm pretty sure you'll find you like women a bit more than you do now, a lot more in fact. Men generally do, you know.'

'I want my dad. Why don't you ever tell me about my dad?'

Lucille looked away out of the window up towards where she thought her mother's bedroom was. There you are, Mum, she thought. Thanks a lot. The truth is all going to come out anyway, whether I want it to or not.

'I don't tell you about your father because until yesterday I hadn't seen him since, well, since before you were born. A long time ago.'

'Did you see my dad yesterday? Why didn't you take me with you?'

Whoops. She'd done it again. Her tongue had let slip again. Yet again. When would she ever learn to keep things to herself?

Never mind, perhaps it was all for the best.

'Because I didn't know I was going to see him, Sean, that's why. But yes, I met with him yesterday.'

'What does he look like?'

'He looks a lot like you. In fact he looks just like a grown up version of you, without the ginger hair. His hair is brown. He's a very good looking man, your father, a very good looking man.' She popped the varnish remover back in her bag, and pulling the rear view mirror around, checked her face.

'Did you love him when you were a girl?'

'I sort of loved him before I became a woman, let's put it that way. But it was really Mummy-Grainne and him who together were responsible for you being born.'

'Did you kiss him?'

Her heart missed a beat.

'Yes, we kissed,' she lied. Well, it wasn't a complete lie. At the beginning of their tawdry little story all those years ago, she remembered now with a wistfulness she would never have dreamt of feeling then, she had experimented once or twice with allowing him to kiss her, purely as a learning experience to see what it was like. And that was all because she had known even then that, unlike blow jobs, kisses were romantic and personal, so by rights they really did belong to Grainne in a way that somehow his penis did not, so she had discouraged kissing. 'Sometimes. That's what lovers do.'

'Yuck. So why didn't I grow in your tummy then?'

'I told you. I can't have babies. Did Richard tell you about what men and women do together when they make a baby?' She was buying time, she was sure he hadn't.

'No. You're my mum.'

'I am not your birth mum, as you know perfectly well and as I've just told you, I'm you're sort-of mum.' She paused and looking at Sean, again felt that old sense of pre-operational shame. Despite the heat of the morning she felt frozen by it, as if her blood had stopped circulating. The hatefulness of this feeling made her want to snap. She bit her lip and went for it.

'And the truth is I'm only a sort-of woman. When I was your age I – I was like you. I had boy equipment, you know, down there.' She darted an angry embarrassed sideways glance in the general area of his crotch and then stared out at the sun-drenched cypresses beyond the car park again. A solitary magpie screeched unpleasantly on a branch before it was chased off by two others.

'You mean you had a willy?' He frowned and smiled at one at the same time, guileless and intrigued.

Time stopped. Lucille reddened, gaze fixed on the trees, heart racing. Then she forced herself to nod her head in humiliation. She couldn't say anything. She just nodded.

'You – you weren't a little girl when you were young?'

'I was! Inside, in my feelings! Granny knew. She was so good to me. But my body was, well, I'm afraid it wasn't right at all. In fact – don't ask me because I will not go into the awful details – but yes, it was like yours. And personally I couldn't bear it. No! I don't mean that yours is horrible, of course I don't. But *mine* was. Or at least it was for me. Because I wasn't really a boy and thankfully, doctors were able to help me and so I had an operation to take the boy bits away and put me right when I was nineteen. And I have been normal ever since. I do like boy bits on boys. Of course I do. That's where they belong. But not on *me* thank you very much! On me they were all wrong.'

Time seemed to restart again. She felt released, looked at him with a friendly smile, the blood flowing freely round her system once more. She could move again. There now. That hadn't been too hard at all. 'On you they are just fine, my darling.'

He nodded matter-of-factly.

'And on my dad. They are fine on my dad too, aren't they?'

'Yes, of course they are. They are fine on him too,' she said.

Sean seemed remarkably unperturbed by her revelation.

'Why doesn't he ever come and see me?'

'He didn't even know of your existence till yesterday.'

'Why not?'

'Because no-one told him.'

'Why not?'

'Well, partly because neither Mummy-Grainne nor I have seen him for more than ten years.'

'I want to see him! Now! Today.'

'Last night you said you didn't want to see him. Anyway we can't see him today.'

'Why not?'

'Well for one thing you are still sitting in the front of the car. And for another it's just not right to go chasing after him the minute I just met up with him again.'

'What about me then? It's my turn now, isn't it!?' He wasn't asking her. 'Isn't it! Isn't it!'

'Get in the back and we'll talk about it.'

He scurried over the seat and strapped himself in. Just like that.

'Isn't it? Now. I want to see him now.'

'We'll see.'

'I fucking hate, 'we'll see'.'

'*Sean*! How dare you use bad language like like that!'

'I fucking hate, 'we'll see'.'

She sighed, helpless. The euphoric sense of release she had gained by telling him about herself was lost as the prison gates of her incompetence as a mother clanged shut again. She started the car and pulled out of the nursing home's well-kept driveway, her mouth set on not getting involved in this. Other eleven year olds didn't talk like this to their mothers. It was horrible. She hated it. But exposed to Richard's free use of bad language at home, it was inevitable Sean would pick it up. She had talked about it over and over again with Richard who always advised serene indifference. If he lost his power to shock, he would become bored with it. That was all very well and indifference she could probably do, but serene she wasn't. And Sean did not seem to be becoming bored with it at all.

'I fucking hate 'we'll see'.' He started banging at the door handle as if he would get out of the moving car if it weren't for the child-proof lock keeping it shut.

She remembered her own desperate need for *her* father when she was a child and just wanted to give way to him. Children should be allowed see their fathers, of course they should. If she took him to see Ron she would be giving them what they both wanted. By the time she turned the car into her own drive, she'd decided that the line of least resistance was best.

She stopped outside the front door. Before she'd even turned the motor off, Sean had jumped back into the front seat beside her and was out of the car leaving the door wide open behind him and running across the driveway. He leaned against the front door bell with a determined, needy look on his face. Lucille sighed. He knew the house was empty, but in a way it *was* good to see him behaving like the child he actually was. As she stepped out of the air-conditioned car to go round to the passenger side and close the door, she still felt like slapping him. He was so completely thoughtless and inconsiderate.

She unlocked the front door.

'Sean, I will ring him now and see what we can do, but if you give me any more trouble whatsoever then it's no deal, okay?'

He ignored her, but she knew that meant he agreed. The actual word, yes, let alone the words, thank you Mum, just weren't in his vocabulary at the moment.

She went straight to the hall phone and dialled the mobile number Ron had given her yesterday. After three rings she heard his voice.

'Hello?'

'Ronnie?'

'Hi!'

He recognised her voice. That was a good sign, but at the same time it made her feel shaky and shy.

'It's me. Lucille,' she said, unnecessarily.

'Lulu! How are you?'

'Hello Ron,' she said more firmly. 'I'm – I'm fine thank you,' she tried to sound formal. No-one had called her Lulu since he used to do so all those years ago. She found herself diving straight into what she had to say to avoid how shy she suddenly felt. 'I've got a bit of a problem, Ronnie. It's your son – he says he's got to see you. Now, he says. Right now or he'll – well, I don't know what he'll do actually.' She tried to laugh, but her shrill giggle didn't sound very amused because she wasn't. 'I told you what he could be like sometimes. Well, it's building up into one of those times now, I'm afraid, So, er, can we meet? Would you mind?'

'Not at all. Of course not. I've been thinking the same thing ever since we said goodbye last night: I've got to see my son.'

Not her then. Of course not. It was understandable. Oh, well, never mind.

'Today?' he asked.

'Yes, today. Please. This afternoon. Can you do it, Ron? I'm sorry. I know I should get Grainne's permission, but he's desperate and when he's desperate he's – he's impossible.'

Beside her Sean started nudging her painfully on the arm. He was nearly the same size as her and his elbow hurt. She flinched and raising an eyebrow at him threatened to put the phone down. Sean stopped hitting her and pulled away with that peculiar forced smile of his, but as usual he didn't give her any eye contact.

'Okay,' said Ron. 'I'm only working on my computer. Where would you like to meet?'

'I don't mind. Anywhere will do. Somewhere a boy can feel not too uncomfortable on a day like this?'

'Holland Park? There's an adventure playground there as far as I can remember, and a café.'

'That sounds fine. When?'

'Say, two clock? At the café? Do you know how to get to it?'

240

He gave her directions which she wrote down and they hung up. Sean nodded. He wandered off into the kitchen for some orange juice from the fridge. She wanted to yell at him to use a glass, but there was no point, he was already slurping it down straight from the carton. She bit her tongue and went upstairs to get changed.

What had she *done*? What had she done?

She had made everything happen too fast, that was all. Nothing serious. She couldn't help the fact that she and Ron had accidentally happened on one another again. Even if volunteering for a PET session to talk about Sean had been a bit silly. But then telling Ron who Sean actually was! And then, after all that, she had gone and told Sean not just about her own past, but about Ron as well. Madness! How could she have?

She sat down in front of her dressing table repairing her face and hair as she winced her way through her catalogue of indiscretions. Dreadful. Simply dreadful. But she'd find a way of making it alright for Sean. Alright enough, anyway. Definitely, she had to. But she had better try and call Grainne before things got completely out of hand. Otherwise she might end up repeating exactly the same mistake as she'd made ten years ago – keeping things secret from Grainne. She must tell her everything, explain what had happened over the last twenty four hours, own up to being a fool.

She delved into her bag for her mobile phone, tapped in the number. No answer, Grainne's phone was switched off. With a hopeless, resigned shrug, she left her a message including Ron's number, and got herself ready to go up to London.

Two hours later with Sean beside her, she joined the queue for a taxi outside Waterloo station. She was maybe a little too dressy in her shiny snakeskin heels and light blue silk dress with the short sleeves. But that was okay. As she and Sean crossed the station concourse most women she passed had taken the measure of her which was always a good sign, and plenty of men had looked at her too. She hardly ever wore this dress because Richard had once said it looked sexier on her than anything else she'd got and she didn't like to encourage him. But Ron was a different matter. She wanted to look her best this afternoon because this was not just about Sean wanting to see Ron. Cool and poised in the slight, but broiling breeze blowing between the station and the taxi rank, she felt content. It was a lovely day and whatever she had done and whatever happened this afternoon, it was going to be interesting.

When the cab set them down at two fifteen outside the Commonwealth Institute on Kensington High Street, Sean complained of the heat. Lucille pointed to the park, and suggested they play a game of walking under the trees and having to stay in the shade all the way to the playground, see if they could find it without treading in any sunshine. Sean glared at her as if she might have forgotten that he was now nearly twelve years old, but said nothing. She bought him an ice cream and they sauntered off separately, but together, always just out of reach of one another. After a minute she decided to take her shoes off, walk on the grass. Even so, within no more than another few minutes she found herself feeling just a little too hot. She didn't want to meet Ron all in a lather. That would never do. She wanted to be fragrant, the most desirable woman in the park. She looked down at her watch. There was plenty of time. She sat down on a bench. Sean scowled, wanting to walk on.

'If you disappear, you'll either find me here or at the café. Follow the signs to it if you get lost,' she said a little tetchily. 'We've got to be there by three.' Why couldn't he ever just be happy to stay with her and keep her company like other children seemed to be with their mums? 'And don't talk to strangers,' she called after him.

She sat back. Above her a single shaft of sunlight dappled down through the canopy of leaves onto her face. She closed her eyes and dozed for a while, briefly opening them again and shifting slightly up the bench as a smelly and dishevelled old woman sat down noisily beside her. On the ground in front of her, the old woman kept on arranging and rearranging her collection of plastic shopping bags into and out of two large black bin liners. Lucille shut her eyes again, but her doziness was disturbed by the rustle of the old woman's repeated fussing with her bags. And her smell. Lucille shielded her eyes and squinted at her. Then she sat up with a start, her heart thumping in her breast.

She knew that hand. Older, grimier, bonier and more veinous it might be, but that prominent freckle just behind the knuckle of the woman's ringless third finger was unmistakable and could only belong to one person.

'Rosie!' she said, breaking into a delighted squeal of recognition.

The old woman glared at her briefly before turning back to her bags and muttering something inaudible.

'Rosie.'

'Oh it's you, Luke. Will you stop bothering me and let me get on with what I'm doing. I've lost your picture.'

'Rose, its me. Lucille,' she said, feeling abashed and hurt like a child. 'Not Luke, Lucille! How are you? I didn't recognise you. You look,' she hesitated. 'You look so old!' There was no other word for it.

'Never mind how I look. It's what I am looking *for* that matters. I can't find it anywhere.'

'Rosie! Don't you recognise me? What's happened to you?' Some of the answers were all too obvious.

When Rose had told her eight years ago that she didn't ever want to see her again, she had repeatedly denied it had anything to do with the fact that Lucille was living with Richard. Despite her hurt, Lucille had tried to stay in touch with her anyway. But Rose never returned her phone calls or her letters. Eventually on Richard's advice she had stopped, (as he put it), persecuting Rose with her need to stay in touch and sadly accepted that Rose had meant what she said. All contact between them had ceased.

'The devil is in the detail, they say. You look too young, so you wouldn't really know that! I'll just have to go through it all again properly. Please don't interfere.'

Lucille winced at Rose's peremptory, school-marmish tone of voice. It was disconcerting because it felt both personal and impersonal at one and the same time. Rose started delving in her bin liners again, pulling out empty plastic shopping bags once more and the occasional old newspaper, one after the other. She was cursing under her breath, muttering something incomprehensible about floating photographs or something. And fire and rain. She seemed quite mad.

'Let me help you. What are you looking for? A picture?'

'I've told you once!' Rose said angrily. 'I'm *not* telling you again. You wouldn't understand. Do you have a swimming costume? If not, then leave me alone. I have to find my child.'

Lucille felt her courage returning.

'Well, you're not going to find him in a rubbish bag, are you?' she said in a careful tone. Quite clearly Rose had become mentally ill.

'These bags contain my belongings, but that which I belong to most of all is gone. I'm *afraid* he's gone anyway, I've got to find out. I dreamt I burned him and drowned him in the Thames. But I don't know. Maybe it wasn't a dream. I may have done. I shall just have to go back to the river, that's all. Search till I find him. Swimming would be good for my arthritis, wouldn't it? Don't I know you?'

'It's me, Lucille, Rose. Lucille! Your – your, I don't know, your friend! I'm your friend, Rosie.'

Rose frowned, picked up everything she had taken out of the bags and stuffed it back in again, saying not another word. Then she stood up.

'I'm a mother. Or I was a mother once. I know I was. I've got to go back to the river. I've got to find him or I'll lose myself again.'

With that, she shuffled off up the path without a backward glance, limping terribly.

Chapter 15.

After landing back in Manchester at midday Grainne picked up her new Toyota and headed for home, relishing the car's air-conditioning as she sat in a motorway traffic jam beneath the cloudless blue sky.

She switched on her mobile phone and rang home to pick up her messages. There were almost thirty. Most of them from clients. The very last one was from Lucille.

'Hello? Grainne? Are you there? You're not, are you? I'm sorry not to be able to speak to you personally because something terrible has happened. No! Don't get alarmed. Not terrible like a bomb or something. What I mean is I have done something bad. Well, no! Not bad exactly. But not good, Grainny! Definitely not good. And it could turn out badly, but it could turn out alright. Oh dear. I should start again really, but your ansaphone wouldn't have enough room on it for me to explain everything! I need to speak to you badly, Grainny. I really do because...' There was a pause then she started speaking so fast that it was hard to hear everything she was saying. 'I met Ron. He's a psychologist. He was giving this lecture I'd been sent to by a marriage counsellor, cos me and Richard haven't been getting on very well recently. I didn't realise it *was* actually Ron till he appeared and started talking. And even then I couldn't believe it! He's changed so much, Grainny. Anyway, I'm gabbling again. The problem is – I didn't mean to but – when we got talking I somehow blurted out that Sean was his son. I'm so sorry, Grainne. But that's just the half of it. What's worse – much worse – is I've told Sean now as well! I don't know why. I couldn't help it. And Sean is insisting on seeing him. Now! Today. I couldn't bear having to put up with his sulks and rages if I said no. I'm feeling very stressed at the moment what with Mum dying and everything. So I rang Ron. He's so gorgeous, Grainny. Really, you wouldn't believe it. Sean and I are meeting up with him this afternoon at three. If you get in within the next twenty minutes, then please, *please* ring me. My mobile's not working so you won't be able to get me after that. I don't really know what to do for the best, Grainne, but we must talk. I'm so nervous. Bye-ee. No! I mean, Ring me Grainny. As soon as you possibly can. Oh, and this is Ron's number if you want to speak to him about it first. I'm sorry about the mess I have caused. Bye-ee.'

Che sera, thought Grainne, playing the message through again and jotting down the number. Then she tried ringing Lucille. No reply. She left a message. Then she dialled directory enquiries and asked for the number of Richard's hospital. Perhaps he would be able to tell her what had happened. She got through to his secretary who said he was busy and would have to ring her back.

Should she ring Ron? What could she say after all this time and exactly how much had Lucille told him? The silly cow. It was so unlike her to blab like that. The shock of seeing Ron must have loosened her tongue. It certainly was a bit of a surprise to hear that he was now a psychologist. Wonders never cease. But if he really was so different, he would hopefully be much more sensible than the man she had last seen eleven or twelve years ago.

The motorway was at a complete standstill. Welcome back to England. She turned on the radio, tuned into the local news station to find out about the traffic. If Richard didn't ring her back within the next few minutes she would just have to ring Ron directly and try and find out what was going on from him.

Without thinking she started ripping at a cuticle with her teeth. When the blood began to flow, she sucked on it angrily.

This was the last thing she wanted. She had just wanted to go home and meditate, quietly reconcile herself to the fact that she was finally back in contact with her family.

Not that she felt any better about that. Not really, because even now after all these years, and after all that truth-telling she and Ma had done together the night before the party, she was still keeping other truths from her. She hadn't told her anything about her work. Not her real work. Deliberately misleading her by gabbling on about her nursing as if it was still her regular and only employment.

So just like before, lies and sex still formed a barrier between herself and her mother. Just as they always had. And they always would. There was really no need for Ma to know what she actually did to earn a living most of the time. What would be the point? Just to upset her? Revenge for not having protected her properly when she was a little girl? No. If there was a childish part of her that did still feel angry with her about that, as an adult she now felt it would be quite out of the question to hurl it back at Ma by hurting her with present day truths she really did not need to know.

Nevertheless, the child in her would always feel betrayed by Ma for once having trusted Uncle Jack.

If she had ever been one to cry she would be bawling her eyes out now. But she never cried.

Ma had asked her about boyfriends, of course, but she had evaded answering her with blarney and blather so slick that Ma didn't even notice. So she had been able to avoid telling her the truth that she never had any patience for men because no man had been able to get past her memories of Uncle Jack. Whenever a man she might have fancied had ever shown an interest in her, images of him would always flashback in her mind's eye. He had been more than a match for every boyfriend she had ever tried to have.

Except maybe for Ron, now she came to think of it. But back in the very early days of their relationship with him she had still been young and naïve enough to believe that love could conquer all.

Sex work was brilliant both for making money and for keeping flashbacks of Uncle Jack at bay. She felt controlled and powerful when performing sex acts with her punters. A true professional, she was blessed with being able to keep her private feelings quite out of what she was doing when she was at work. Memories of Uncle Jack became mere phantasms wispily floating around at the back of her mind when she bent over a prone client on the table to finish off his massage with whatever extra he was paying for. Whereas in her private life he would always intrude. Always. A huge and ever-present malevolent monster, continually spoiling any closeness she ever managed to build up between herself and the one or two men she had tried to love. Nevertheless she sometimes wondered whether she would have been unattracted to men anyway, regardless of Uncle Jack. She had often wondered whether she was lesbian, definitely preferring the company of women, but it wasn't sexual.

Her work had another positive spin-off. Doing something she could feel in control of, had been one of the main reasons why self-harm and subsequently anorexia had been so attractive when she had been younger. But both behaviours had had visibly damaging results. Or as she experienced it, damagingly *visible* results. In contrast, her work as a professional masseuse behind closed doors and in the safety of a well organised health club provided her with exactly the same kind of buzz as cutting or starving herself used to give her, without any visible harmful effects on her whatsoever. The buzz was unique to the act of doing wrong, attacking her sense of integrity and well-being. That was what she craved. And she always would. So why shouldn't she take money for it? And what if it could all be traced back to the effect of Uncle Jack? Prostitution provided her with an income which as a nurse she could only dream about. And it wasn't as if she was so desperate that she ever did anything she didn't want to do. She never resorted to wearing basques or stockings or any of that nonsense for her punters, despite not being so young anymore. She did what she did in her sports gear. They could like it or lump it. The club charged her an exorbitant fee for the use of her room, it was true, but that was a price well worth paying. Not only for turning a blind eye to what she actually did there, but also for providing her with respectable cover and immediate help if an emergency arose. There was an alarm button under her massage table wired up to the security office behind reception. In six years she had never once had to use it. She was going to be thirty five soon and she'd come to accept that despite her work, which anyway wouldn't last beyond the life of her looks, hers was always going to be a celibate life.

She smiled at the irony of that, as the radio traffic announcer talked about a six mile queue on the M6. Perhaps she would ring Ron after all. But what would she say? Hello Ron, this is the mother of your child. Then what? What would be the point? To tell him she didn't mind if he wanted to see his child? What right was it of hers *to* mind? She had seen nearly as little of Sean as he had. And if he was the transformed figure Lucille seemed to think he was, it was probably better that the boy got an experience of his father than of no parent at all.

She thought about turning the engine off. At once the cars ahead of her inched forward a few metres. The battered white van immediatey in front of her reminded her of all the times Uncle Jack had done his thing with her in the back of his Transit on a farm track up in the hills, as battered old white vans always did. There was nowhere he hadn't abused her and nowhere she had ever been able to go to get away from the memories of it. But she was better now at recognising them as they came up out of the blue to haunt her. And better at pushing them away again.

And seeing the man himself for the first time in all these years at Ma's party had definitely made a difference. She'd insisted to Ma that she wanted to see him, stopped her from ringing Auntie Bobbie to cancel his invitation. And she was glad. What a snivelling, self-piteous old creep he was now, stuck in that rickety old wheelchair of his, looking grey, undernourished and surprisingly small. That was the most shocking thing. He'd always loomed so large in her psychological life that he seemed to be everywhere, but when she met him again he'd turned out to be a damp sock of a man now, huddled beneath his smelly old blankets. As threatening as a drowned rat. In contrast, Auntie Bobbie, who had been so petite two decades ago, had turned into a great galleon of a woman, pushing him around with a saintly smile on her over-fed, innocent face. Maybe I'm not the only one who never grew up because of Uncle Jack, thought Grainne. At the party Bobbie had dutifully sat beside him the whole night, continuously, but daintily stuffing herself and beaming genially at all and sundry. She fed Jack by hand every now and again too, finding kind words for anybody who could be bothered to chat with her. Many had. But not Grainne. After politely greeting them both and spending a maddening minute listening to Uncle Jack whinging about his inability to do anything for himself anymore nowadays, she had made her excuses and greeted someone else.

She was glad she had seen him though, and that his life should now be a squalid, long drawn out kind of living death. There was some justice perhaps, of a kind. Seeing him had laid some of the ghostly images from her past, if not the feelings. They would never go. They were a part of her and always would be. But the huge nightmare figure of her childhood had now been replaced by a pathetic wretch of a man.

The radio was becoming repetitive and she turned it off. At the same moment her phone rang.

'Richard! Thanks for ringing me back. How are you?'

'All the better for hearing your voice, Grainne,' replied the old smoothie. 'We haven't seen you for years. I hope all is well? How are you and what can I do for you?'

'I'm fine Richard, thanks. But I had a slightly hysterical call from Lucille about Sean.'

'What? Is something wrong?'

'No-o. I don't think so anyway. She said she had arranged for Sean to meet his father this afternoon and wanted to talk with me about it first.'

'Did she though? I know nothing about it, I'm afraid. I sometimes wonder whether I know half the things Lucille gets up to nowadays. She certainly met him yesterday at some training course she was on about human development. He's in the training and consultancy game, you know. Doing very well, I understand. I'm afraid it sounded like claptrap to me. But Lucille said she found some of the ideas inspirational and enjoyed it very much.'

'Well that's important I think. If you're not enjoying something it's not worth doing it at all, is it Richard?'

What clichés she was able to conjure when the need arose. But she had sensed some edge to his complaint about not knowing half of what Lucille did, and felt she needed to defend her friend, support her by giving him back a dose of his own medicine, something double edged. Lucille may be your wife, she thought, but she's my friend and we liars have to support one another. The excited tone in Lucille's voice on her telephone message suggested she'd found Ron a lot more interesting than her husband. Maybe it was partly because he was a doctor and she was a nurse, but Grainne had always felt that Richard was a bit of a slimeball. For the life of her, she couldn't understand what Lucille had ever seen in him.

'I quite agree with you, as a hedonist at heart myself,' he said in his effortlessly superior way. 'But why are you calling me about it?'

'I thought you might be able to tell me what's happened, if you wouldn't mind, please Richard.'

'I'm not sure I can. All she told me was that the lecturer on her course yesterday turned out to be er, what's his name – Ron, your ex. And that's it really. Except they went out together in the evening afterwards so that she could tell him more about Sean and he could give her the benefit of his, um, advice about how to handle him.'

'She didn't say anything about meeting him with Sean today then?'
'Nothing.'

Did he sound jealous? Oh well, it was none of her business anyway.

'Richard I wonder if I could ask a very big favour? Would you mind if I came down and stayed overnight for a day or two? Two days at most. I want to be back at work on Monday, but I feel if Sean is going to meet his father today then it really is time that he met his mother again too. Don't you?'

'Well, I see what you are saying.'

'And do you agree?'

'I suppose I do as a matter of fact.'

'So you wouldn't mind if I stayed a couple of nights then?'

'Of course I wouldn't. I'd be delighted. And please do. It's what Lucille and I have wanted for years, as I am sure she has often told you. We've got plenty of room. When would you get here?'

'I flew in from Belfast an hour ago and since I got out of the airport I have been sitting in a traffic jam, so I don't honestly know. But I've got my things with me so I could just drive on once it starts moving again. I could be in Oxshott between seven and eight this evening? Would that be alright?'

'I would certainly be in by that time,' he replied. 'I don't know about Lucille and Sean of course. I imagine he might want to stay with his father if they get on alright. On the other hand, he may get moody and tongue-tied and just want to leave, knowing Sean. But never mind all that. Do you know how to get here? No of course you don't.'

She got her pen out from her bag again, wrote his instructions down on the inside cover of her road atlas. Then she thanked him and hung up. She might as well ring Ron after all. Why not? Presumably he was going through something quite similar, being about to meet their son for the first time.

She hadn't seen Sean herself since he was a tiny toddler, although she remembered the enormous wrench involved in separating herself from him like it was yesterday. It had been mentally equivalent to the physical pain of giving birth to him fifteen months before, except unlike labour she had been in charge of the process. And the struggle not to see him, had lasted much longer. It hurt terribly. And for the first few weeks after leaving him with Lucille, while she received hospital treatment down in Beckenham for her anorexia, it was all she could do not to give up the fight there and then, drop everything and just go back over to Lucille's and retrieve him. It had taken every perverse drop of determination in her blood not to do that, the determination that up till then she had been focusing on eating and on not eating. Her skin had literally crawled for him, her whole body – what little there was of it by then – itching to take him back. Then the itch became physical. Eczema attacked her everywhere, but particularly across her breasts and belly. But Grainne knew it was all for the best, because she didn't want to harm Sean by selfishly trying to stay attached to him. So it was just another part of the process of separation from him. It took about three years, but eventually she was successful in fighting off the feelings of wanting him back, and the process was complete.

Mostly.

There were periods of emotional relapse, particularly after her discharge from hospital when again it sometimes took all the love she had for him not to go and see him and take him back from Lucille. But eventually it became second nature to deny her feelings. Just as her anorexia had made hunger become more satisfying than eating, so her love for Sean had made not looking after him better than having him back in her arms. She even began to be proud that for once in her life she'd genuinely been able to do something good for someone else. Genuinely and without being paid. So even though Lucille rang her every day once she was out of hospital, begging her to come and see him and saying he was pining and whimpering for her all the time, she was able to be firm and tell her that it was much the best thing for him in the long term: if she had nothing to do with him she could not directly do him any emotional harm. Lucille had told her she was talking nonsense, that Sean needed *her* more than anyone else, but Grainne finessed this emotional appeal when Lucille rang up one evening choking back tears.

At first Grainne had not noticed what a state she was in.

'Grainne, you've got to take him back,' Lucille said.

'What's this, Luce, you need another telephone counselling session?'

She'd replied jokily, expecting Lucille who always used to like a laugh, to join in with her.

'You must have got my messages. I came by with him this afternoon to see you, but you didn't answer your door. I know you were in, Grainne. How can you do this to your own baby?'

'Lucille! Get this! Right? I don't care if you can't understand it, but once and for all you have to *hear* me.' She paused deliberately for effect, then raised her voice and speaking slowly and clearly said, 'I can't and I won't have him back.'

There was an awful silence between them then which Grainne eventually broke.

'I'm sorry I didn't let you in, but it would have hurt all of us if I had.'

'He needs you Grainne. No matter what I try to do with him it's not good enough because *'I'm* not *you*. I *have* heard what you've said, and I will look after him because I love him. But you haven't heard me. It's you he wants.'

'Well he's wrong to want me, and you can show him that, Luce. He's too young to know any better himself. Show him he's wrong. I would only do him harm.'

'*This* is harming him! I don't want to show him he's wrong. Because he isn't! It would be a lie. I'm doing everything I can, but only because you won't! And because I love him. Not to show him he's wrong and certainly not because I can look after him better than you. Because I can't. And you're all wrong to think I can, Grainne. I do my best, but all he does is cry. Or scream. I take him in my arms and he lets me hold him, but the crying and the screaming never stop. It never stops except when he's asleep. And even then, he whimpers. Other babies his age are smiling and into everything, but whenever I take him out or to a mother and toddler group or shopping or anything, we have to leave again because no matter what I do I can't stop his howling. I can't go anywhere with him. I can't see anyone. And I'm sure it's all about wanting to be back with you. Completely sure, Grainne. Can you hear me? He's your baby, Grainne. Your own sweet little baby. It's you he wants and it's you he needs.'

Grainne felt her whole being longing to embrace Sean as Lucille spoke. But as ever, she ignored such feelings. If she loved him, she had to stay away from him. Her personality was too damaged, too warped to do him anything but harm. The pained silence between them returned before she replied.

'Have you finished, Lucille? Have you said everything you've got to say?'

'Yes. Yes I have.'

'Good. You're right. But I am his mother. So I know, in a way that you cannot, that also you are *wrong*! He may want me back, but it really would be damaging for him to live with me. Because I can't help it – however much I love him – there is a part of me that hates him. And I know Lucie, I KNOW I would harm him. So please, please, please don't give up on him for me. I beg you. You must be his mother now because you are my best friend and I know you won't harm him. You will give him love and it may take a while, but eventually he'll know it. And he will grow out of this crying one day soon. I'm sure of it. You see, I am actually still ill, if I am honest. I may have been discharged from hospital, but the truth is I still spend my whole time either thinking or forcing myself not to think about calories, nothing else. I couldn't possibly think about babies. So it would be disastrous for Sean if I were to have him back, disastrous. Don't you see?'

'Rose thinks I should take him to see a child psychiatrist,' Lucille said tentatively. 'One who specialises in Sean's kind of problems, not just the paediatrician he sees at the moment. I think she's right. I mean Dr Stevens is a very nice lady, but nothing is changing, nothing is getting any better. Would you mind, Grainne?'

Grainne had wanted to stay distant, express no opinion at all other than the one she had already, that Lucille had him in his care so she should make the decisions without consulting her, but she couldn't stop herself saying,

'No! Don't do that. That really wouldn't help at all. I worked with one once, when I was training. They can't see anything without diagnosing some non-existent psychological illness. There is nothing wrong with Sean. Nothing – that he didn't already have, Lucille, cos of how I treated him in the womb and in his first months of life. I think you're doing a wonderful job with him, nobody else would have given up her work to look after a friend's baby for her . But you've only had him for a few months so it's only natural that he should still be crying all the time at the moment. That's not mad, is it? It's normal. Any little toddler of fifteen months would be the same under the circumstances. But he'll get over it. I know he will. He doesn't need a psychiatrist.'

'He will by the time you've had your way with him,' replied Lucille, almost shouting. Grainne was impressed, but then as she'd known she would, Lucille retreated back into softness. 'No I don't mean that! I'm sorry Grainny. It's just so difficult. I don't think I can manage anymore.'

'He'll just have to go into care then,' said Grainne coldly. *She* was not going to soften. It would only bring heartache for all concerned. 'Social Services can find him some foster carers and arrange for him to be adopted. Or he can go into a home for autistic children or something, cos nobody would want to adopt him, would they?'

'Grainne!' Lucille shrieked. 'Stop talking like that about your own little boy! I *love* him. Nobody else could love him, except you, the best person of all, if you only would.' She paused, but Grainne deliberately did not respond. It was in Sean's long term interest that he must not suffer the burden of having her as his mother. It was imperative. He absolutely must not.

She heard Lucille sniffing, then blowing her nose.

'At least come and see him.'

'That would only prolong the agony. For all of us,' she replied, adding more softly, 'it will get better. I know it will.'

Perhaps Lucille heard the implacability in her voice.

'Maybe, Grainny. Maybe you're right. Maybe he will stop crying eventually. You can't cry all your life, can you?'

Well, not with tears, thought Grainne now, inching her car forward another couple of metres.

She had rung Lucille up nearly every day for the first six months after she came out of hospital to offer her support – from a distance – and to find out how Sean was doing. Eventually Lucille's bulletins did become more optimistic. He did find time for things other than crying.

By the time he was five years old, Grainne hardly spoke to Lucille more than once every month or two. When she did, Lucille would describe a boy who never sat still unless he was so concentrated on something that he could not attend to anything else, but also a boy who did not cry at all now about anything, ever. An odd boy. A boy who Lucille did in fact take to a child psychiatrist when he was seven after she'd become the third Mrs McElvey and had had enough experience looking after Sean to become more confident about taking parental decisions like that without first consulting Grainne. A boy who presented what the psychiatrist prosaically called a mixed picture, between Attention Deficit and Hyperactivity Disorder and Asbergers Syndrome. Lucille had rung her to tell her about it afterwards. Disorders and syndromes were not strictly speaking illnesses, the psychiatrist had told her, and they were therefore untreatable. Nevertheless and confusingly he had prescribed a combination of carbemazapine and methylphenidate and pronounced that what was of most benefit to children like Sean was knowing they had the love of their family and a stable predictable structure to their lives. He had said patronisingly and without any real enquiry, after eliciting that she was married to a doctor, that he was confident Lucille was able to offer him both of those things.

It happened to be true, as Grainne had always known of course.

She slipped back out of her reverie to inch the car forward another couple of metres. She dialled Ron's number.

'Hello?'

She didn't recognise his voice. But it had to be him.

'Hi, Ron.'

'Who is this?'

'She with whom you once shared a life, Ron. Grainne. Remember me?'

'Grainne!? Grainne! How are you? First Lulu. Now you. And after all this time. It's nice to hear your voice. How are you?'

Was this really Ron? The timbre and accent were much the same but his vocal delivery was absolutely unrecognisable – brisk, alert, confident and socially adept. The man she left eleven years ago had not possessed a single one of those attributes. So he really could be anybody.

'Not too bad. I've been worse, Ron, since we last spoke. What about yourself?'

'I'm – I've never been better. I'm just about to meet up with Lucille and – and er, the son you never told me about. Sean.'

'Oh, good. I'm so glad you haven't met up with them just yet. I feel I owe you an explanation about Sean. Before you see him I mean. I should really have given you one a long time ago, I know, but I chickened out. That's why I'm ringing.'

'What kind of explanation?' His tone had changed, he sounded uninterested. 'Lucille has already told me enough, I think, as far as I am concerned anyway. But, of course, you don't know what she said and you would obviously have different things to say yourself. I understand that. As regards the details at least, if not the headlines. But it's not really necessary.'

He was so articulate. She felt befuddled and a little daunted. Already she could feel that this man now was as different from the one she used to know as chalk from cheese. It felt weird. But she would persevere with an attempt at normal conversation, or as normal as a conversation could be between two people under such circumstances.

'What did she say?' Grainne asked.

'Is this the right time or place?'

'I don't mind if you don't mind, Ron. Anyway I actually don't know where I am. Stuck in a motorway traffic jam somewhere a few miles from Manchester. Where are you?'

He laughed politely with her.

'That's a coincidence. I'm out on the street too. On foot though. I'm just coming out of Kensington High street tube station and it's quite difficult to hear you amidst the traffic noise and all the hustle and bustle here. I can hardly move there's so many people milling around. The sunshine must bring everybody out. So it may be the right time for this conversation, Grainne, but it's not really the right place. Not for me. What do you think? Shall we talk later?'

Was he asking her or telling her? She felt very controlled either way, something she never allowed any man to do.

For a moment she had a vivid memory of the old dependent Ron who used to confer with her about everything, was incapable of taking a single decision for himself and couldn't control the flow of his own urine into a toilet bowl. Lucille was right, this man was different.

'Maybe just the headlines then?' she said. ''Cos you're right, of course you are. I would like to meet up with you too, Ron, and explain properly. Give you my version of the details. Not just about Sean but about me too if you like. Why I went. That kind of thing. Did Lucille tell you about that too?'

It was curious. Even though they were now obviously completely different people, she could sense they were both still carrying feelings around from their mutual past as if what was between them had only happened yesterday. What made it more curious was the fact that by the time they had parted all those years ago their relationship had actually been almost non-existent. Neither of them had really cared what the other said or did by then. So why should they care now? It didn't make any sense.

'To be honest, Grainne, I don't really need to rake over the ashes of ancient history. Who said, the past is another country? No. I can't remember either. But that's how it is for me now. So I can't really remember everything she's told me.'

He was lying. She could hear the defensiveness in his voice, but the Fuck Off in it was equally audible. On the other hand they were actually strangers now, it was true, so perhaps she was wrong. Perhaps it was just her imagination that there was still a feeling of things being unresolved between them.

Ron seemed to sense that this reply had left her feeling rebuffed. He sounded as if he wanted to retrieve any hurt he might just have done her when he said,

'What I do remember Lucille told me, is that it was her fault that you suddenly decided to leave me all those years ago, because she told you about what she and I had been doing together. But as I said to her that meant that it was actually my fault too, because it is surely true that whatever we did, we did do together.'

Grainne was silent. He was definitely pushing her away. But at least he was being truthful. Why didn't the truth ever set her free like it was supposed to do – like it did in the movies?

But why, too, did he still sound almost defiant after all these years?

'She also told me that the very day she left to go and live with that woman who paid for her operation, you discovered you were pregnant. She told me you moved into a nurses residence for a while, and that after Sean was born you decided not to contact me because you felt I was too ill and unreliable to be able to cope with being a father – that it wouldn't be good for the child. Does that about sum it up?'

Grainne nodded. She hadn't noticed that the van in front of her had moved on nearly fifty metres. Two cars had taken advantage of the gap she had created and nipped inside. The car behind her hooted.

'Are you still there?'

'Oh! I'm sorry. Yes, I'm still here, Ron, and yes, I suppose you've summed things up very well indeed.' As an afterthought she added, 'as Lucille must have told them to you.' If he hadn't sounded sore about her leaving him, he definitely sounded unhappy about not having been told about Sean. She would have been too, if the boot had been on the other foot.

'You were probably right,' he said. She thought he added something else, but could not hear him properly. The sounds of the London street around him were certainly busier and more energetic than the traffic out here on the motorway. That was for sure.

'What was that?'

'I said, you were right to think I wouldn't have been able to function effectively as a father, but you still should have told me about him.'

'I know I should have, Ron, but at that time I couldn't cope myself. I was trying to do anything I could, short of actual abortion, to get rid of him. I didn't want a baby.'

'So why didn't you have an abortion?'

'I don't know, I really don't. I was so confused. I mean I don't want to be offensive, but I didn't feel I had a man I could rely on, so it would have been perfectly rational to have had one. Residual religious hang-ups, maybe? I don't know. I knew I wasn't fit to be a mother and wouldn't be able to look after a baby. But I honestly don't know. It was a feeling. I just felt it would be wrong to abort him. But I'm sorry. You are actually quite right. This isn't the time or place to be talking about these things. Can I see you? Can we meet? What do you think?'

'I don't really think that would be a very good idea at all. Perhaps we'll meet up one day. You never know. I certainly don't believe there is anything more I need to know now. No offence.'

They hung up. Fuck you, she thought.

Grainne still didn't like him, and he was clearly still a selfish bastard whatever Lucille might believe about him being changed and whatever feelings she might have for him. Grainne noticed she was so livid her heart was racing.

The traffic around her, in contrast, remained at an absolute standstill.

Chapter 16.

Ron returned his mobile phone to the pocket of his jacket which he was carrying over his shoulder as he made his way through the milling crowds of shoppers and tourists down towards Holland Park. The heat of the afternoon on the busy street was torrid. As soon as he could he crossed the road to the shaded side of the street. He had dressed to be cool in his lightest camel-coloured linen suit but still felt himself sweating. He slowed down. Perhaps it was speaking to Grainne again that had put him into a sweat. Even after all this time she still had the power to make him feel stupid. For a brief terrifying moment as they had been talking he had even found himself experiencing a dash of that old sense of paranoia he used to call his cancer before the Olanzapine had kicked in.

That had been a nightmare. He hadn't wanted the medication at all, but the psychiatrist had insisted, talked about forcing him to take it if necessary, under a section of the mental health act. There was no doubt though that it had helped. His brief stay in a psychiatric acute admissions ward had also been salutary. In fact he looked back on it now as a defining moment. Thereafter he had been consistently determined to take a rational pragmatic trajectory through his life, always planning the next step in his rehabilitation, if not his rebirth into someone he could be proud of.

He turned right through the gates into Holland Park. There was no hurry. He still had more than half an hour before he was due to meet Lucille. He would sit down in the shade under the trees and think about what he wanted to achieve from their meeting. He always liked to set himself a target. It was only rational.

Then he noticed that the blonde on the bench up ahead was her.

She was blowing her nose as he approached and didn't notice him until he was right up close. He smiled a greeting, sat down beside her and said hello in a quiet, friendly voice as she glanced up at him from behind her tissue with a look that was almost resentful. How could that be? He had done nothing for her to resent. Not recently anyway, and not yet. Her eyes were red. She looked like she had been crying.

'What's the matter? What's happened? Can I help?' He asked in the practiced, solicitous manner laced with hypnotic repetition he always deployed professionally.

'It's Rose. Look.' She pointed at an old bag lady quite a distance away now disappearing round the corner in the general direction of the café.

He studied Lucille's face, not comprehending, and her eyes filled with tears again. Almost as if his looking at her triggered her failure to hold them back. Or was he giving himself too much power? He would find out in a minute.

'I owe my life to her,' she said, 'and now she's living on the streets and doesn't recognise me. I feel so sad, so sorry for her and so hurt. She refused to acknowledge me just now even though she was sitting right beside me, just where you are now. She did recognise me though, I *know* she did. But she blanked me completely, said she had lost her identity with her child and I wouldn't understand. It was a – a bit upsetting.'

She blew her nose again, got a mirror out of her bag and carefully wiped around her eyes.

'Oh this was not what I was expecting at all,' she said, giving him a nervous glance, then peering at herself mournfully again before putting the smudged tissue and mirror back into her bag.

His impressions from yesterday were confirmed. She was very attractive.

'Rose?' He said. 'Do you mean the woman who took you in and paid for your surgery?'

She nodded.

'Are you sure? Yes of course you are. I'm sorry. So, she's a bag lady, is she? I dimly remember spending a not unpleasant evening with her once, after falling over and breaking my wrist. She was very kind.'

'She's lovely, absolutely lovely. But now she's walking the streets of London trying to find something. I don't know what. Herself, I think, for pity's sake. I've got to help her. I've got to.'

'I don't see how you can. She would have to want you to and allow you to and from what you say that's er, unlikely. I guess at some level she must have made a choice to live like this.'

'How can you say such a thing?' Lucille's voice became shrill. 'She's completely confused and she's definitely not at all happy. You of all people ought to know that that's not always a choice.' Her eyes were flashing with anger. He liked it.

'No, you're right of course, it's not always a choice. But at some level, if she recognised you, but refused to do so openly, then there must be at least some element of choosing not to, don't you think?' He was all reason.

'I don't know. And I don't care. All I know is I must help her. She helped me when I needed it. I wouldn't be me if it wasn't for her. I'm so sorry, Ron, I really, really am, but unless you want to come with me. I'm afraid I'll have to say goodbye now. Perhaps we can arrange for you and Sean to meet on another day, if you don't mind. But I have got to go after Rose now and try and persuade her to come home with me. I've simply got to. I can't wait. She might disappear otherwise, and I might never see her again. I must help her. I must.'

She didn't wait for him to reply and set off immediately after the old tramp who had continued her slow waddle away out of sight by now. Ron looked at Lucille for a moment uncertain whether he wanted the hassle, then with his eyes on her arse he jumped up and ran after her. What the hell! He also had a son to meet and it was important to go with the flow of what was happening now he was out here.

He caught up with Lucille in a few strides. As he did so, she stumbled. She was walking too fast. He instinctively put an arm out and caught her before she could hit the ground. She thanked him, doubly, for coming with her and for catching her, continued to hold on to him for a little while as they walked on.

'It's just that after my mother and my – Sean – no-one has ever meant so much to me as Rose,' she explained breathlessly. 'No-one. I just can't let her go like this without trying to do something to help. Do you know what I mean?' She disengaged from him, her brow furrowed, purposeful, insisting he understand.

'I do. Of course I do,' he replied. 'But where is Sean?'

'Well, I told him to meet us at the café at three, and I am sure he'll be there. He's so little in some ways as you'll see – in emotional ways – but in other ways, such as time and place and reading maps, that kind of thing, he's better than an adult. Certainly better than me. I can never find my way anywhere. But we must hurry. I mustn't lose Rose.'

They rounded a bend in the path and then pulled up short. There was Rose not thirty metres away. She was talking to a ginger haired lad in a T-shirt and trainers.

Lucille squeezed his arm, looking at them both for a moment, a beatific smile on her face. Then she said softly, 'That's your son, Ron, talking to Rose now. That's Sean. I wonder how they found each other. He normally never talks to strangers. And he hasn't seen Rose since he was three or four years old. He would never have recognised her. But look at them, they're talking together like two old friends. She must have recognised him, even though he's three times the size he was when she last saw him.'

Ron made to go on over to them, but Lucille held on to his arm and squeezed again, gently pulling him back.

'Look, isn't that nice? Why don't we sit down here and watch them for a while? It's so wonderful to see Rosie again! And Sean is such a fine little boy, isn't he? Well, not so little, I know. He's almost as big as me now.' She laughed. 'And you can see from here that he looks just like you. He even carries himself in the same way you do. It's so obvious. I don't know how I never noticed it before.'

'Yes, I can see the resemblance, but from here it's his orange hair that gets to me. Just like Grainne's was. Or I dare say is.'

He patted his other jacket pocket where he had put the computer game he'd bought for the boy. Whatever was he going to say to him? He had never had anything to do with children. But he was going to have to start somewhere. And then continue and never actually finish. Never give

259

him a permanent goodbye. At least that's what he'd promised Lucille yesterday, because he did know about the subject of child development. Academically, at any rate. It just would not be right to disappear out of the boy's life again once he had introduced himself to him. It slightly complicated his plan to seduce and then dump Lucille, but no matter. He would deal with that when the time came. Anyway he might even change his mind about that. For a while at least – if she fucked as well as she looked, he might want to keep on with her for a while.

'It seems very clear to me, looking at him, that you've done a great job mothering him,' he said, stroking her hand which was still attached to his arm. She simpered, nodding her head, didn't remove it. Flattery would get him everywhere.

'I have really, haven't I?' She said. 'He's been so difficult. Ron, though, you'd never believe it sometimes. Look at him now. A more perfect little boy it would be hard to imagine. But he bullied me – I know it sounds silly, but it's true – he bullied me into ringing you up and arranging this meeting. Today, I mean.' She paused, shaking her head which drew his attention to her hair which was full and lustrous in the afternoon sunlight. He was enjoying this. 'I wish I knew what to say to Rose,' she said in a small voice. 'She shouldn't be living rough on the streets. But it's obvious she is, isn't it?' She carried on staring at her with a sad face until suddenly her eyes lit up and she said, 'I don't know how to put it to her, but I know what I'd like. I'd like her to stay with me. I'd love it if she stayed with me. Until she can feel she's found her identity again, if that's what it's about. She helped me find mine. It's the least I can do to offer her that.'

'Why don't you just say so, then? Tell her that's what you'd like to do?'

'Because she treated me just now like I don't exist.' She shrugged. 'And if I don't exist, how can I possibly ask her to stay with me?'

'What would your husband feel about her coming to live with you both, supposing she agreed to?' Ron asked. 'Would he mind?'

'Well he was *her* husband once too, so I think he would want to show her some compassion,' Lucille replied more briskly. 'Under the circumstances. In fact I am sure he would.'

Her husband would clearly do whatever she asked of him then.

'He was *her* husband too?'

'She was his first wife.'

Lucille's face lit up again as she saw Rose delving into one of her bags with Sean standing close beside her with an expectant, interested expression on his face as she did so. 'Look at them. Just like two old friends. I think she wants to give him a present or something. I do hope he isn't rude to her.'

Ron looked across at his son watching the old woman turn to another bag and begin searching in that. He could see something self-conscious about the way the boy was concentrating on what Rose was doing. It meant, of course, that Sean was probably aware of him sitting over here beside his mother. And that he was shy perhaps, awkward about acknowledging the fact. In a minute, once Rose had moved on, or while Lucille tried to talk to her again, he would stroll over and introduce himself to the boy. It was the strangest feeling imaginable, but he could certainly see the resemblance with himself. He could also see Grainne's hair.

He returned his attention to Lucille. She was easier to look at. He could see she was aware of his gaze and didn't really want it. Not just now. He stood up, suggested they join Rose and Sean. It was the right thing to have said. She nodded and they started walking over. As they approached her the old woman began making strange noises.

* * *

Rose McElvey couldn't find her kitchen devil. First her child had gone, then her identity went missing and now her knife wasn't anywhere to be found. It was intolerable. Absolutely intolerable.

She gritted her teeth, then started grinding them noisily as she felt a scream of frustration beginning to build up inside. She tried to smile at the boy.

'Yes, the most amazing thing,' she said. 'So please don't go *just* yet. Somewhere in one of these bags, it is. I just don't know which one. I'll find it in a second. I used to be such a tidy person, you know. Everything should have its place, don't you think?'

'Yes I do,' Sean replied. 'What's yours?'

'What ever do you mean?' Rose replied, a little taken aback by the child's strange directness. She forced a smile trying to retrieve the atmosphere of a moment ago.

She had approached him just now with the promise of something special. Although she had lost her sense of self, she knew it had something to do with children and the need to dispatch them to a better place in order to protect them.

Her hip was giving her such trouble. Really she needed to sit down in order to search through her bags properly. Never mind. She'd just have to grin and bear it.

'What is your place? I mean, where is it? Do you live here?' The boy asked her.

'No, no. Not very often. Sometimes. '*What* is my place?' is a much more interesting question.' She had remembered now. 'To help bring about the greater good of the many. I am here to sacrifice the few – some of them anyway – for the sake of the many. It's a battle of Britain. Are you confused? Runaways, dear. I'm talking about runaways.'

'You don't make any sense.'

261

She could feel he was getting restless and wanted to leave. She hurried her riffling through the next bag. Where was it? Where was it?

'I mean,' she said, focusing on making herself crystal clear to the boy. 'That I have to give something amazing to the children and young people I specially choose to help me help all the other runaways everywhere else.'

'And I am specially chosen?'

'That's right, dear. Like my little boy was. A bit younger than you he was at the time. A part of my very self, though, my very self.'

She didn't care how much she gave away. This child wouldn't understand what she was on about. Anyway she wanted to be caught. Now she was losing her marbles. Put away somewhere safe. That young woman just now had disturbed her equilibrium. Lucille. Yes, she remembered her now. She remembered her very well. She had been her lodger for two or three years a decade ago. She had given herself to her as well. Her very self. Like a mother. In order to look after her and help her to be *her*self. That's what mothers were for. To help their children safely become themselves.

That was it! She could remember everything now. It wasn't a dream. Perhaps seeing Lucille again just now had prompted her memory to start functioning again. A mother! She had actually set Luke's picture on fire in a forlorn attempt to finally let him go. And to let her motherhood go. But her very self, like the little fire on his photograph, had slipped off the plank of wood and sunk into the Thames too. Drowned. And she had killed two, or was it three, street kids as well. All to no avail. There had been no public outcry or political commitment to improving children's services. Not as far as she knew. She had watched the news religiously on television through shop windows but there never seemed to be an item about what she'd done. The lack of public concern was outrageous. She'd scrutinised newspapers people had left in bins or lying on benches, but nothing. Not a thing. Her crusade would have to be intensified.

'I don't believe you,' the boy said, moving closer beside her and peering into the bag she was going through. 'I don't believe you have got anything in there at all.'

Memory was flooding her now in a tidal surge. I don't believe you. That was what Luke so often said in his last few weeks when she had tried to reassure him that all would be well. Then, when she had amended it to saying she would do everything she could to *try* to make things alright he had said he still didn't believe her. It had been heartrending hearing him talk like an embittered old man. But then it had been both her humiliation and exaltation that he had become so acceptant shortly before he died. Wiser and more mature than most grown ups, his realisation that he was hurting her by saying he didn't believe her had made her so proud of him. He had wanted to be kind to her despite how helpless and inadequate to the task of keeping him alive she and Richard had proved to be. Ten years old. For him to know at ten years old that there was nothing that could be done for him and then to absolve her of the blame for that, had somehow made her feel both more grateful and more guilty than anything else. But it was the love he showed them both which had been so blinding.

'I don't believe you,' this little boy said again.

As these words echoed back across the years, Rose knew with a sudden cold clarity that she had been insane these last few months. Quite, quite Mad.

Fat tears started streaming down her grubby cheeks. She had meant well. She had always meant well. She had attacked young people living rough for a good cause. But now she felt horribly human again. No cause, however good, could ever justify evil means. She had truly been evil, a child-killer so corrupted and depraved that she had been about to stab this well looked-after little boy in his nice clean clothes.

She had become a monster.

She wanted to bawl out loud with the guilt and the shame and the pointlessness of it all even as she continued looking for the knife. When she found it she would throw it away. No, better still she would turn herself in to the police and hand it over as evidence. If they still thought she was dotty, she would slit her own throat. Discreetly. Alone in some hole in the dark somewhere. But where was the damn thing? Where was it?

'What are you crying for?' the boy asked.

She didn't say anything. She wanted him to go away now.

Then she found the knife tucked into the middle of an Evening Standard, tightly wrapped inside three Asda bags. She removed the package from the newspaper and started unwrapping it.

Pulling the knife free, she held it up in the air to look at it, wiping grimy strands of dank grey hair out of her face. It glinted in the sunshine with an intensity and radiance equal to her realisation that she had been mad. For months if not years. She turned the knife over, holding it point down to stop it blinding her. At that moment there was a piercing scream.

* * *

'Sean!' Lucille shrieked. 'Get away from her! NOW!'

Sean didn't move.

Everything went into slow time.

Lucille watched Rose raise the knife and for a moment, which felt like forever, was frozen, paralysed by the horror of what she was seeing. Then she heard herself screaming again and saw Ron hurtling forward in far too slow motion towards the woman who had been a mother to her and the boy who had been a son.

Rose turned and saw Ron looming out of the sunshine and shadows towards her. She instinctively raised her hands in a fear which somehow wasn't really frightened, was somehow almost welcoming. Lucille saw Sean begin to step aside as if to walk away from something that wasn't really happening as his father came bounding up, heaved him into the air and almost hurled him out of the way. In the same movement she saw that Ron had crashed into Rose, his weight and momentum knocking her to the ground and causing her to land on her left arm with her hand still clutching the knife, driving her hard down on to it. Instantly reacting to being skewered, Rose's whole body then jerked and quivered and she rolled over onto her back, the knife clearly visible, sticking out from the top of her left thigh.

Lucille choked back another scream. Then, whilst her heart still felt frozen, her body came out of paralysis. Stumbling in her silly heels again, she kicked them off and ran towards Rose lying in a crumpled heap on the ground. Ron was now down on one knee with Sean and she heard him introducing himself to him and apologising for the drama of his sudden arrival on the scene, almost as if nothing had happened.

But it had.

Rose was lying on her back in the pathway smiling up at the leaves and sky above with the knife sickeningly stuck in her hip at a forty five degree angle through her dirty serge skirt.

Lucille knelt down in the dirt beside her, confused, almost faint with the mix of shock, anxiety and love she was feeling. This woman whom she'd loved like a mother and who now looked so much older than her fifty-something years, covered in dirt and grime and smelling of piss and booze and dustbins, was as pale as death. Sweat beaded her brow. Perhaps she *was* dying. Lucie couldn't see any sign of blood, not yet anyway. Were there any main arteries down the outside of the hip? She just didn't know. Ron might. Ron better.

But he was still talking to Sean.

'I'm glad you two have met, but can you come over here please, Ron, and help me. Rose is hurt. I think she's seriously hurt.' She stamped on the panic in her voice.

She looked down at Rose who was now staring back up at her.

'Lucille. My darling! What are you doing here?' she said, in tone as warm, familiar and everyday as the cups of tea they used to share together.

'Rosie! We'll call an ambulance. Get you to hospital.'

'Don't do that. Take me to a police station or a priest or preferably both. I have to confess, to be reconciled. I was a Catholic once you know.

'You're hurt, Rosie.'

'I'm not, my love. I'm fine. It doesn't hurt at all. Truly. I shall get up in a moment. Why ever did that rude man knock me over?'

'We thought you – we – we – we thought Sean w-was – oh! I can hardly speak! We were frightened Rose, the way you were holding up your knife.'

'You thought I might hurt the child? Very sensible, then. Very sensible indeed. I think I'll get up again now dear, if you don't mind.'

'You couldn't do anything at the moment and I really think you shouldn't move. She shouldn't, should she, Ron? The knife is sticking right into her. What shall we do? We need to get help.'

Ron strode over, squatted down beside her.

'Yes,' he said, standing up again. He went over to his jacket which was still lying on the ground a little way away. He'd dropped it just now in the rush to rescue Sean from Rose's knife attack. He pulled out his mobile phone from an inside pocket.

'Don't!' Rose brayed with a volume incredible for someone lying hurt on the ground.

'You're bleeding like a – you're bleeding badly, and we need an ambulance. How it will get up here I'm not sure.'

'Like a pig, young man? Yes. Well, it's just superficial and I think I must be the judge of whether I need to see a doctor. I have a bad hip anyway. I don't think a little flesh wound is going to make any difference to that. If you could help me up now I would be very grateful. And I must ask you again NOT to phone for an ambulance.'

She tried to move and farted. She didn't try to suppress or disguise the wince of pain either of these actions induced. Lucille bit her lip to stop herself crying out.

'No.' He switched on his mobile and started to punch 999 into it. 'I'm sorry, but I have to get help. You need urgent medical attention.'

'Would you please STOP that!' Rose boomed from the ground. 'Right now! I won't go in an ambulance and anyway you might well have to do some explaining about this little accident, yourself. You surely wouldn't want that, would you? At the very least you'd be inconvenienced. I'm sure I can get the knife out if you would just let me stand up.'

Rose's imperious tone would brook no argument. She put her hand to hip and touched the knife. Her skirt was now dark and wet and her fingers immediately became bright and bloody. Lucille looked away feeling sick, then forced herself to face what was happening again, fearing there would be even more blood if Rose pulled the knife out. But it was true. It was not in very deep, only in an inch or two at most, maybe three.

'It's gone into the fleshy part of my hip back towards my bum,' said Rose. 'It is only a flesh wound, for heaven's sake. A bit painful now, it's true, but not very deep. I am going to remove it. No. Don't try to stop me. It's my hip. And it's my knife.'

Lucille could hear the shrill coarsened rage of the streets in Rose's voice, but she could also hear her old friend, her old friend who always used to say 'for heaven's sake', whenever she was even the tiniest bit exasperated.

But when Rose moved to grasp hold of the knife's handle, Ron gently took her wrist and prevented her, his face set hard.

'She's alright, Ron. She's herself now. She knows me again. She's quite safe. You are, aren't you, Rose?'

'Of course I am.'

Ron nodded, unconvinced and continued to hold the older woman's wrist.

'Lucille! Are you going to allow this thug to restrain me like this? It's an outrage.'

Lucille suppressed an hysterical giggle at the awfulness of the situation. Not really knowing what was right, but wanting to go with her feelings she made a random choice.

'Ron, please let her go.'

'No. I can't.' He smiled at her and did look seriously regretful. She felt he must have some good reason, didn't mean to be obstructive for no reason.

'Why not? It's not right to go on holding her when she's said she's safe now. Is it?' she added uncertainly.

'We don't know what she might have done to herself. I mean she might have gone through an artery,' he said. 'Do you know more than basic first aid? Or anything about anatomy?' She shook her head. 'Neither do I. All I know is I wouldn't know how to staunch a wound like this. We must get help urgently. Till then I don't think she should move.'

'I am not inanimate so please do not refer to me in the third person. Tell him to let go of me, Lucille please.'

Watching the three of them on the ground, Sean snorted disconsolately.

'Richard is a doctor,' he said. 'He'd know what to do.'

'This is an emergency, Sean. We need immediate help,' Ron said. 'But thank you for the idea.'

'No! It *is* a good idea!' Lucille heard herself screeching, wanting to stop the arguments. 'If, that is, you really won't let us call an ambulance, Rose.'

'I won't. I won't go in an ambulance and that's that.'

'Well I'll see if I can get hold of Richard then. Thursday afternoons he's always doing outpatients so it's easy enough to reach him. Can I use your phone please, Ron?' Lucille held out her hand and when he passed it to her she got up and dialled Richard's number. It was engaged. She went over to her shoes lying in the dirt stood them up again, slipped them back on. She looked around nervously as she pressed the redial button, wondering what people would think. It was amazing that on such a hot busy afternoon no-one else in the park had yet noticed what was going on. Then again, she supposed, all this had happened in virtually no time at all.

The number was still engaged. Come on, Richard, come on! Get off the phone and speak to me.

'Will you let go,' Rose repeated from down below, glaring at Ron.

'Will you promise to just lie here and leave the knife alone while we find out what to do for the best?' Ron asked her, matching her cold hostility tone for tone.

'Of course I do.'

'Alright then. Fair enough.' He let her wrist go as Lucille got through to Richard's secretary. 'You once called an ambulance for me, you know. Long time ago now. I'd slipped in the rain and broke my wrist. Remember?'

Rose closed her eyes.

'I'm afraid not,' she murmured sadly. 'There's so much I've forgotten.'

Ron remained sitting on the ground beside her. He could very well have just saved Sean's life. At the cost of Rose's. Lucille tapped a foot impatiently as she waited to be put through to Richard. She could see that some of Rose's blood had stained the right trouser leg of Ron's crumpled linen suit over the knee. That could be more difficult to get out than the varnish on her skirt this morning, she thought. He glanced up, caught her looking down at him, gave her an encouraging smile just as Richard came onto the line.

At the very same moment Rose closed her eyes with a fixed grin on her face, then yelped like a vixen. She had taken advantage of Ron's momentarily diverted attention to pull the knife out of her hip. It now lay glistening in a shaft of sunlight on the ground beside her.

'That's better,' she said with a satisfied smile, eyes still closed.

Ron picked up the knife, shook his head with an ironic grimace, looked very worried indeed which in turn worried Lucille.

'Tell him what she's just done now as well,' he said.

Lucille nodded, began explaining in detail to Richard what had happened. She listened carefully as he advised her what to do. It was such a relief to be given a script. She nodded over and over again till she felt she'd got what he was saying, then hurriedly repeated it back to him to make sure, and hung up.

'Rosie, I'm sorry, but Richard says we've got to look at your wound, see if it's gaping, and that we must try to stop it bleeding. We have *got* to look at it before you can move, he said. Ron, perhaps you and Sean could – I don't know – perhaps you could just look the other way, while I take a look.' She shuddered. 'Then we'll know what we have to do.'

She waited for an expensive woman with two small children and a poodle to pass hurriedly by. The woman was not curious at all, had clearly marked Rose down for what she was and adopted the attitude of someone who has no interest in such people. Ron moved Rose's bags beside her so that to a limited extent she and Lucille had some privacy. Then Lucille gently pulled Rose's skirt up over her hip on her right side. She wasn't wearing knickers, which somehow wasn't surprising, and her bony legs were literally black and blue all over, with dirt, bruises and varicose veining. Her right knee was swollen and bent with arthritis. She smelled frightful. She couldn't have had a bath in months.

Although the wound seemed deep and Rose's skirt was soaked with blood, it was definitely longer than it was wide and did seem to only be seeping now. Taking a tissue from the small pack in her bag, Lucille carefully wiped around it as gently as she could, feeling slightly sick at how horrible this was and relieved that it wasn't worse. It didn't seem to be gaping. Mercifully. Richard had said she would have had to take her to hospital if it was, which would have been tricky. Nevertheless she wondered if it would start to bleed heavily again once they got Rose up onto her feet. She pulled the rest of the tissues out of the pack and folded them in half. Then she placed them over the cut and asked Rose to keep her hand on them while she went to look for something to hold them in place. Rose nodded. Lucille stood up, telling Sean and Ron she was going to the cafe to see if she could find anything useful there. Perhaps they would even have a first aid kit. She needed to find a bandage or something to hold the tissues in place over the wound whilst they got her out of the park and into a taxi. She told herself she must not panic. That would be silly. There'd be a first aid kit at the cafe, sticking plasters and bandages as well probably. There had to be.

Anyway, she thought, brushing the dirt from the back of her dress where she had been sitting on it, she would do whatever was necessary. As soon as they were in a cab she'd make sure the driver stopped at the first chemist they passed and buy some antiseptic, plasters and bandage. She would do anything for Rose. Anything.

To be fair to him, Richard had understood that on the phone just now, and agreed that Rose could come and stay with them for a while, said he would attend to her himself as soon as he got in. He had agreed to leave work immediately. Lucille wondered whether he had been just a bit too keen to see his ex-wife's hip bone structure again. Well, if so he was in for a very unpleasant experience.

She asked Ron to ring for a cab to take them to Oxshott. It didn't matter how much it would cost, she said. He nodded, saying he'd call for a black cab because there was more room inside. The nearest exit from here was Holland Park road, he'd ask for the cab driver to pick them up there outside the gate in fifteen minutes.

Lucille headed for the café. Sean said he was coming with her, but she firmly told him over her shoulder that he couldn't, she would be back in a few minutes, he should stay with Rose and his father.

'I don't like you,' the boy said to him in an amazingly matter-of-fact manner. Ron raised his eyebrows and nodded his head to indicate he didn't care and wasn't surprised.

'I should think not. We've only just met,' he replied.

Ron felt an odd irrational little tweak of something he could almost identify as paternal pride. It was indeed a strange thing to have suddenly become a father.

'I was going to kill you,' Rose said to the boy, equally matter-of-fact from her horizontal position on the ground. 'I'd changed my mind by the time I got my knife out but that *was* what I was originally going to do. '

'You wouldn't have been able to,' said the boy. 'You're just a slow old woman.'

Rose laughed. 'You're probably right.' she said.

'Why?' Ron asked her.

'I'm not sure I really know,' she replied sadly. 'Grief isn't madness I know, but denying it is. The thing is, I didn't even know I'd *been* denying it. Maybe I drink too much. Or too little. I don't know.'

'I'm not frightened of you,' the boy said in an almost kindly way. 'But you talk rubbish. I think I am going to go and find my mum.'

'She asked you to stay here with us,' said Ron.

'Fuck off,' Sean replied archly, as if inviting an outraged adult response. But he didn't set off after Lucille.

'Who are you talking to like that, dear? Do you know?' Rose asked.

The boy looked disarmed.

'Him,' he said.

'Shouldn't you call him by his name?'

'Fuck off, Ron.'

'I've heard that said before somewhere,' Rose commented evenly.

'I haven't,' said Ron, suppressing his anger. He must bear in mind the boy was damaged. Sarcasm would go straight past him.

'I thought your mum just said this man is your father. Shouldn't you be calling him, Dad?' Rose asked.

'Fuck off. Dad.'

'That's better,' she pronounced from below in a school-mistressy voice.

'I'm not sure about that actually,' said Ron.

'Well, of course I don't myself condone his bad language either,' said Rose from the ground. 'But I always feel that if you are going to be rude to someone than you should do it politely.'

'You're mad,' said Sean seriously.

'I have been,' she agreed. 'But I'm not sure I am anymore. I may be sane. Which could be worse! Do you know what sane means?'

'Of course I do.'

'If I was sane that would be a big problem for you,' Rose said, farting again. 'Because then you would not know what to make of me. You would feel you had to hate me when you don't. Not really. Like you don't really hate your father. You just don't know him.'

Ron was amazed at how she had picked up what was going on from the snippets of conversation she had had heard.

'I knew you when you were a small child,' she said. 'You won't be pleased to hear that in my humble opinion you haven't changed a bit. Not one little bit. Still completely clueless when it comes to understanding other people.'

'You're mad,' repeated the boy, less certainly.

'You didn't realise you were hurting your father's feelings when you told him you didn't like him. And he didn't either. I understand these things. I understand people like you who cannot feel what it is like for other people.'

'You smell and I'm going to find my mother.'

'Where?' Rose asked. 'She'll never be where you look for her. Not all your life long.'

Ron watched his son frown, perplexed, as if it just wasn't in the script that he should be talking with someone even stranger than himself.

'Why not?'

'Mums never are for some children. They may be where you find them, but they are never where you look.'

'You' re just being silly, wasting my time.'

'That's right, dear. Well, not wasting it I hope, but keeping you here a little longer with my silliness while we wait for your mother to come back.'

'I don't like people being stupid.'

'I can tell. That's why you are so clueless.'

Ron observed feelings he could recognise in the expressions on his son's face. They veered between perplexity and derision.

'You're mother will be back in a minute,' he said. 'Look here she comes now.'

Sean ignored him. It was going to be a very difficult business getting to know this boy. Let alone like him, he was clearly humourless, antisocial and clever, and Rose was right of course, emotionally clueless as well. It would take a long time for them to find a way of relating to one another. Still, if Sean had insisted on meeting him today there must have been some desire or motivation there.

He would have to use all his own experience as an adopted child to feel his way into a relationship with him, by trial and error. His own sense of hurt and resentment at seven years old when he found himself plonked into yet another family who said he was theirs, still rankled after more than thirty years.

He watched Lucille hurrying back now with an anxious expression on her face and a steaming bowl in her hands, nearly tripping herself over again in her rush to get back.

'Sorry I was so long. I'm wearing the wrong shoes for running around like this,' she apologised to Rose, trying not to shake as she put the bowl of hot boiled water carefully down on the ground between them, then pushing loose strands of hair behind her ears in a practical, purposive way. Ron noticed the round blue earrings she wore sparkling in the dappled sunlight. 'They did have some antiseptic wipes and some plasters,and they gave me this clean tea towel which they wetted for me so that I can clean you up a bit, Rosie, which is great isn't it ?'

She stood up to refold the towel and when she had done so, she ruffled Sean's hair with a light, fond touch, clearly some kind of a mother. Not even a very extraordinary kind of mother as she removed a small twig from his hair. In contrast as she knelt down on both knees in the dirt beside Rose again, she was like a daughter, looking after the old woman with tenderness and concern. She was certainly strange, very strange, to a man with no parents and until now, no children either.

As he watched her set to work, Lucille's new found confidence with her bowl and her bandage lulled him into believing the old crone would be alright after all. Lucille glanced up at him, caught him looking at her and returned his stare with an anxious smile. Her priority was Rose. She made a face at him, intimating that she wanted his help with Sean again while she attended to Rose. He nodded and putting an arm out to the boy, gestured that they should both look the other way, maybe talk together.

'I don't want to. I'm going to watch,' Sean said, pulling away from him and deliberately making a meal of looking down at Lucille and Rose on the ground. 'I'm going to be a doctor when I grow up.'

'Well then you'll know that doctors and nurses use screens to stop strangers seeing what they are doing to their patients. And you and I need to be a sort of screen so that those people coming towards us from over there don't see anything they shouldn't whilst your mum cleans up the lady's wound. You and I have to respect and protect her privacy from the eyes of passers by. That's our job.'

'You can't respect a bag lady,' Sean said, but he turned around anyway.

'It's what I am, dear,' said Rose in a cheery voice from down below behind them.

Ron was pleased he had finally seemed to have had some effect on the boy who was now glaring at the elderly couple slowly advancing along the path towards them.

The boy immediately turned round again to watch what Lucille was doing. She was in the midst of hiking Rose's skirt up again and rearranging it around her so that she was as decent as possible whilst she attended to washing and cleaning the wound in her hip. Lucille glanced up, gave Sean a warning frown.

'Oh don't mind him,' said Rose. 'Let him look if he wants to. It's such a warm day I shouldn't think there's anyone lying down in this park who hasn't gathered her skirts up to catch a bit of sun!'

'I know! Why don't you two go and wait for the cab? We don't want it driving off without us.'

Ron heard the entreaty in her voice and looked at his son.

'Will you be alright?' he asked her. 'Rose may need supporting to get to the gate.'

'I'll be fine,' said Rose.

Seeing the old woman's knife still lying on the ground, Ron picked it up and dropped it into one of her black bin liners, which seemed to be stuffed full of empty plastic shopping bags. Then he picked the bin liners up. Despite their apparent bulkiness they were remarkably light, he could carry them both in one hand.

'I'll take these for you then,' he said. 'Are you sure you'll be alright with her?'

'Certain,' Lucille replied.

'Come on Sean. Let's go.'

The boy didn't move. Lucille glared at him. Ron raised an eyebrow with what he hoped was a friendly paternal smile. Sean, patently reluctant, started to move off with him.

*　　　*　　　*

The Boundless Book of Rules had been written to cope with a solitary life. First at home and then on the streets. It didn't really apply when any kind of relationship was being offered to her, so Rose felt confused as she watched Lucille's small, intent face focusing on cleaning her up. She was being tentative and gentle. Rose felt cared for, which was utterly strange after all these years, but not unpleasant. Not even a little bit. She was just unaccustomed to it, that was all.

The Boundless Book of Rules decreed that she shouldn't talk about anything personal for fear of having feelings she wouldn't be able to bear. And for years now she hadn't allowed herself to be personal with anyone. She had consequently had no feelings whatsoever. But now she found herself feeling warmth for this girl . She hadn't meant to hurt her all those years ago when she'd told her she would prefer never to see her again. When Lucille and Richard decided to live together, she hadn't been able to cope with her feelings of bitterness, betrayal and jealousy. She had known what she felt was unreasonable. Richard had, after all, long been remarried, and Lucille had always been quite open with her about how captivated she was by him, never tried to deceive her about it. Nevertheless the thought of her having a relationship with him had been distressing somehow. Almost incestuous in some curious way, and without wishing ill on them, Rose had decided it would be best if she had no more to do with either of them.

Some months later, like a biblical revelation, The Book of Rules had further decreed that if she continued to follow its precepts religiously she could dwell permanently in a world devoid of emotion, a world of sensations, which unlike feelings could be managed and controlled. Sensations like hunger, thirst, tiredness, pain. In return she need never again – ever! – suffer the intensity of feelings like joy or sadness, love or loss. At first it had been quite difficult blocking out such things. She had had to work obsessively hard to fill every moment of her time with sensations, activities or thoughts to prevent any horrible messy feelings from sneaking up and overwhelming her. But after a while, like meditation, she had got better and better at it, so that eventually it became second nature to her. As long as she stayed away from the scene of her first and most dreadful crime – the crime of not having been a good enough mother to her son.

'How are you, dear? You're looking wonderful,' she said, trying not to wince as Lucille dabbed delicately at the wound.

'I'm alright Rosie, better than you anyway. I'm sorry if that hurt. I think this wound is terribly deep. But I am taking you home with Sean and me, and I am going to look after you for a while. Richard's going to try and come home early so he can have a look at you.'

'If I let him.'

'If you let him, yes. And please do, because it looks really bad.'

'Maybe. I am not sure about staying with you though. Thank you very much, my darling. I'm quite happy with the life I lead.'

'You don't look it. You look pale and ill and like someone in her sixties not fifties. You need a rest, and you need to be looked after. You're nothing but skin and bone. You need a good meal. Lots of good meals. You used to be so lovely and round and plump.' Lucille wrinkled her nose as she wiped the wound with an antiseptic wipe. 'You also need a bath.'

They laughed together, both desperately trying to close in on their old intimacy.

'I have done terrible things, Lucille.'

'I don't care. You've done wonderful things too.'

'I was worried about the children on the street. So I killed one or two of them – poor things – to draw attention to their plight. It didn't work though. I feel so dreadful about it. I have to turn myself in. I was so surprised there wasn't an outcry about that last little lass. She was still some mother's child, but nobody cared.'

273

'Perhaps you just imagined it,' Lucille replied as she dried the skin surrounding her wound with a clean tissue.

'No, I didn't! Did you *imagine* I was holding my kitchen devil over Sean? No! Of course you didn't. I have to go to the police.'

'When you are feeling better you can, can't you? If you really want to. But I really don't see what good it would do. Perhaps it would be better to do something to make up for it? It would be awful to go to prison. I'm sure that wouldn't help at all.'

'Or Broadmoor – somewhere like that. Yes, maybe. I think *that's* the right place. Then whether I did what I did or imagined I did wouldn't really matter.'

The embarrassed, hesitant little laugh this prompted them to share wasn't just gallows humour. It was an attempt by both of them to reconnect.

'What matters right now is to get you better, darling Rose! Then you can decide what to do.'

'Aren't you worried I'll have another go at Sean?'

'Oh! No-o. That never occurred to me at all,' said Lucille, applying a large sticking plaster just a little too roughly to her hip. Rose winced. 'Oh, I'm so sorry!' She bit her lower lip in silence, concentrating on applying the dressing. Rose glared at her, shaking her head sadly. Hadn't the stupid girl heard what she'd just said?

'No, Rose. I do believe you when you say you changed your mind. And I know you regret whatever you were doing. And I know you are a lovely person really, and wouldn't harm a fly. So... No! I'm not worried about that at all. I shouldn't be, should I? Should I?'

'I'm not who I was.'

'You are *just* who you were. I know you are Rosie. I recognise you. You're just older that's all. But you haven't changed a bit. Not in yourself.'

'How do you know? Look at me.'

'I just know, that's all. I know you. You were – you *are* my best friend. I don't care what you look like or what you've done. You gave me my life. I wouldn't be here now if it wasn't for you.'

Lucille looked almost tearful as she spoke. Rose regarded her soberly. It was clear she was still as dizzy as ever when it came to making snap judgements, and it was also clear that she was ruled by her emotions. The very opposite of herself. But as it happened she was right. There was no way she felt like harming Sean or anybody else now. Something had happened to her. Lucille had happened to her. Again.

'Help me get up, poppet,' she said. 'Take me home.'

Their hobbled progression through the park was painfully slow. Rose leaning all her weight on Lucille who went barefoot with one arm underneath Rose, the other carrying her shoes. The pain from the occasional stone beneath her feet was more bearable than worrying she would send them both tumbling, as long as they went slowly, which suited them both. When they finally got to the street twenty minutes later, the taxi was waiting with Sean already inside on a fold-down seat staring straight ahead ignoring everybody. The cabbie was reading a newspaper, obviously quite content his meter was running. The man who had knocked her over, Ron – she thought she vaguely recognised him – came over to help them. Rose disengaged from Lucille and let him ease her inside. She was proud of the way she managed to fall into her seat with the grace of a queen despite her considerable pain.

'Come and sit beside me, darling,' she said to Lucille patting the seat next to her. 'Oh what a shame! You've spoiled your lovely blue dress with my blood.'

She watched Lucille look down at the dark stain across the front of what was obviously an expensive silk frock. Lucille smiled

'I don't care,' she said. 'I never liked it much anyway.'

'I think she's still bleeding quite heavily,' said Ron standing beside her at the open door of the taxi and peering in. He pointed at Rose's left foot. She tried to lift it up and pull it back, but the pain in her hip wouldn't allow it so she made ineffectual pulling movements trying to push her long skirt down a little a further to cover her foot. She failed, and felt the small, but unmistakeable trickle on her ankle which Lucille and Ron were looking at, slowly building up along the frayed, colourless edge of her shoe. She felt angry. Too much was suddenly going on which she didn't feel in control of.

'You're right, Ronnie. I'm sorry Rose, but I think we need to get this treated properly as soon as possible,' said Lucille. 'I don't think it can wait for Richard.' She asked the cabbie where it would be best to drop them off.

'Depends how badly hurt she is, doesn't it,' said the cabbie. 'As the crow flies Queen Mary's is directly on the way over to the A3, but I think it's only got a cuts and minor injuries service now. Otherwise it's the Chelsea and Westminster or Charing Cross. Take your pick. I'd advise Charing Cross.'

'Queen Mary's,' said Rose emphatically. 'All I need is a bit of stitching.'

'What do you think, Ron?' Lucille asked the man. He shook his great stupid head. Oh, yes. Rose could remember properly now who this buffoon was. He was that unpleasant oaf who'd pretended to kill Lucille's dog. Lucille herself gave him an equally stupid smile and nodded her agreement with him. Rose hated being disagreed with. 'Charing Cross please,' said Lucille looking at him. The father of the boy, the man who had sent her flying, nodded his assent. Ronald. He used to be a fat young man with a beard. Rather stupid, she recalled. Well clearly that hadn't changed although he had lost his beard, his belly and his youth.

Rose harrumphed and looked out the window as the cab pulled away. She didn't like this. She didn't like it at all. At the same time it was curiously pleasant to feel looked after. And she did feel sane. Incredibly sane and incredibly guilty.

Chapter 17.

'Dr McElvey? How do you do? My name is Ronald Symes. Your wife asked me if I wouldn't mind bringing your step-son home. Did she call you? We caught a train from Waterloo. It seemed to stop at every station, but, well, here we are.'

'Welcome,' said Richard. 'We are most appreciative, thank you.'

As usual the boy swept in without any acknowledgement of his existence at all and as usual went straight upstairs.

'Hi Sean,' Richard said loudly to the boy's back. 'Yes, yes. Thank you. Come in, do,' he added, stretching out a hand and shaking the other man's. 'Lucille told me about her amazing chance encounter with you yesterday.'

Oh, God. Had the appalling degree of his jealousy and suspicion revealed itself behind this over-avuncular greeting? He pulled his trousers up onto his convex waist, trying to pull it in a little.

'These bin bags belong to Rose,' said Ronald Symes who seemed to have noticed nothing and gestured towards the couple of large black plastic bags on the ground beside him.

'Here, let me take them. We can leave them here in the corner of the hallway so that they're there for her when she gets here. I'm not sure which of the spare rooms Lucille would want to put her in, so we'll just wait for her to decide when they get here.' He flashed Ronald Symes his polished Consultant Smile – all impartial efficiency and aptness.

Ron was taller than him, he noticed. Younger too. A definite rival. Potentially at least.

After they had lined the bags up against the wall, he showed the other man into the drawing room and invited him to take a seat. 'Lucille called me from A and E. just a few moments ago actually. Welcome to our humble abode.'

As self-deprecation went, it would have worked a little better had his abode actually *been* a bit more humble. He realised he was showing off. It was completely unnecessary, and probably a clear signal that he felt as insecure as some stupid old walrus who knew he could be ousted by a younger, fitter male like this one. A seven bedroomed, detached house in Surrey with four en-suite bathrooms couldn't even begin to be described as humble. But in a ghastly hypocritical inversion of the facts, he was actually ashamed of his relative wealth and power, which was why he always tried socially to avoid anybody with less or more money than himself. That meant virtually everybody, of course. They only made him feel embarrassed or contemptuous respectively. He knew nobody around here at all. He and Lucille had been to one or two dinner parties and Christmas drinks do's with some of their neighbours at which he had trotted out his old fashioned champagne socialism and won himself no friends, but that was it. Lucille was different, of course, she seemed to know everyone around here.

He had just now put the phone down after hearing from her on the Accident and Emergency pay phone that Rose was still waiting to be seen. She had been triaged soon after they had got to Charing Cross and then been told that there was an average three hour wait for less urgent cases. That was three and a half hours ago. She still hadn't been seen by a doctor. Lucille had been beside herself down the phone complaining they were discriminating against Rose because she was a 'street-person', but she told him that Rose herself had been completely calm about the delay, saying it would give them both a proper opportunity to talk . Lucille told him they'd not actually stopped chatting for the whole three hours as they sat waiting to be seen, but now Rose had fallen asleep in her chair which was why she was ringing to let him know what was going on. She asked him whether Ron had brought Sean back yet, and told him to be friendly to him and offer him a drink. Then she suddenly had to go. They were ready to see Rose and she had to wake her up. His attempt at a fond and tender goodbye to her was spoken into the ether. She had already put the receiver down. So he didn't have time to tell her that in a couple of hours, maybe sooner, Grainne would be descending upon them too.

Still at least they could then all entertain each other. As ever, he wished he had more control over other people. He would certainly have organised all these reunions a bit differently had he known they were going to happen. Spread them out a bit. Time always seemed to conspire to make things awkward. In all fairness though, if Grainne and this man happened to want to see their son on exactly the same day after all these years, he wouldn't in principle want to stand in their way. It was just a shame it had to be in his house.

Rose sounded nothing like the woman he had married more than a quarter of a century ago. He hadn't had a single thought about her, or to his shame, about Luke, for years.

'Can I offer you a drink? Gin and tonic? Whisky?'

'That would be nice, thanks,' Ron replied, clearly wanting to size him up. 'A very small Irish please, if you've got it, with lots of water. Thank you. Have you heard from Lucille yet?'

'Yes. She rang a few minutes ago. Rose is being seen right now. So other things being equal, they'll be back down here within the next hour or so, I expect.'

'Good. They'll both be pretty exhausted. It's been a very warm day, hasn't it? A very warm summer in fact.'

Ah, the social niceties. Fine, thought Richard, small talk I am comfortable with. As long as they avoided discussing anything too deep or personal all would be well. Last night after the rare, but still delightful enough, experience of making love, he had questioned Lucille about how Ron had reacted to being told he was a father. In reply she seemed to speak about him in such a confident and knowing manner that his jealous hackles had immediately risen. She'd noticed the furrow between his brows and had actually reached up to stroke it away which had pleased him because it was an abnormally tender response from her, but it also made him feel profoundly suspicious. She, of course, had insisted that he had nothing whatever to be jealous of and never had had. But he felt she protested too much. He tried to look on the bright side. If nothing else, it would certainly be interesting to see Rose again after all this time, for a little while at least. The truth was their marriage had been so much more of a meeting of minds than his marriages to either Lucille or Mary had ever been.

'Ice?'

'That would be great. Thanks.'

He passed Ron the tumbler and invited him to sit down.

'How was Sean?'

'Yes, well it's hard for me to say, never having known him before. But what I would say is that after what Lulu told me about him yesterday, I was not unpleasantly surprised. In fact I was pleased to note that he's fiercely loyal to her, which is a good quality, I think. And he is clearly very bright.'

Richard nodded. And you're overly precise, didactic. He was familiar with such sententiousness, suffered from it himself often enough. He could deal with that. But, what was this man doing, referring to her as 'Lulu'? What kind of over-familiarity was that? Lucille had not told him anything about the relationship between them all those years ago, but clearly they had been easy enough with one another for him to refer to her as Lulu.

He didn't like it.

But he didn't want not to like it, because he had to be careful not to let his jealousy get out of hand. He knew how these things could develop into horribly self-fulfilling prophecies – if you were jealous, fate gave you things to be jealous about. He couldn't help thinking everyone was better than him and that he didn't deserve any of the good fortune he had been given. It was a ridiculous way to feel when his success in life had been a product of his own hard work and acheivement, when he was one of the few scientifically trained people he knew who had actually had a classical education too, when he had received distinctions and praise for his work throughout his life. His mother had used to chide him about this neurotic self-deprecation because it had been a characteristic of his personality since earliest childhood. She had done her best to iron it out of him when he was young by becoming increasingly irritated with him about it as the years went by, so that by the time he had reached his early twenties he had driven it underground and no-one had a clue that that was how he really felt.

Not even Lucille. She had an inkling, sure, because he had told her, but she hadn't believed him, said he couldn't be a successful consultant gastroenterologist and still believe everyone was better than him, it just wasn't possible, so it must be an affectation. He knew what he felt, even if his feelings failed to correspond to the objective facts of the matter. Everyone else was better than him, and there it was.

Ron was already making him feel inadequate with his full head of brown hair and his foppish linen suit. Richard could never wear linen suits. Not at work anyway. His credibility would be seriously compromised if he went around the wards looking pre-crumpled, already dressed for the weekend.

'Sean *is* a bright boy,' he said in an agreeably avuncular tone, wanting Ron to let him play at being the genial host. 'Knocks the pants off me at chess. And as for computer games, well, I'm afraid he won't even play one with me anymore, because he's so good at them. To be absolutely fair to him though, he has tried to share some of my interests. I have an interest in duplication, in trying to see what's been stolen or copied, and from whom, in literature, painting or music. Of course it's unreasonable to expect a small boy to be fascinated by the question, for example, of whether that Lloyd-Webber chap ripped off Haydn's Seven Last Words for his Jesus Christ Superstar, or whether Chagall's keening cows and donkeys are directly lifted from the Nativitata of Simone dei Crocifisse in the Uffizi, or whatever. But I think duplication in the arts does also intrigue him in a way. He *hates* not understanding things. Even things he doesn't find intrinsically interesting.

Ronald Symes' polite nods of understanding reinforced his own sense of embarrassment and pretentiousness. The problem was that because he was so lonely, he would seize any opportunity to share and expound upon his puerile enthusiasms. He had better be as honest as he could about that if he wasn't to come over as a complete plonker.

'Having a hobby compensates for my humdrum daily working life, you know: endless ward rounds, endoscopy slides, intestinal pathology, fruitless meetings with managers about finances. The train-train de la vie. Sean doesn't know what the hell I'm on about most of the time. Lucille indulges me without really sharing my enthusiasm. Do you have any hobbies, Dr Symes?'

What a tedious, self-important old windbag he had become. No wonder he had no friends, he thought, watching Sean's father move from digesting all this waffle to contemplating his own interests.

'Ronald, or Ron. Please. I don't, actually. I used to enjoy tinkering with motorbikes when I was a younger man, but now...' He shrugged, shook his head. 'No, I don't. But I know I should do, because I do actually agree

280

with you. It's very important to have hobbies and interests outside of one's work. If you want to have a life.'

Was he hiding something? Was womanising his hobby? There was definitely something a bit shifty about him. Or was he having a little dig at him, suggesting that without the comparative analysis of duplication to be interested in, he wouldn't actually have a life?

'But I'm really not sure,' Ron went on. 'That what people call plagiarism isn't sometimes just the coincidental expression of something, you know, er, archetypal across different periods of time in different places,'

So he was capable of a priggish pomposity almost equal to his own then, a kindred spirit of a kind. He hoped it didn't mean that he also had more than a passing interest in Lucille. In an act of will Richard suppressed this jealous thought, concentrated instead on what the man had just said.

'Nothing new under the sun? That kind of thing?' he asked, feeling more animated. Despite his modish appearance and his shiftiness, Ron's reply had just demonstrated he might be someone with whom it would be possible to enjoy an interesting conversation. Such people were rare.

'That kind of thing exactly. Great art, authentically great art cannot be copied I think. But to be completely honest, I wouldn't really know. I know nothing about either music or painting. I read a bit though.' He smiled apologetically.

Richard always liked a little humility, admired it too. It was what he himself aspired to, if only he were able to express it more genuinely. Ron's self-deprecation certainly raised him further up in his estimation. Perhaps he would allow himself to be a bit more personal with him after all.

'It's going to be slightly embarrassing for me when Lucille gets back here with Rose,' he said. 'Rose was my first wife you know.' He poured himself a glass of mineral water. He didn't like drinking alcohol during the week. 'Did Lucille tell you that? I've been married twice before actually.' It came out like a confession, something he was ashamed of. Whatever else three marriages showed, it certainly evidenced some kind of problem in maintaining relationships.

'I understand. Lucille was one of my first girlfriends,' Ron replied equably, as if finding his level. 'But I've never been married.'

What? They'd actually been an item then? Why had she never told him?

Richard felt his spine go rigid and his chest go tight. An incipient headache which he had been fighting off all day took possession of his brow and then moved in an iron band around his head to the back of his neck. He ignored it, tried to get a grip, calm himself down. After all, why *should* she have told him? She said last night she hadn't seen this man for eleven or twelve years. But she should at least have mentioned that their relationship had once been intimate. She should have. If marriage was about two people sharing everything, not just sex, as she had seemed to be saying to that awful Counsellor woman a few weeks ago, then surely she should have told him last night that not only was Ron the boy's father, but he was also an old boyfriend of hers. But she hadn't.

Why not?

Because she didn't want him to know, of course. And why would she not want him to know unless she was covering something up? But if that was the case, why had Ron just gone and revealed that their relationship had in fact once been close? It didn't make sense.

Perhaps there was nothing to feel worried about after all. Perhaps their relationship had been so brief and of such negligible importance that she hadn't considered it worth mentioning. He must stop feeling jealous. He really must.

But he didn't know how. That was the problem. He could only pretend.

'Oh, really? As a matter of fact I do recall her telling me you and she had had a relationship at one time,' he lied. 'We're still very much in love and lucky enough to be able to share most things with one another,' he said, almost without meaning to. It just came out.

God almighty. He *was* such a plonker. There were lies, barefaced lies and bollocks. And if ever he had said anything that sounded like bollocks then that was it. He'd been so phoney, even a child would have known he was lying. And not a minute ago he had just had the complacency and hubris to be telling himself he was a good liar for God's sake!

'That's a great gift in any relationship – the ability to talk openly with one another about everything,' said Ron with an even smile.

'I understand you're an expert,' said Richard trying to suppress the bitterness in his voice. 'On what is good for people I mean.' He paused momentarily, took a deep breath. 'I suppose I really should stop trying to pull the wool over the eyes of an expert. Lucille told you, of course, how it was she came to be on a, er, what do you call it, a psycho-educational training course?'

'She did actually, yes. She said the two of you had been to see a couple counsellor together. It's my belief that if two people can be sufficiently bothered about one another to go and get counselling for their relationship then they probably don't need it; there must be something good going on between them. I don't mean to be patronising.'

'No, no. Of course not.' But he *was* patronising him. He was ten or fifteen years younger than him, and had never been married. What could he possibly know about it? But then again it would be nice to think there was still something good going on between Lucille and himself. Certainly the way she had made love last night suggested that not all was lost between them. He could only hope.

'Lucille seems very well,' Ron said. 'Much happier than when I knew her. There used to be a harder, more desperate quality about her which isn't there anymore. Nice.'

He *was* patronising him. No question about it. Fucking impertinence talking in such an over-familiar way about his wife, but understandable, he supposed reluctantly.

'Tell me about yourself er, Ronald. I'm Richard by the way. How did you come to be, erm, a popular psychologist?' There, that felt a bit more equitable. He too could be patronising.

'Well, I suppose in the same way as you became a specialist yourself. Study. Hard work, that kind of thing.'

'Mm, yes, of course. But what I meant was what made you interested in it?'

'Well, Lucille played her part in that actually. She and my girlfriend at the time both − I don't know how to put this − they both gave me their notice, shall we say, within twenty four hours of one another. I was a bit upset about that, mulled it over for a year or more and could not really come to any clear conclusions about the part I had played in my own downfall. In fact I came to murkier and murkier conclusions, so I decided to take myself in hand. Learn a little about how human beings tick, in the hope that I could maybe make some sense of it one day. I'm still not sure I've even begun. But, well,' he shrugged. 'That's what happened.'

'That's really interesting and very honest,' Richard smiled, his jealousy tap now full on and overflowing. I don't mean to pry, of course, so please don't answer if you don't feel you want to. 'But,' he cleared his throat. 'As you mentioned her, how did you actually *feel* about Lucille leaving you? Just as a matter of interest, you know.'

'I didn't really have any feelings about *her* leaving, she wasn't girl enough for me then. And anyway I knew for some weeks before that she was going and why.' His smile was open, he didn't seem to be lying or manipulative. 'And as a matter of fact you are not prying. She's *your* wife now and you have been living together for far longer than I ever knew her. So you are bound to be interested. We were friends. That's all. She had run away from home and ended up lodging with us for a year or so. Longer than that − more like a year and a half it was. We became an item of sorts − just for a few weeks − before she moved out in order to, as she put it to me last night, be made normal.'

'Ah,' said Richard, 'that was under Rose's wing, wasn't it? In my old house. I took a pittance from her for my half of its value, you know. God knows what it must be worth now.'

'It was never serious between us, if that's what you want to know. She was young and desperate, I think. She must have been desperate. To have been making out with me. And I was confused about where my brain was located. In my brain, my penis or the bottom of a glass. What went on between Lulu and myself was born more out of circumstance than choice. If I could run my time over again I would have left her well alone actually, put more energy into repairing my relationship with Sean's mother. But I wasn't up to it.'

'So the other woman, I mean the woman you were actually living with was Grainne?'

Ron nodded.

'Lucille's told you about it then?'

'A bit.'

'In fact, as you can gather, it was Lulu who was the 'other woman' really. Grainne was my partner. My biggest shock yesterday was not so much seeing Lucille – as hearing about Sean from her, that he was my child. Grainne's and mine, I mean. That did come as a surprise.'

'It is curious the way chance can intervene in our lives. Serendipitous even,' said Richard musingly.

Ronald seemed to be narrowing his eyes, as if alert to what he might be about to say next.

'There does seem to be a parallel: just as they parted from you within a day of each other, it looks like you are about to meet up with both of them again within a day of each other,' continued Richard.

'Why? What do you mean?'

'Grainne is coming down here this evening. She phoned me earlier this afternoon.' He looked at his watch. 'In fact I am expecting her at much the same time as Lucille and Rose. So we might both be catching up with our ex-partners tonight. Grainne wants to see Sean. She felt if he was meeting his father then he ought to meet his mother as well and she invited herself down to stay for a few days. Which was fair enough, don't you think?'

Richard observed Ronald grimacing as if the prospect wasn't one he was exactly over the moon about, but he nodded his head anyway. It was reassuring to observe that the equanimous Ron could lose some of his poise too. And he could well understand why he would be reluctant to see Grainne. He himself didn't actually want to see Rose again out of choice either, as it happened, but some things you just had to do.

'I also spoke to her earlier,' said Ron. Richard suppressed the pleasure he felt on hearing the angry edge to the younger man's voice. This Master of Cool was clearly feeling the heat. 'I told her I would prefer not to see her. Not just now. I wasn't – I mean, I am not – ready. It's not the right time. It's enough for me at the moment coming to terms with having a son.'

I like a man who has got his priorities right, thought Richard, feeling much more relaxed. He didn't need to be jealous after all.

Like the winner of a stag fight that somehow hadn't happened, Richard felt magnanimity towards Ronald sweeping in as his jealousy slunk off. It would be back.

'There's never a right time for anything. Or to put it more positively: every time necessarily has to be the right time, I find. Because we don't really have any choice about it, do we? Can I make you another whisky?' He took Ronald's tumbler and refilled it with a more generous pouring of Jamesons, remarking, 'Voltaire ripped Liebniz off when he had Candide say this is the best of all possible worlds. He ridiculed the idea, because really he knew how important it was for people to at least consider it. And to feel clever. It makes us feel rather grand, don't you think, to realise that *any* time – in the best of all possible worlds – has to be the right time. Even the worst of times.'

'I'm not used to people giving me ideas to consider,' Ronald replied, returning to the polite, more measured way of speaking he had started with. 'I see what you're saying, and I'm sure you are probably right, but I am afraid what I feel is that it's not actually the right time, right now, for me and Grainne to meet up again. And I think, if you don't mind, that when I've finished this drink I'll just say goodbye to you and Sean and be on my way.'

'Fine, fine. Suit yourself. I quite understand. I would feel the same way. Time can be a terrible thing. My son Luke would be coming up... what? Twenty five by now. He died fifteen years ago, when he was only ten. That wasn't the right time at all, except that at least he was saved a lot more suffering.' He looked directly into Ron's eyes. 'So I do understand – only too well – when someone tells me they feel the time is *not* right for something. Of course I do. Actually I used to be so much more angry about it then than I am nowadays. I would rant and rant at all the flaws built into Life's Rich Tapestry. Death, Disease, Injustice and so on. The problem of evil. You know. Aquinas and all that. In fact, after Luke died I felt that if this flawed world reflected the face of God then God was also flawed. And I hated Him, Her, It or Us, with an evangelical fervour. But now I find that when I do suffer from the occasional attack of Belief-in-God-itis, it is always with an admixture of pity and sadness rather than rage. I feel sorry for the creator of so much sadness.'

He had often trotted out this little diatribe. It made him feel better. Like a prayer. It was a comfort somehow, to patronise God.

He was aware he was feeling a little short of breath and took a few deeper inhalations to compensate. They didn't seem to make much difference which was irritating. He wished his headache would go away too. He also felt extremely hot, even though the early evening temperature was quite a few degrees down on what it had been earlier in the day. He took off his jacket and undid his tie, draping them over the back of the tasteless green and white chinz sofa Lucille had bought him for Christmas

285

last year because she had read in a magazine that they were 'his' colours. He undid the top buttons of his shirt. What with the phone ringing and the doorbell going, he hadn't even found time to freshen up and change since coming in from work half an hour ago. It had been a busy day and the evening didn't promise to be any easier - one thing after another. He wiped some sweat from his brow with the back of his hand, thinking he must try to lose some weight and get fit. He was going to be fifty five soon. He would have to develop a healthier lifestyle, join Lucille in the gym perhaps.

Ron laughed. Richard glared at him. It grated to be laughed at.

'Pity for a flawed god in leafy Oxshott in, er, Surrey isn't it? Yes, Surrey. I'm sorry. But to me it rings slightly un–

'Unconvincing? Unnecessary?'

'I was going to say unnerving actually.'

Ron gave him a disarming inoffensive smile. He didn't seem to have any axe to grind, changed the subject completely.

'It *is* very nice around here, though, almost too nice.'

'You're quite right, of course. And you mean twee, don't you. It is ridiculous for someone like me to be whinging about the infinite, and berating the nature of existence. My only excuse is that looking at stomach ulcers and bowel cancers every day does lead to a certain amount of morbid preoccupation with life's, um, constraints.'

Outside at the bottom of the garden Richard saw a roe deer pass discreetly into the woods behind the rhododendrons beyond his well-manicured lawns, as if trying to avoid the stench of all his conceited twaddle. He strode over to the French windows and fumbling, opened them wide. That was a bit better. Fresh air was what he needed right now. He took a few deep breaths. His chest and head both felt so tight he thought he might very well faint. Birds were beginning their summer evening discussions in the trees outside.

'Yes, I can imagine, especially if you are going through marital difficulties as well.'

Richard wanted to rear up in umbrage and state he'd never suggested he was going through any such thing; but his headache had now become so over-powering he frankly couldn't care what the man said. He just wanted to get rid of him.

'Again, you are quite right,' he replied, wanting to collapse. 'But I have no right to feel sorry for myself.'

What was it about these psychobabblers that somehow you end up sharing your private business with them? It was time the man left. Before he himself keeled over onto the floor.

'Now, if you don't want to bump into Grainne,' he said briskly. 'I suggest you let me call a minicab to take you to the station. I'd drive you myself but I feel I'd better be here in case any of them arrive.'

Actually he was suddenly unable to do anything except sit down. He did so heavily, almost falling into his ghastly chintz sofa.

'That's okay, thank you,' Ron replied. 'Are you alright? You don't look very well.'

'I'm fine thanks. Just a bit exhausted I think. Maybe I've got a virus coming on. I get at least one a year. Hospitals are dangerous places for picking up bugs.'

Just then the sound of tyres on the gravel driveway heralded an arrival.

'But if you wouldn't mind getting the door I'd be very grateful,' Richard said, picking up the phone from the coffee table beside him. 'I'll call you a cab right now.'

Ron nodded and left the room for the front door. Richard dialled the cab company, but it was engaged.

He put the phone down again and listened to the sound of Ronald opening his front door. He felt weak, as if he couldn't have got up out of his chair even if he'd wanted to. He heard Lucille's voice exclaiming delightedly at Ronald having opened the door and knew immediately that he had been right the first time. He did have a rival.

'Ron! I'm so pleased you're still here,' he heard her saying. Then: 'Where's Richard?' in a patently less excited tone of voice.

'He may have taken a bit poorly,' he heard Ronald reply. 'He's in your sitting room lying down on the striped sofa.'

'I'm here, Lucille, h-h-h-hello,' Richard called, hurriedly trying the cab company again. He kept on miss-hitting the keys on the phone and fumbled to clear his errors. What was the matter with him, he wondered angrily. 'I'm afraid I'm not fee-l-l-l-ing a hundred percent.'

She came into view, stopping at the doorway to the drawing room to put down her handbag on the side table and give him a wave. The sight of her made him feel a bit better. He'd always liked her in that light blue dress. Of course he had a rival. How could he not have? There would always be rivals. Not least because he was so much older than her. That was the problem between them. He was too old. It was the problem right now.

He felt so tired.

'Oh my poor darling,' she returned inoffensively and with no interest in him whatsoever. 'Rose is still in the car,' she said. She swept back out of the room in Lady of the Manor mode, and he heard her say to Ron who was still out in the hall, 'Ron, would you be an angel – again! – and help me help Rose out of the taxi? She fell asleep again as soon as we started on the journey down here. And she's still asleep now. She must have been so exhausted. I think it's all been a bit much for her. But the good thing is I don't think she is in any pain. She *said* she wasn't anyway. Isn't that great? And she only needed four stitches and a tetanus injection.

After all that waiting! I thought it was going to be far, far worse. I want to get her indoors, run her a bath, make her something nice to eat and tuck her up in bed so that she can have a proper night's sleep. She told me she hasn't slept on a mattress since she had a Crisis at Christmas bed at the end of last year. Isn't that terrible?'

Richard watched them through the window as they walked hurriedly across the drive to the taxi. Rose was in the back. Lucille opened the door and bent in to talk to her. Standing behind her on the asphalt Ron discreetly adjusted himself, his eyes quite clearly on her backside and legs. Stop being jealous, Richard told himself, there really is no need.

He felt the tightness in his chest intensify and the iron band squeezing his head tightened its grip still further and with such force that he knew now something serious was happening.

He sat back on the sofa with his eyes closed and hoped that the pain would pass. At fifty five he was not really yet mature enough to join the stroke brigade, he knew that. But he also knew there were always and plenty of exceptions to general rules. So it was possible.

He wasn't a hypochondriac but he felt cold with fear.

Stop panicking, he told himself, this is just me in a rage that my little tart of a wife has contrived to bring an old boyfriend down here. This is not, repeat, not ischaemic. It is *not* an infarction. I'll be fine. I just don't want to see all these people, that's all. So I'm just behaving like some woman in a nineteenth century romance having an attack of the vapours. That's all this is, an anxiety attack.

He tried the phone again and this time managed to hit the right key first time every time. That's better, he thought, as he got through to the minicab company on the second ring.

'H-hello-lo? I wonderderder....er I der der...er.'

Oh my god. I'm aphasic, he thought. I'm fucking aphasic.

He tried to talk again. 'Uh, mmm, uhm, mmm uh.' He heard the man on the other end of the line speak impatiently to someone else in the room with him and then hang up.

The sound of the dialling tone was deafening.

He tried to put the phone down beside him but didn't feel even the tiniest bit able to coordinate doing so. Then it fell out of his hand onto the sofa anyway and from there with a soft clunk onto the shag-piled floor.

He felt frightened. He felt like screaming. But he couldn't even get a sound from of his mouth.

He heard the sound of a car door closing and the taxi pulling out of the drive. Lucille and Ron were talking to Rose as they helped her into the house. So Ron wasn't leaving straightaway after all, he thought with disinterest and detachment. Not even the slightest bit jealous anymore. He heard Rose's voice, still recognisable if more gravelly after all these years, saying how nice this was of Lucille; and Lucille asking Ron if he

288

would pick up her bags and follow them up to the room at the top of the stairs. He heard her helping Rose slowly up the stairs, telling her that he himself had been taken ill; she didn't want to expose her to any germs she said, just in case; they could meet one another again tomorrow when surely both of them would be feeling a little more up to it.

Richard tried again to sit up and call out to them, but nothing happened.

Outside, a pair of blackbirds were talking to one another across the lawn. He looked out at the evening sun streaming down on to the grass and noticed he felt curiously peaceful. Whatever was happening there was nothing he could do about it except go along with the process. Who knew? Perhaps it was just a temporal lobe thing, a fit. Or maybe an example of what the psychiatrists used to call conversion hysteria. He had after all been using Ron like a therapist during their conversation together just now. He was a troubled man. Whatever, he could not help feeling quite calm now as his whole field of peripheral vision darkened so that it was as if he was looking out at his drawing room through a blurry, black tunnel.

He heard the sound of another car pulling into the drive.

A minute or an hour later, a slight ginger woman with cropped hair, dressed in a light green track suit was standing in the doorway. He dimly recognised her and wanted to smile, but could only feel the left side of his mouth trying to tremble.

'Your front door was wide open so I came in. Richard?'

He tried to speak.

'Richard? Are you alright?'

For the life of him he could not reply. He was still unable to move. But he could hear her voice perfectly, clearer than the mother of all bells.

PART THREE

This Was Now

(Ten years later still.)

Chapter 18.

Lucille McElvey drew the gold-tasselled curtain cord in her living room and opened herself up to the dawn of another July day. She sipped at a cup of tea and looked out the window. The seafront at Eastbourne had hardly changed in decades. She wished she could go out walking on it. Soon, she promised herself, the day after tomorrow perhaps. The further west you promenaded, the higher you went, till eventually you reached the cliffs at Beachy Head. She loved that.

Although she went jogging along the front at this hour three mornings a week, she hadn't been up to Beachy Head for ages because it took too long. She liked to walk it energetically on her own, all the way up to the top. She enjoyed cold, tourist-free, blustery days in winter best, when the grey sea was flecked white with anger and she couldn't tell where it ended and the sky began. Hair tied back in a scrunchie, wrapped snug in her light-blue, goretex anorak, she would put on her training shoes and step out deliberately to enjoy the feeling of drizzle on her face and wind buffeting her body, lapping up the freedom to walk in it by herself. On her own. Just for a couple of hours up to the top and back, now and again licking the wind-borne salt spray from her lips and having to keep moving to keep warm. At the top it was wonderful to feel both safe and vulnerable, cradled for a few minutes by the physicality of earth, air and sea colliding; at once tiny, but hugely alive in the teeth of the wind. And then exhilarated, she'd turn back down once more out of the gale, skin glowing. It almost made going home again feel good.

Her simple aim each time was to steal a few merciful hours away from the choking oppressive constriction of her twenty four hour role as Richard's live-in nurse and carer.

But it wasn't winter now. At the moment the relative cool of the early morning belonged to the milkman, the odd delivery van and the occasional purposive commuter. In a few hours time, the hot and sticky summer tourist season would be patterning the seafront with children and families, ice-cream vans and traffic wardens. Lucille smiled to herself. In a couple of days she would be able to join them, get out of here and take a walk up to the top without having to feel guilty or worry about Richard. It would be a blessed relief.

She wasn't a wife anymore. She wasn't a widow either. Her whole day every day was taken up with caring; with washing, dressing and completely looking after someone who could do nothing for himself.

Well, virtually nothing. But she honestly didn't feel bitter and twisted, she just felt trapped, that was all. As a consequence, the overwhelming sense of the otherness of men, their hardness, their stink, their certainty, and the way they were always *at* her, which, heaven help her, she used to find so captivating and strange, was now no longer even the slightest bit mysterious. And in Richard's case anyway, because looking at her with the eyes of a man was nowadays the *only* thing he was capable of, not even the slightest bit alluring anymore either.

At least she no longer had to actually put the food she cooked for him into his mouth, which was a relief. Four years ago he had miraculously rediscovered a limited amount of left-sided hand-to-mouth coordination, although he was still completely paralysed down the right. She only wished he could discover hand-to-willy coordination too. Somehow that still eluded him. It was dispiriting – if she let it be – having to fetch it out for him every hour, so that he could urinate into his plastic bottle. If she didn't, he would invariably wet himself despite the disposable nappies she kept him in, and she would end up having to undress him, wash him and change him all over again, which was even more depressing.

She took another sip of tea.

Today it was still and damp, both here over the town and out there over the Channel. Beachy Head was shrouded in mist; but over the sea a carpet of sunlight was sitting on top of the departing low white cloud, rapidly evaporating it. Lucille watched its surface burning off in fluffy white plumes as she thought about her day ahead. Every now and again a beam of pure sunlight managed to pierce through, lighting up the otherwise grey water in a pool of brightness, goading the cloud to disperse altogether or move still further away.

It might turn out to be a lovely morning. After all, it was still mid-summer.

She was having her hair done later, then meeting a friend. It could be a nice day, all being well. No, it *would* be nice. She was determined on it.

Soon Richard would start stirring, making little grunting and grinding noises around the occasional lost syllable, and the even more occasional slowly enunciated word. Poor old thing. He was convinced he could talk. It didn't help to dispel this illusion that she could actually understand his emotional meaning a lot of the time. She loved him and she lived with him, so she couldn't help tuning into what he was feeling, sometimes despite herself. He called her, 'Schul', which she thought was probably the nearest he could get to the first syllable of her name, only he enunciated it backwards with an extraneous 'ch'.

At least she had her own room which she could get away to at night for a few sweet hours of solitude before sleep stole her again in preparation for the next day's drudgery. Each evening after she had washed him and shaved him, checked him and treated him for bed sores, changed his colostomy bag, put him in the hoist to move him from his chair to his bed, tucked him up and switched out his light, she would look after herself. Having a bath or a shower each evening and then making a little pot of tea was the last and nicest ritual of the day. Settling down, cosy in her dressing gown alone in front of the television with Hello, or Bella, something glitzy and stupid, she would indulge in the bliss of time and space for herself. Top Tips for Boobs and Bums or Scrumptious Summer Puddings or whatever it might be could be safely enjoyed without reality intruding anymore. Then she went to bed with something to make her think, which always sent her straight to sleep.

She didn't feel she was necessarily obsessive about it, not really, but her admiration for the sense of order and anodyne sterility that living with Rose had given her twenty years ago was still such an influence. So if Richard's room unfortunately reeked, however faintly and no matter how hard she tried to remove it, of the ongoing battle between excreta and disinfectant, hers smelled of orange blossom, her favourite scent, and scrupulous cleanliness.

It was completely white. The soft shag-pile carpet and the linen curtains, her duvet, dressing table and fitted Louvre cupboards were all white. It was a place where the aches and pains of the day were just a bad dream. She wanted to keep it that way. Virginal, pristine, to remind her of the childhood bliss of being with Mum. She loved pleasing Mum who loved pleasing her. It brought a smile to her heart even now, just remembering the care Mum took doing her hair with pretty grips and ribbons for her while dad was out and then hugging her over and over again for being her beautiful little girl.

And it was only in her bedroom now that she ever came even a little bit close to that feeling again. So she kept it perfectly clean, dusted the surfaces every day, changed her bed linen every week, and washed the curtains once a month. In the eight years they had been living here she had never once wheeled Richard into it. It was sacrosanct. Hers alone. The place where she could unwind and find again what Mum, who used to do Hatha yoga, called her Inner Sense of Peace.

Ron always came to stay with her for a few days while Richard was away with Rose, and for a while she had tried sleeping with him in here. But it hadn't done. Her bed was too small for two people and Ron was so large that unless she nestled herself in his arms all night long, which after a while became uncomfortable, she either felt crushed or in danger of being nudged out of bed altogether and dumped unceremoniously onto the floor. So unless she had fallen asleep herself after they made love, she tried to insist he go and sleep on the sofa in the lounge.

She somehow couldn't bring herself to make up Richard's bed for him, even though Richard had always encouraged her to, because it too was sacrosanct. He had always been a jealous husband before, but Richard had told her, via grunts, nods and careful eye contact, that he loved her, and that because he loved her he wanted her to take Ron as her lover, if that was what she wanted. There was no way she could have had an affair with him under Richard's actual roof. Not till they moved to Eastbourne, and then only when Richard was away.

Ron himself had proved something of a disappointment, sadly deteriorated since he had given up trying to be a father to Sean. He was not the man who had left her and who she had been pining for at all. It wasn't that she didn't still look forward to his visits. She did.

It was mostly sexual, but that was alright. In fact it was fine. She didn't mind. He remained rather attractive, she thought, for a man of fifty one or fifty two. Not in a conventional way, not with his hooked nose, tired eyes, slightly receding chin and the lines running down his cheeks from his brows to his jaw; but his awkward ruggedness and the way he looked at her still made her catch her breath as it hooked her desire. She wasn't young herself anymore and had grown up enough to realise that with the possible exception of her embarrassing past, she wasn't actually very remarkable either. Her interests were ordinary, her pleasures simple. So seeing Ron for a few days every time Richard went to stay with Rose, always helped her feel at least she wasn't *completely* uninteresting either. So what, if half the time nowadays she only had sex with him because she knew that nothing else would prevent him from being all over her all night, and she needed her sleep? She still enjoyed it, and was genuinely touched that he continued to want her, despite how much they had both changed. His lovemaking was still hungry and imaginative. In return she did her best to please him too, felt happy with how easily pleased he was and didn't want to lose him again.

His visits helped her not to feel completely alone with the hard facts of her life. They connected her with her past, gave her a sense of continuity. So although she wouldn't have dreamed of telling him in so many words, or not very often anyway, because it would have given him too much power, she didn't mind using her body to show him how glad she was he could be bothered to make time for her by coming down here to see her for a few days. And it wasn't all one way. Not really. Like Richard, Ron needed so much comfort, love and understanding himself. And it was nice giving him that too. In fact it was perfect, her favourite thing of all, if the truth be told. Better than sex, even.

Because of all things, simply giving love and being a comfort was what most made her feel *right* in herself and true to who she was, a feeling all too rare since Mum had gone. Richard needed her patience and devotion, but Ron needed to be listened to, to be understood, to be reassured, and to be provided with sex. She could give him all of those things easily except, sometimes, the understanding. Sometimes that could be difficult but she was always prepared to try.

She wasn't completely stupid. She knew that as long as she could feel she was needed and had something to give, then she could also feel that she really existed, that she was actually a person. Not something nebulous and insubstantial like the fragment of a dream, or a memory from childhood of her mother smiling at her as she helped her bake a cake, or hang up her clothes on the washing line, or do the shopping, or whatever.

She finished her tea, took the cup to the kitchen and rinsed it. Richard needed comfort to get through each day, and she needed her little comforts too – a cup of tea first thing in the morning and last thing at night was very soothing.

Ron was coming down this weekend, perhaps tomorrow or maybe Saturday. She must remember to get a bit more food in . He could eat her out of house and home, that man.

Ten years ago when he had first swept her off her feet with his dauntingly long words and his Ph.d, he used to talk the hind legs off a donkey, both before and after they made love. That had been a comfort too. He had been such fun, playful, teasing, considerate.

Despite how hard it was caring for Richard, and despite the awful loss that not caring for Sean for the last ten years had left her with, she did feel lucky. Like her preoperational past, thinking about Sean was too painful nowadays. Sean had been living with Grainne ever since she brought Rosie home for what turned out to be some weeks, that hot summer afternoon when they met up again in Holland Park and Rose somehow got stabbed in the hip with her kitchen knife. It was amazing to think that was already ten years ago now.

Giving Sean back to his real mother had been one of the most difficult things in her whole life, not just because Lucille had been left aching for him, but also because it had been so shocking to find that contrary to what she had always believed, she hadn't actually wanted to give him back to her at all. For ten years she had gone around believing it was the only answer, but when the time eventually came when she had to give him up and return him to Grainne, it hurt so much that she wanted to faint, repeatedly coming up in cold sweats and feeling all dizzy in the last few days before he actually left with her. And after he had gone, she used to get up and sit down again all the time for the loss of him, gawping like a fish out of water, and sometimes gasping for breath like one too. These panic attacks kept coming, every day for weeks, if not months afterwards.

In fact his leaving left her nearly as bereft as the death of Mum had.

She couldn't think about that either without feeling overwhelmed. Sean's going had been a terrible shock, but at least he was still alive and it had to have been the best thing in the world for him that he should be with his mother. Lucille had really forced herself to believe that. And she had believed it, and still did. But Mum's death, for all that she had been expecting it for so long, hadn't just taken her away from her, it had also

297

taken away a very real, very solid part of *herself* as well; left her feeling in some ways like *she* didn't really exist anymore either, which she hadn't expected at all. At the funeral, which she had attended wearing the white designer dress Dad had bought for Mum some years before and feeling in it, just as Mum had said she would, like a sailing boat, it was all she could do not to want to sail away with her. The pain of losing her felt more physical than mental, like a hot wind which would flay her, take her skin from her if she didn't go with it – with Mum – to wherever it was dead people went.

She couldn't go with her of course, but some months after burying her, she suffered a brief, severe attack of what the doctor said was psoriasis, shed all her skin painfully over a period of a few days. It had hurt like nothing else before or since and at the time she had been extremely worried about what permanent damage it might do to her still relatively flawless skin. She poured bottles of moisturisers and medicated body lotions onto her raw and peeling body. A week later, almost as fast as it had come, the psoriasis was gone again, and a couple of weeks after that her skin was nice and peachy again, as if nothing had happened.

From then on it became a little bit easier feeling motherless and insubstantial once more.

Even so, a year after she moved to Eastbourne, when Ron suddenly and unaccountably sold his flat in Clapham, with no notice, let alone any discussion with her about it, Lucille had not just felt confused, she'd felt hurt and slighted. He hadn't told her anything. Just disconnected his phone one day and disappeared without trace, not even leaving a forwarding address. She'd felt distraught, rendered even more insignificant and insubstantial, if that were possible. With Sean gone and Rose long ago having returned to her home in Balham, the loneliness of her life as Richard's carer pressed right in on her. The truth was her occasional weekends with Ron in Clapham had been her only consolation after relocating to Eastbourne, so their sudden and unexplained cessation was beyond what she could bear or understand when she allowed herself any feelings. So she had tried not to allow herself any feelings at all, just got on with the job of looking after Richard.

Ron did eventually send her a polite letter which didn't include an invitation to come up and see him. It simply informed her of his new address and telephone number, offered belated apologies for the suddenness of his departure six months earlier, said he'd had to go and live in the Midlands so he could be near his son, and told her he'd got a job at a minor independent school as a psychology teacher.

She'd known all this anyway by the time he got in touch with her, because Grainne had told her. She hoped he might have at least had the consideration to ask how she was in his letter, but he made no enquiry about her whatsoever. Nor did he ask in his letter her how she might be feeling about his having gone like that without telling her, taking it for granted that she would understand. The boy needed a father. That was all.

And that *was* all. Not a word, either, about his feelings for her, or the lack of them. In fact not another word from him for a further eighteen months, during which she came to slow painful terms with never seeing him again. At first she had tried to contact him, but whenever she phoned he always had the answer-phone on, never returned her calls and ignored all the letters she sent.

She couldn't understand what she had done to be treated in such a way. She'd been reaching out to him, he should have responded. *She* would have, if things had been the other way round.

It wasn't as if she hadn't been able to understand his need to see more of his child. She had missed Sean terribly herself because despite contact being occasional but regular at first, it had inevitably tailed off over time. The distance between Eastbourne and Leicester was just too much. Sean himself had not been the kind of boy to telephone her very often although when he did, he said the sweetest things which just made her cry. Grainne herself often rang her for advice and to tell her how Sean was doing during the first few months as mother and son got to know each other and their relationship inevitably came up against occasional teething problems. After a while her phone calls, which only reopened her own wounds, became further and fewer between. Grainne wasn't insensitive, she knew how difficult it was for her.

They had talked about it honestly and planned it all carefully, both women wanting to do what was best for Sean. So while her heart felt it was suffering palpitations, Lucille's head had not been able to disagree with Grainne's contention that as part of the process of transition it would be better for Sean to have less to do with her, for a while anyway, so that she could forge a proper maternal relationship with him without any competition or help from his erstwhile foster-mother. Grainne meant 'forge' like a sword, she said, not 'forge' like in fake. Lucille had been quite able to see her point, but still felt cut by it. She'd tried to hide this, trilling her encouragement and support, hugging them both, telling them everything would be alright, more than that, it would be wonderful, and agreed that Sean should be persuaded to think of her as his *Auntie* Lucille, rather than his mum; and that's what she always signed herself as on her birthday and Christmas cards to him thereafter. Sean, sweet boy, refused to play ball, continuing to call her Mum on the few occasions they saw one another and showing her more affection than he ever had while they'd been living together under the same roof. Perhaps he could tell that her heart wasn't really in it when she tried to discourage him. She did miss him more than she could bear sometimes.

Ron following him out of her life too had sometimes felt like the end.

Then, two years after he disappeared, and just when she thought she had finally got over him, Ron was back, standing on her doorstep, grinning like a bastard and asking to come in. He was living in London again, he said, thought he'd come down and see her. On the off-chance.

Oh really?

As fate would have it, Richard was away in London staying with Rose for a couple of weeks over Easter to give Lucille respite. She had automatically, if reluctantly, let him in with a little shrug, confused and shaky. Shock, anger and desire, all at the same time, were in the mix, as were anxiety, curiosity and memories.

The only explanation he offered for his reappearance was that it was better now if he just saw Sean occasionally at weekends. Now he was properly a teenager and didn't therefore need so much contact with his father. He spoke in the tone of someone who was an authority on such matters. Lucille knew there was a lot more to it than that. Grainne had often told her on the phone about his unsuccessful, sometimes laughable endeavours at being a father, but she didn't say anything, just nodded her head in solemn understanding.

His attempts to inveigle his way back into her affections were so cack-handed, so amateurish that, despite her bitterness, she didn't know whether to laugh or cry with finding she still wanted him.

And with wondering what had happened to him because he had changed again.

He told her how much he had missed her and how beautiful she was. She found herself shaking her head and smiling at one and the same time. He just wasn't the man he used to be two years previously. In fact he was more like the man she knew in the dim and distant past, the one who used to live with Grainne back when she – back when. He had even put some of his old weight back on. She warned herself to be careful. He was also a man who had proved he really didn't care about her feelings at all.

So it was upsetting to find she still fancied him, couldn't help enjoying his attention and wanting more of it, even as she reminded herself that he wasn't to be trusted. As he tried to sweet-talk her, she did what she could to avoid noticing the pleasing bulge in his trousers and the hungry look in his eye. But she liked being found attractive by him, she always had, and she couldn't help what she felt. The more he went on, the more it was as if the hurt he had done her by disappearing more than two years before just didn't have to matter anymore. He was back and that was all there was to it.

What made him even more difficult to resist was the fact that despite what was happening in his pants, his cockiness and arrogance all seemed to be gone. He seemed so much nicer now, so much less egotistical. Humbled somehow. Grainne and Sean must have seen to that. He'd lost none of his directness though, stroking her arm and her hair and openly admitting his interest in her now was about getting his end away and feeling less lonely. That put her off at first, right off. But then, when he told her he only wanted sex because he'd lost his confidence as a person and didn't think he was actually capable anymore of managing a proper relationship with anyone, she could understand, had been there herself once, and found herself beginning not just to want him, but to love him again too.

He just wanted a little sex and companionship. That was all. The fact that he was honest enough to say so wasn't *just* brazen and shameless. It also happened to be true. She could feel it. And that made it okay somehow, even as she knew it probably shouldn't. A little sex and companionship was all anybody wanted when it came down to it. She certainly wouldn't mind some. Despite all the hurt his leaving her had left her with before.

Her heart went out to him completely and she knew herself to be seduced once more as he acknowledged both the cruelty of his departure two years earlier, and his insensitivity in not remaining in touch subsequently. He hadn't known how to tell her, he said. The best thing seemed to be to just do it, cut all ties, because his interpersonal skills were purely notional, academic. He could only talk about them, teach them. He didn't actually have any himself at all.

She couldn't disagree. He *had* been cruel. Relationships with other people clearly did ask too much of him emotionally. She told him he was right, but found herself making sure that her body language spoke only of forgiveness and desire. He said he cared for others, for Sean, for her, but he was unable to actually *be* caring in how he behaved with them.

She wouldn't herself go as far as saying that, she told him in all seriousness, sensing he was about to make a move and crossing her legs towards him as they sat together on the sofa. Sure enough, he moved closer, kept on looking from her face to her knees and back again via the rest of her body as they talked. She was glad she had just been about to go out shopping when he rang her doorbell and was looking fairly presentable. She told him she understood, knew he was not intentionally horrible anyway. He shifted closer still, put his arm on the back of the sofa behind her and began toying with the nape of her neck under her hair, then slipped his huge fingers under her top and onto her shoulder. She smiled her pleasure at him. She couldn't help it. He said he now recognised that he was both incompetent and destructive. She wanted to pull away, wanted to seem to be a little harder to get, for her own self respect, and really did want to listen to more of him speaking the truth like this, it was so refreshing after all the different kinds of gobbledygook he used to come out with in the past. But hearing such honesty from him, as his strong fingers went back to stroking her neck through her hair, massaging it and making her wanting to move against them like a cat, she couldn't help it, all she wanted was to feel him on top of her with his sex inside her. He could save the talking for later. Sighing, she leaned in towards him and rested her head under his arm and then he did stop talking. Before she knew it she felt his hand come down onto her breast and then his other hand was under her skirt and they were kissing.

As he moved her into a horizontal position on the sofa and undid his belt she didn't lose her sense of pride and self respect altogether. A part of her wanted to resist, but couldn't, that was all. She felt so lonely too. There had been nobody else – no other man, that is – while he was gone. Besides, just as she had sensed he would, he made love to her with an empathy and understanding which belied what he had just said about being incompetent and destructive.

When he was spent and took her in his arms she breathed in the smell of him and wasn't surprised to find herself telling him, against all reason, how much she'd missed him. She told him over and over again about all the different ways she had felt it over the last two years, as he kept on planting little kisses on the top of her head. Then she found herself feeling both angry and tearful at how glad she was he was back, and wanted to beat her fist down on his chest. Instead she twiddled the hair on it between her fingers feeling confused. Certain of only one thing: this was so much better than being alone.

So they agreed they would become lovers once more, but again on a part-time basis. She did have her limits despite her shameful surrender. He would stay with her for up to a week, but no more than that, each time Richard went away to stay with Rose, which happened three times a year. Other than that they would not see each other very much at all, except for the occasional dinner date or brief overnight stay at his place. It was a good solution. He might have changed, become more honest, but he was still unpredictable, and for all her need of him she didn't want to be hurt again.

So theirs became a simple, if strangely compartmentalised little relationship. She talked, mostly. He listened, mostly. And they had sex together. She specially loved being with him after they had had sex, because then he didn't really want anything from her anymore. They'd chat in the dark for hours sometimes, with her doing most of the talking, of course, and in response he would occasionally grunt. The fact, that unlike Richard he could actually speak if he wanted, meant she didn't mind if he didn't. She loved settling herself beside him after he had finished with her, and he liked latching onto a nipple again like a great big baby, occasionally grunting as she gabbled on about whatever it was she was thinking or feeling at the time and stroking his head. Content, she would natter happily into the small hours of the night. Sometimes they'd have sex again. Eventually she would realise the rhythm of his breath meant he had fallen asleep, and would stop talking, tapping his stubbly cheek to encourage his mouth to fall open before she moved. She couldn't help feeling important then, loving the sensation of being what he needed, even if he did find her too boring to be bothered to stay awake for, and even if the damp patch of semen was making her sticky and uncomfortable. On such nights she would stare up at the ceiling quietly aglow, then slip silently away to the bidet in the bathroom, put on a clean night dress and go and sleep on the sofa in the living room.

*   *   *

Four hours after opening her living room curtains and having her early morning cup of tea, she and Richard were making their way up King Edward's Parade through a brisk July morning. She was meeting Paula for coffee and cake at the tacky turquoise grandeur of the old Arcadian Palace hotel. Plump frumpy Paula was a fifty year old, self-confessed chocoholic with a predilection for too much pink and black which sometimes made her look like a Licorice Allsort. But she had the sweetest nature, and the sharpest business brain. Lucille often told her how much she loved the way she looked, the way she displayed such a serene lack of interest in conforming to any trends whatsoever. Paula proved appearances, whether kept up or otherwise, can be completely deceptive. Lucille didn't tell her that of course. Paula wasn't insensitive. And sweet though she was, she was no Licorice Allsort either. Lucille had actually met her years ago in Oxshott when she had briefly employed her as her financial adviser. She had proved really invaluable at helping her to sort out her affairs after Richard's stroke and had been a good friend ever since.

And Lucille's affairs had certainly needed sorting. Richard had cashed in all his life cover, had no accident or sickness insurance, nor stocks or shares or anything. He had invested all he had in the house, which nevertheless had continued to need to be paid for. It had been Paula who had told her about purpose-built, fully equipped, self-contained flats for the elderly and disabled over in Eastbourne where she herself lived. And eventually Lucille had sold up, paid off the mortgage and bought this flat for less than a third of the price she got for their home in Oxshott even though it had a sea view. Ever since then she had lived off the interest, his pension, attendance allowance and long term sick and disabled benefits.

Not that she had had to live *too* frugally. She could still afford to have her hair done every other week, and if she saw something she fancied in the shops she could usually find the money for it, if she wanted to. But she just did not need another fancy frock or a nice new skirt for changing urine-soaked sheets in every morning. She needed an unattractive, nylon housecoat, rubber gloves and a bottomless well of patience. So she tended to live in jeans and a T-shirt most days. Nice enough jeans and pretty enough tops. But as a carer – capital C – you had to be realistic, and you had to be practical.

She was forty years old, but felt she looked maybe three, even four years younger. It was still important to try to keep herself looking nice and pamper herself when she could. But both her previous lives, as a lady of leisure in Surrey, and before that as a sex-obsessed girl in South London, were now almost as difficult to remember as that dim and distant period she thought of as The Childhood. She lived in the present nowadays as far as possible. Her only indulgence was having her hair done. If you didn't have pretty hair and shoes – topped and tailed, Mum used to say – then everything else about the way you looked wouldn't be quite right, and you couldn't really feel good about yourself. That's what she felt.

She had just come from the salon ten minutes ago, her shorter, dark, now auburn hair curling inwards in nice big waves around her face in what she felt was a quite satisfactory mix of the soft and the stylish. Teased up and full on top, it tapered down around her cheeks and neck in a sort-of bob, so that her mother's lovely collection of costume earrings and necklaces, which she had recently retrieved from the back of a drawer, could be shown to more effect. You had to make adjustments for the reality of middle age.

As usual she'd left Richard parked by the reception desk to sit with Jackie, the seventeen year old apprentice, whose trapped, hungry looks and sultry pouts reminded her of herself at that age. Richard grunted and groaned, barked and moaned in his occasionally successful efforts to actively overcome his dysphasia enough to help Jackie with her Sun crossword. Lucille could tell the girl herself really wasn't that interested in it. It was sweet of her to put up with his bellowing and barking solutions to her in that distorted way of his which even the most patient of people would find maddening if they had to live with it for any length of time. In response to his grunts, Jackie would make comically uncomprehending faces at all and sundry, including Richard, till eventually she understood what he was saying. He would then guffaw his delight without a trace of irony or sarcasm. Surprisingly, given her sulkiness, his laughs always made Jackie howl with laughter too, and from her chair in the salon Lucille would smile at her reflection. It was good for both of them to get out of the flat sometimes.

Whatever she might look like at home in her jeans and housecoat, she always tried to look her best pushing his chair behind him when they were out. It would have been mortifying if the grimness of her reality ever

304

revealed itself as she walked around the streets of Eastbourne with Richard, also dressed to the nines, propped up in front of her. She always pushed him along in his electric wheelchair with a serene, self-contained expression on her perfectly made-up face, defying anyone to imagine she found her life even the slightest bit difficult. Again, it was a matter of pride.

So if his head lolled forward, or his mouth dribbled as they walked along the front, or if there was a tell-tale trickle dripping from his inside trouser leg, she would invariably take it in her stride, turning a delicate heel and discreetly straightening him up or covering him; mentally covering up her own humiliation about what it said about her inadequacy as a carer; simply carrying on as if she actually didn't have a care in the world. Mercifully, such accidents were rare because over the years she had developed a reliable system for managing him. She had become an expert at it.

'Thank you, darling, but as you know, I've always been a bit silly about colours,' she said to Paula who had arrived at the Arcadian five minutes before her, and who complimented her on her slightly short, slightly swirly, new coat with a satisfying gawp. It was *very* purple and lined with satin, lovely to put on and take off and glamorous to wear. They kissed. Lucille glowed. She did love meeting Paula, whose directness might be bracing, but who also said the sweetest things. And when she did so, you knew she meant them.

She looked around the leafy interior of the Arcadian and smiled. They liked meeting here because it managed to be both tacky and tasteful at the same time, full of enormous terracotta-potted palms and exotic plastic creepers adorned with masses of lovely bright flowers, as if a mid twentieth century Hollywooden fantasy of the tropics had been transposed to east Sussex. The colour of the plush carpet was like golden sand. You could sit down in the warmth of the hotel, ignore the north easterly winds sweeping in across the English Channel from Siberia, or wherever it was, and imagine you were Zelda waiting for F. Scott Fitzgerald.

It wasn't actually a bad day today outside now, and Paula had chosen a small table by the window, which stretched from floor to ceiling, so they could look out to sea. Lucille locked the wheels of Richard's chair, undid the buttons of his coat and propped him up a bit more. She slipped out of her own coat and laid it carefully over a chair beside her before sitting herself down and ordering a pot of Lapsang Souchong.

Dressed in a cerise skirt, a dark red v-neck top and plum heels which she wasn't altogether sure weren't a bit frumpy with the skirt though they matched her bag quite nicely, she was confident she was the picture of a quietly elegant lady with the money and leisure time to properly look after herself and her disabled husband.

And it wasn't a sham. Not really, even if leisure time was rare and her resources had ever so slowly continued to dwindle over the years, despite Paula's best advices. Anyway, even if it was a sham, it actually didn't matter. At home, and in her relationships it would have mattered very much, of course it would, if what she really felt had been hidden behind appearance and illusion, but she didn't hide her feelings at all; neither with Richard nor Ron, or the few women down here she had been able to make friends with, most of whom were Carers like herself. But out in the world, it was different. She didn't want strangers to know how she was really feeling or how ghastly her life actually was. She wanted to briefly enjoy creating the illusion, even believing herself for an hour or two, that her life was no harder or worse than anybody else's.

'No brains at all really,' she said with a broad smile. 'I can't help it, even now after all these years – all I care about is appearances. So I'm ever so glad you like my coat, darling.'

'Your Silly-Me-I'm-Just-a-Little-Airhead shite would seem much less of an affectation if you only made more of an effort at getting things wrong,' Paula said, grinning. 'You know, toothpaste down your front perhaps, or Richard in different coloured socks, something like that. Anything which might actually *show* you were an Airhead. But if there's any air in you at all, my darling, I'm afraid it's all hot.'

An unshaven, bow-tied young waiter arrived pushing a small cake trolley. He couldn't yet be out of his teens, thought Lucille feeling old, he certainly must be younger than Sean.

In an over-familiar, obvious way, beginning and ending with her legs, he gave her a slow, speculative once-over as he provided Paula and herself with a mechanical and desultory rundown of the various pastries, sponges and meringues he had on board. Pushing her skirt down toward the top of her knee and concentrating on the cakes, she ignored him of course, but was secretly gratified.

'I really shouldn't,' she said to Paula, who had already pointed out the chocolate fudge cake to the waiter. 'I can hardly get into anything less than a fourteen anymo–.'

'Don't be silly, don't be boring and please don't be rude, Lucie!' interrupted Paula. 'For a woman in her forties–

'Rude? Me? Paula, I've never known a woman as rude as *you*, never! And I am forty. Just forty! I'm not forty-one for more than two months yet.'

'Well, I'm forty five, so believe me I know what I am talking about. For someone in her forties you have a figure to die for. You're just trying to rub in how overweight I am.' She smiled at her fondly. 'Bitch.'

'Bitch yourself!' She smiled. 'I don't know how I put up with you. I really don't.'

'Don't interrupt me please. I'm on a roll,' Paula said, pushing her rimless spectacles up her nose. With her other hand she reached up for her piece of cake from the waiter before he had even found time to place it on the table in front of her. 'Or should that be a slice?' she said, looking at it and licking her lips. 'Where was I? Oh yes! Trying to make me feel even fatter than I am already. Which is horrible! And it won't work, cos I don't care! I'm starving,' she added, glancing from the waiter to Lucille and back again before tucking into it. She didn't miss much, Paula didn't.

Lucille looked up at the youthful waiter with her most dazzling smile as he passed her a slice of angel cake. He paid no attention to it whatsoever.

That was more like it. She long ago realised that whenever a man half her age looked at her at all suggestively he either had to be dangerous or have serious developmental problems. Older men were another matter altogether. She knew that in some strange kind of way she would always be looking for her father, because his face often flashed up before her when she was least expecting it, so she did still enjoy being on the end of *their* glances; when she wasn't too exhausted or too absorbed in attending to Richard's needs to notice them. But sex with them? The very thought made her shudder. An appreciative glance, like the one she shared with the doorman just now when he helped her push Richard in through the revolving doors, was quite enough.

The waiter turned to Richard, who grunted his assent as the young man's long finger passed over the cheesecake. Richard could speak quite a few words now with a certain amount of clarity. Maybe as many as fifty. With her, at least, he had definitely over the years become quite skilled at making his wishes known and having his needs met. It was an absolute godsend that he could use the first finger of his left hand to indicate yes and no. Once for yes. Twice for no. He could also still chew and swallow perfectly and had therefore put on a fair bit of weight. And he had always been a big man anyway. That was why they needed the hoist. There would have been no way she could have looked after him without it.

She hated him for having had a stroke and brought them down to this. But she would always love him till the day he died, even if she wasn't altogether sure why. Perhaps it just came down to the fact that he was hers, he needed her and she was loyal. The urbane and charming man of the world that he had been before, and whom she had been rapidly falling in hate with ten years ago, had long departed. She had been distraught about the death of her mother, and distressed about Sean being taken away from her, but the awful truth was the timing of Richard's first stroke had in some ways been perfect. By becoming an invalid he had provided her with someone to look after and care for again just when the previous recipients of her passion to look after and care for others had been taken away from her.

'Richard has more needs than a child. I'm sorry, Richard, I don't mean to be horrible. You know I don't. But it's true. And when I've finished looking after him I've got nothing left for anything else, except to make sure I don't look the way I feel! So if I don't go straight to bed myself, I collapse in front of the TV in a face mask or curlers or something. You know! Something – anything! – to look after myself, to help me feel better about myself, wind down and get ready for the morning. It doesn't actually matter that I am not going to see another soul the next day. It really doesn't.'

She wasn't trying to fool either of them, but sometimes lies were true.

'So why bother then?' Paula asked between chompings.

'For me. Out of habit. I don't know. It's what I do, part of my routine. Routines are such a comfort when you're alone. I have to remind myself I exist in my own right, I'm not just a carer, you know? *You* are special, individual. And you know you are. That's why you don't really mind so much about what you look like, isn't it? But I'm not. No! Don't look at me like that. All that's special about me is my past. Otherwise I am as ordinary as anything. There is not one special thing about me at all. I lie by myself and feel scared to be alone at night with Richard bubbling and snoring next door. I'm just like anybody else. And what I feel – what I have always felt – is my appearance is all I have got. And now I'm,' she paused with deliberate drama, then broke into a surrendering smile. 'Now I'm... in my forties – okay? – it's fast beginning to disappear, if it hasn't gone already. Then what will I do?'

She made a silly face, but did actually feel quite glum about it.

'Accept it?' Paula suggested. 'I mean, we can't lie to ourselves all of our lives.' She removed a little pat of chocolate icing from the arm of her snow-white fleece. 'Accept yourself? For who you are?' She looked at the small dark brown stain it had left behind, shrugged away a grimace. 'Never mind. Can't be helped. It's not a WORM,' she said cheerfully wiggling a pinkie. They both laughed. 'Not like what you're talking about. Not yet. As WORMS go, you know, you're really wriggling!'

Whenever they met together over coffee and cakes, their conversation always turned at some point to WORMs, their acronym for What Really Matters. WORMs put everything into perspective. From fashion to compassion for victims of illness and disease, and back again, from the meaning of life to the understanding of incomprehensible husbands, WORMs could always be invoked to guide their conversations. They could chat for hours about WORMs and when they did so the cakes always somehow tasted better, the tea so much more sippable.

This was probably half the reason why Lucille had put on nearly four pounds over the past ten years. Two whole kilos. It wasn't much, but for Lucille it had meant sometimes going up a dress size. In some shops she was a twelve and in others a fourteen. The other thing causing this weight-gain had to do with the strength she had built up looking after Richard. She had to be fit. Two or three times a day she needed all her physical strength to manage him, simply because of the fact that he was now more than twice the weight she was, and he needed turning over. Thank heavens for small mercies, such as the fact that he could just about move his legs forward or upward one at time. And for large mercies like the hoist.

She didn't actually look muscley, thank goodness. Not all ripples and sinews, like Grainne. However fashionable that might be nowadays for some women, for a person like her who took comfort in a conventional, unthreatening femininity, it would actually have been a bit unnerving. In fact after twenty two years of oestrogen and progesterone coursing through her system she felt that from a distance her shape would have to be described as a classical English Pear. Especially now that her breasts and her bottom were a bit bigger. The truth was that close up and naked she was actually the tiniest bit saggy in both the boob and bum areas. So because she was otherwise still quite slender, she felt that naked she actually more resembled a dried up old prune, than a pear. But from a distance and in her clothes there was no doubt about it, she was somewhere between a Williams and a Queen Charlotte. At least she still had good skin.

There was just no understanding some people. Especially herself. What she did know, was that despite everything and incomprehensible though it was, she did now feel ever so much more confident than she ever had in her twenties and thirties, let alone in the misshapen days of her childhood. The most comforting thing was the simple everyday fact of her anonymity, just an ordinary woman living in Eastbourne who most people didn't even look at twice.

She turned to see how Richard was doing with his cheesecake. He was clearly enjoying himself listening to them talk. He liked going out with her and meeting her friends. Anything to break up the monotony of his life.

'Laffit,' he said with his bizarre, lop-sided smile.

'Sorry darling?'

'Lllaffit. Llaffit...Laffit!' He paused in the face of their uncomprehending frowns and sounding irritated, tried again. 'Lab-bit.'

'Labbit? Labbit. Rabbit?' She nodded, turned to Paula. 'Rabbit! We're rabbiting apparently. He likes it though, don't you darling? It makes him feel superior. He's never had any time at all for what I called 'trying to understand' and what he used to call 'guff' or 'psychobabble'. I know just what he'd say now if he could. He'd say it is stupid trying to accept yourself when you've got no choice anyway. You would, wouldn't you Richard?' She didn't wait for him to grunt his assent. 'I think that's why he absolutely refused to allow the rehabilitation team to offer him any counselling. Even though I was having some!'

He closed his eyes and reopened them. It was his way of nodding. She knew he could in fact have very slowly nodded at her if she had waited for him to do so, but it took him a full minute to complete the process of moving his head up and down once, and neither of them had the patience for that so he had learned to use his eyelids in lieu of his head. In fact when they were on their own together she did the same thing – a slow blink meant yes between the two of them.

Bits of cake were dislodging themselves from the corners of his mouth. Lucille reached over with her napkin and wiped him tenderly. She was feeling particularly affectionate towards him just now, because tomorrow she would be driving him over to stay with Rosie for a couple of weeks.

Ever since they moved down to Eastbourne, Rose had had him go and stay with her three times a year to give them both a break. These Respite Fortnights, as Rose called them, had taken on an almost sacred quality for Lucille. She was able to quietly enjoy feeling free for fourteen days. She liked Ron visiting, but never for more than a week. She prized her freedom too much. In both of the last two years during the summer fortnight, she had taken a long weekend holiday abroad by herself. Although on each occasion the pleasure of being alone in Paris, then Barcelona had palled just a little, after a day or two in cities where everyone her age seemed to be paired off with someone else.

'It's going to be so wonderful to be free for a couple of weeks. It's like being let out of a cage. Richard understands. We share the same cage really.'

He beamed a painfully slow, painfully small and solemn nod of agreement for Paula from behind his cheesecake. As he did so, Lucille watched Paula's cheerful round face light up, as large and round as her glasses.

'In fact,' Lucille said, through an embarrassed and frightened little giggle. 'He'd like me to kill him.' She felt herself wincing. 'True, isn't it, Richard?' He blinked and grunted in obvious confirmation. 'Can you believe it?' She looked wide-eyed at Paula.

She needed Paula to believe it, both because it was true and because it was upsetting.

'Believe it, Paula, please.'

Paula looked at Richard who managed to hold her glance and give her another slow blinking nod, otherwise keeping his stare at her up throughout. Knowing him as she did, Lucille could see every fibre of his being behind that stare, longing beyond anything to die.

'Yes I can, really, I *do* believe it. I'd feel the same way myself. It's a terrible life for both of you.'

'It's not *too* bad! But last night was a bit miserable, to be honest. We were watching this TV programme about genes and evolution. Did you see it? No? Oh. Well, it was saying all living beings from, I don't know – from fishes to humans – have to die in order that others may live.

Something like that, anyway. And Richard managed to say 'like Jesus', although it came out more like 'Lie Sejus'. It was a shock because he was never a Christian! He had no time for Christianity at all. So I asked him if he wanted to go to a church and he got so agitated and angry that for a minute I thought he was having another stroke. Trust me to get him all wrong. I've always been great at that! So I sat with him and then after five or ten minutes of trying his hardest, he managed to say 'Kill me''.

I thought he meant it as a joke at first, that it would kill him to go inside a church, so I thought nothing of it, just carried on with the ironing. But he said it again and again. He wouldn't stop, till I started getting ratty with him and telling him to shut up. Then I was so ashamed of myself about that, for losing it with him when he can't help it, so I went out to the kitchen and made some tea. He stopped for a while then, but later when I was getting him ready for bed he started up again, over and over again, till I couldn't help it, my scalp started tingling, and I realised I was crying as well. I really don't want to start again now, as a matter of fact. I really don't. But for some reason my whole stupid head feels full of horrible feelings just at the moment.'

Picking up her napkin, she discreetly dabbed the corners of her eyes, looking around at the other people in the room as she did so. She did not want to mess up her face again. She had come up all blotchy after the tears last night, as she always did when she cried. Taking a few deep breaths and avoiding Paula's sympathetic expression which would have just set her off again, she diverted herself by cooing over a little three year old girl who had wandered over to their table pushing a doll in a toy push-chair. The doll had slipped down in its seat and was in danger of falling right out. She helped the little girl sit it up straight again, asked her what her dolly's name was, clucking admiration of its red and white checked dress. In her Benettons and curls, the child looked at her with wordless disdain, then proudly steered the push-chair back to her mother's table across the floor.

'Talking of hair,' said Paula putting a hand up to her badly-done chignon and trying to push some loose strands back into it, 'yours is always so pretty. I bet you've just come straight from the salon again, haven't you? It's really nice.'

Lucille nodded impatiently, took a sip of tea and broke off a little corner of cake with her fork. But instead of lifting the cake to her mouth she put the fork down again.

'I keep on telling you I could do yours, if you'd like me to,' she said. She touched Paula's arm. 'I'm sorry. It *is* sweet of you to try and change the subject and everything. But in the end it's how you feel that matters, isn't it? Not how you look. That's why you were saying I should accept myself, wasn't it? My hair has been every colour of the rainbow and every style over the years, but who cares? Only me, and only for as long as I do!

And then it's gone. I know it's obvious, and I know everyone always says it, but love is the most personal thing there is and the only thing that sticks. I'm beginning to realise that now. To realise there are more important things, like – like I love this old hulk of mine.' She looked at Richard. 'I do. I wasn't upset because of what he was asking me to do, but because – I'm so ashamed – because,' she leaned closer towards Paula and lowered her voice to a whisper. 'Because just then, I did want to kill him. You know? I really wanted to just put him to bed and smother him. It was like all the work I've put into looking after him all these years meant nothing to him. Not that *that* mattered. Not really. He has a right to his feelings, doesn't he? What mattered was *I* wanted to kill him. I really did.'

She blurted this out, smiling and crying at once with the relief of telling. Paula reached over and put a warm pudgy hand on top of hers, patting it and stroking it, but that made Lucille want to cry even more so she withdrew her hand and quietly blew her nose.

'I'm sure he understands,' Paula said.

'I know he does! But I would *never*! You know that, don't you ? He's disappointed in me. He really would like me to.' She looked at Richard and then back at Paula. 'I would never kill anything or anyone.'

Paula stared sympathetically at her, nodding her head. Then her eyes twinkled as she grinned.

'You know what they say, Lucille: everybody is capable of murder given the right conditions.'

Richard twitched, which Lucille was all too well aware meant that he was excited. She watched him carefully for a moment. Yes, the veins on his temples were racing and he was clearly trying to nod his agreement with Paula.

'Thinking about it makes me feel ill. I can't even kill insects. But last night when he kept on repeating it, I found myself wanting to say, 'yes, alright I will!', so very, very much, that I just felt like running away, packing my bags and leaving, there and then!' She made a hopeless little face. 'But Richard needed his wee bottle.'

She smiled at Paula, but it felt like a grimace and Paula didn't smile back.

'We need a break, both of us. We really do. He's off to Rosie's again tomorrow, thank goodness! I'm taking him up first thing, and I can't wait. You can't either, can you, Richard?' She reached over and parted his hair with her hand. She couldn't help it. She loved him. You had to either love and stay with, or hate and leave someone as needy as him. There was no happy medium. Not for her. Love had to be just one corner, her corner, of the eternal triangle between hate and indifference. And it had to be protected.

'Wanting Richard gone for a couple of weeks is very different from losing him forever, isn't it?' Lucille continued. 'It's just that ten years has been such a long time. For both of us. After the first stroke his consultant told me that once someone's had one cranial bleed they are more than likely to have others and to die within a couple of years at most. At most! And that's what we both expected to happen. Yet here he is still alive, and virtually unchanged since his stroke, except bigger and fatter and older. He's sixty five soon. All the same I really wouldn't want anyone to kill him.'

The atmosphere between them had relaxed again, the tension gone. They both laughed merrily. Then Lucille felt herself going pink and gave a tiny, almost imperceptible nod before saying,

'I didn't really want to, you know, *actually* kill him. But I'm just so tired of all my routines. And my boring little life. And he is so tired of his. The more he went on at me last night, the more I felt like doing what he asked! It was scary. I couldn't sleep afterwards. I just lay in bed shaking and scared of my own feelings. I mean if he was going to get better it would be a different matter, but he's not.' She let her gaze drift wistfully off out the window over the sea for a moment then switched on her reliably cheery smile. 'Let's have some more tea! I'm so sorry to be doing all this whinging, Paulie. Just like last time we met. I always seem to be moaning.'

On the way home the selfish feeling persisted as Lucille negotiated the usual round of struggles: getting Richard's wheelchair across the roads before the lights changed; remaining patient when people didn't make allowances for her on the pavements; thanking them when they did; pacing herself and taking little breaks, little momentary pauses to avoid her hands and arms getting sore or becoming too exhausted or uncomfortably hot. But she was good at it. She had had years of practice.

You have to accept what you've got in life, she told herself, Paula was right. But accepting what life had dished out to her had been impossible, and If Richard could have an operation now and be cured, she would not hesitate to do everything humanly possible to arrange it for him, spend every penny she had left. To be true to Richard, in terms of her own life, her own identity and her own truth, she understood his wish to die as deeply as if it were her own.

Chapter 19.

'Oh, and Lucille?'

'Yes?'

'One more thing, dear. I've run out of olive oil for cooking. Could you stop and get me some, do you think, before you arrive?'

Rose said goodbye and carefully put the phone down enjoying the sensation of slotting it in place. She did so enjoy ritual. In terms of day to day living nothing else gave her so much reason to carry on; every completed ritual giving her an incentive for starting another one. So where once it had been a prison now it was a pleasure. It contained her like a mother. It looked after her. It prevented her from getting out of hand or wandering off onto the streets again. Where once it had locked her in, now it was the key to every door. Not that she went out very much anymore anyway. Not unless she had to. Internet shopping was an absolute godsend. You could compare prices all day, compiling such detailed lists – heavenly!

For the next two weeks she was going to have to modify her usual routines and habits. She wouldn't, of course, be able to spend hours comparing supermarket prices against her weekly income from pension and benefits before doing her weekly shop. That was too solitary an activity when she had company. Lucille and Richard would be here in less than an hour and it would take at least that long to get everything set and ready for him, so she better hurry up and start by getting on with transforming her sitting room into a bedroom.

But she was stuck.

No, not stuck, she reminded herself. Choosing to remain stationary. *As* if stuck.

Silly woman! Remaining stationary in order to properly ritualise the preparing of the room. Because rituals were now wonderful things. They provided opportunities, not constraints, for putting thoughts into actions.

Now, the thought/question was: how to get from the kitchen into the sitting room. Answer: Simple! You sit up; take a last sip of tea; slide your chair back, and arching your spine you push your chair carefully backwards using the back of your knees and rising up out of it in one movement, using the heel of your hand to help you by pushing it down on the table top to lever yourself up, thus incidentally preventing yourself from needing another replacement for your hip replacement. You then rotate yourself carefully around and make a bee line at a snail's pace for the door into the hall.

Simple.

She took a deep breath then followed this prescription, and from the hall followed her usual ritual for going into her sitting room. This involved brushing the door frame with her left hand and using her right wrist and forearm, but *not* her hand to push the door open. Once actually in the room she stopped, took stock and pulled out another mental plan she hadn't used since the spring. It was the blueprint she had been using for Richard's visits for years now. Taking another deep breath, she opened the windows, then began pulling the sofa-bed away from the wall. It was supposed to be lightweight, but it still felt terribly heavy to her. Despite the considerable, if not complete, easing of pain and the increase in mobility that her artificial hips had given her, she was still wary of doing herself an injury. So she tugged and pulled at the sofa-bed gingerly, pulling it out bit by bit and turning it round so that it was now alongside the wall rather than having its back to it. This would give her more space to move around the room and get Richard in and out of his wheelchair each day. Lucille would be bringing the portable Hercules with its hydraulics to help her lift him in and out and she had to make room for that as well, otherwise he would end up being stuck in bed for the whole two weeks which would never do.

Rose made her way very slowly, step by step, up the stairs taking her downstairs, banister-side path up to the landing. She knew this didn't make sense, but it made her feel good in a sensible, practical kind of way to try and wear out the carpet evenly. For as long as she could remember, it was the carpet on the stairs that she had always been most worried about.

Anyway it was a minor enough concern and a harmless enough ritual which without constraining her in any way, gratified her need for order. That was the important thing. As well as connecting her up with her past. She had always had up and down paths on the stairs ever since she was a little girl. And she did like to try and hold onto a sense of continuity in her life, having effectively 'lost' so many years, first to grief and then to wandering around the streets of London. So she valued the patterns that had persisted across the time of her life. Besides, most of her actual memories were long forgotten. Lucille and Richard's existence directly attested to the fact that she did actually have a past, but it was her pleasure and prerogative to try to link her past and her present together, to feel *consistent*, by way of old patterns of behaviour and action.

The house itself was full of memories for her.

She tried to keep it in perfect condition, but the years of renting it out whilst she had been away had taken their toll. There was something impersonal about the place now. It was no longer a home, it was somehow a 'holiday home', and had a false feeling about it which she could smell under everything – a musty, almost institutional smell, from having been cleaned for nearly ten years by agency cleaners who did not love the place, and from having been lived in by so many passing strangers. Irritatingly, the smell wouldn't leave no matter what she did, but as it wasn't worth having the whole place gutted or redecorated she just had to try and make do. Each month she chose a different room to thoroughly spring clean. By the time she got back to the first room again ten months later, the musty uncared-for smell was always back, even though she tried to throw open all the doors and windows at least once a week as long as the weather wasn't too bad. Yesterday, with some annoyance, she had suddenly realised why this was so. She had been wrong all the time about the permanent unpleasant aroma. It wasn't the smell of passing holiday-makers and industrial strength disinfectant, it was the smell of her. The reek of old lady. And it was so unfair: she wasn't an old lady yet. Sixty one wasn't old. Not really.

She got a fresh duvet cover and a pillow case out of the airing cupboard, and waddled back downstairs again, this time taking the track she usually used for going up. It was odd how going downstairs was so much harder than going up. Never mind. She was feeling quite content. It was always a pleasure having Richard come to stay. It made her feel useful, gave her something to do and someone to talk to. It was particularly pleasant talking with no expectation of any reply. Of course he did occasionally struggle to respond to her and when this happened she tried to rein in her impatience and listen to him, as a courtesy, if nothing else. They did have a history together, after all, even if it was mostly ancient.

And it was nice to see the third Mrs McElvey so regularly as well.

She could not now fully understand why she had dropped poor little Lucille so unceremoniously, stopped speaking to her altogether after she and Richard had first started having a relationship together. What on earth had possessed her? Lucille was like a daughter to her. Like family. So often in both her personal and professional life, Rose had observed how family relationships themselves somehow always managed to resist the passage of time, went on being exactly the same, oblivious to all the changes life inevitably brought to the people having them. So the pain of cutting off contact with Lucille had been that much more intense than it might otherwise have been had she had been merely a friend. Closer in fact to the pain she'd felt about losing Luke.

And now here she was with them both again, as if neither of them had ever gone, as if there had been no breach between them at all, and as if she herself had never been away living on the streets for years. She still occasionally had to remind herself of the fact that she was not Lucille's mother and also of the fact she really did not mind about her relationship with Richard after all this time. Not really. It just didn't matter anymore. What mattered was compassion. Which was why, at least as far as she was concerned, they had all been friends again for years.

More than friends.

Last week Rose found a solicitor in the yellow pages, had him come round to the house and redrafted her will, leaving everything to Lucille. There was no one else. And there was certainly no point in leaving any of it to Richard. Lucie would probably need every penny to look after him properly as the years went by, poor thing. If he survived. Or to pay for some respite care two or three times a year once she herself had dropped off the perch and couldn't offer it any more. So because she no longer had any savings, she decided that her home and its contents would all go to Lucille.

You had to plan for your eventual demise. Of course you did. If you didn't realise that by the time you were in your early sixties, you must already be suffering from some kind of dementia.

Rose felt every single day of her age. She had had two hip replacement operations in the last seven years and had lived a very sober lifestyle for the last ten. But still her body gave her aches and pains. A legacy, she thought, of all those years of sleeping rough. And sometimes her head hurt because still she didn't know if she had in fact really killed those poor children during the last few weeks of her life on the streets. Her certainty about whether what she had done, and what she remembered, was real, began to crumble after she went with a reluctant and disapproving Lucille to the police to confess.

That was a long time ago now too. A month, maybe two at most, after recovering from accidentally stabbing herself all those years ago. She had still been staying with Lucille at the time, convalescing. The poor girl had been so transparently happy looking after Richard and herself, and had done so with so much love, it was obvious that she was giving them the care she was no longer able to give to Sean.

The police hadn't believed her. And neither Ron nor Lucille had been prepared to tell the police about her attack on Sean. They both said they had overreacted to the sight of her holding up her knife. At her own request, she and Lucille had met formally with a female detective constable and a uniformed policeman at Fulham police station. She'd refused to have a solicitor present, had shown them her bread knife, and described precisely how she had killed the girl in the park next to the New Kings road. But they told her she must have imagined it because no fifteen year old white girl by the name of Francesca from New Malden had ever been reported missing on or around the date she mentioned and certainly no incident of the kind she described had been reported. The parks were regularly patrolled, Eelbrook Common particularly so, because of the number of drunks pouring out onto it from the pub across the road, they said. If she had indeed committed a murder they would have known about it. They didn't, so she hadn't.

Perhaps it would be wise to consult a psychiatrist, the patronising and absurdly young little detective constable had suggested. Rose still felt herself seething at the memory of the female constable's frizzy blonde hair and hard, weasely face looking at her with professional pity, contempt and boredom, as she explained there was insufficient evidence to warrant an investigation. Rose had also tried to tell them about the sleeping crackhead and the brick, but she couldn't remember where precisely that had actually happened. Again, there had been no reports of any such incident having occurred anywhere in London on or around the dates she thought she had committed the 'murder'. No evidence, which meant there were no grounds for investigation. The woman DC told her that she was probably imagining things, which was why she wasn't going to arrest her for wasting police time, and glancing at Lucille, advised that she should let her daughter take her to see the doctor. Perhaps there was a medicine she could take, and if she was still struggling with chronic alcoholism there were specialist centres where she could get some help.

Well of course she had *already* stopped drinking after her attack on Sean and moving in to stay with Lucille. But she didn't tell them that. And if she had been mad before, curiously that too had seemed to have come to a sudden stop that day in Holland Park when her relationship with Lucille had recommenced. So there had been no question of seeing a doctor by then.

Nor ever since.

*   *   *

For the next three quarters of an hour Rose hoovered, dusted, emptied bins and got everything ready. When the front door bell rang she felt as prepared as she could be to receive them.

She opened the door. Lucille flew into her arms. As they disengaged, Rose removed a bit of fluff from Lucie's neat little white cardigan and looked at her, silently beaming. Only one other person had ever evoked such warm love from her .

'Oh Rosie, it's so good to see you!' Lucille's voice rang and her eyes shone. As ever, Rose couldn't help feeling deeply touched.

Lucille put a plastic Waitrose bag on the table. She looked inside. 'Extra extra virgin – good! And what's this? A box of dark chocolates too. Lovely. Thank you, darling.' She gave Lucille another kiss then said, 'Come on! Let me help you get Richard out of the car.'

She followed Lucille out to her cavernous, specially modified Nissan and stood around uselessly as she opened the doors at the back, and lowered the tailgate. Holding the skirt of her old-fashioned, lemony smock up out of the way, Lucille climbed in and undid the catches holding his chair in place.

'How are you, Richard?' said Rose, looking at him slumped huge and flaccid in his chair, like a sixty five year old emperor in state..

'....'eyeyeyeyee-ee-ine,' he eventually grunted, laboriously achieving something approximating a slow wave of his left hand. From beside him in the car, Lucille grinned, nodding her head.

'He is actually! I can't understand why he goes on and on about wanting to die all the time.'

Lucille had brushed his hair and somehow managed to get a ridiculously bright blue and yellow striped sweat shirt on to him. He was so enormous, and Lucille so slight beside him stepping lightly back on to the ground to lower him down, that not for the first time Rose really was amazed at how she managed. She scratched her head in puzzlement. As she did so, Richard's keen intelligent eyes looked right through her, seeing her thoughts. He slowly achieved a lop-sided smile as his chair equally slowly descended to the ground.

'Oh, you do *that*, do you?' She said to him warmly. 'You selfish old git! But it's good to see you too.' She bent and gave him a quick hug.

Rose helped Lucille lever his chair over the lip of the front door and into the kitchen. She must remember to get the ramp for the front door from the garden shed. She put on the kettle and remarked on how well Lucille was looking. And she was too. Pretty, and something she had often seemed incapable of avoiding in the past, not too plastered in make-up, just a little lipstick and a touch of eye-liner. She looked nice, less insecure, like someone who didn't need to always make an impression any more. Her hair was pretty and her shoes were perhaps a bit too flimsy and precarious for clambering in and out of big four wheel drives, but her overall appearance was that of a woman who didn't need her femininity to be 'in your face' anymore.

'I'm feeling good too, Rosie. Great, in fact. Thanks to you. I always love the first day of my holidays! It's so exciting to know I'm going to be free to do what I like for two whole weeks. Not that I do much,' she laughed. 'But you know what I mean.'

Rose nodded, smiling. She filled the teapot. With Richard's wheelchair drawn up between them, they sat down at her old kitchen table.

'He started a couple of nights ago, saying he wants me to kill him. I told him don't be silly, you're going to stay with Rose, but he just ignored me completely and has carried on saying it now for the whole of the last two days, till I do feel like throttling him, actually. I really do. Just to put us both out of our misery.' The brittle little laugh which followed this statement sounded like a knife. Rose could hear the serrated edge on it.

'He's eligible to live in a nursing home,' Rose said. This was no laughing matter. 'You really don't have to put up with that sort of thing from him.' She gave Richard a disapproving glare. Naturally he didn't seem to mind at all.

'But I don't want him to go into a nursing home. You know I don't. It wouldn't be right.'

And from her tone of voice she didn't want think about it either, thought Rose.

'Do you like the sweat-shirt I bought him from BHS yesterday?' Lucille asked. 'It's nice and big, easy to get on and off.'

'It's very bright and colourful,' Rose replied carefully. 'But I wouldn't want one myself.'

They laughed together, even Richard tried to join in.

'I wanted to try and cheer him up - what you wear *can* make a difference sometimes.'

'Of course it can,' Rose replied, no-nonsense. She herself was wearing her usual combination of large denim shirt worn loose over comfortable dark baggy jeans, one of four identical pairs.

She noticed Richard was looking at Lucille. It was clear the old letch still fancied her, even if they couldn't actually have that kind of relationship any more, and even if he had actively encouraged the appalling Ronald. When Lucille had first told her about that, it made a positive difference to how Rose perceived Richard. She rediscovered a respect for him she hadn't really felt since before her own marriage to him had begun to go wrong.

'How's Sean? Such a nice boy. Tell him he ought to come down and see me.'

'It's ages since I last saw him myself. He phoned me last week actually, saying he was going off windsurfing near the Giants Causeway in Northern Ireland for the weekend. He's got some relatives near there apparently. I told him to make sure he packed a jumper. He probably won't, but there you are,' she smiled and without the slightest trace of irony said, 'Boys will be boys.'

'I hope you *do* tell him to come and see me.'

'Of course I do, but I hardly see him myself anymore, since he started at Durham last year, I don't think Grainne's seen very much of him either. At least he rings me occasionally, which I really think is good for a boy of twenty who was once clinically diagnosed as having no social skills whatever, don't you? I love hearing from him.'

Rose could hear the distant echo of a deep longing for him in Lucille's voice. The echo of a mother's pain. It had been a sundering, a little death for Grainne to take Sean away from her. And heaven knew what it must have been like for the boy. It had been rather selfish of Grainne, Rose thought. It was very difficult to understand how Lucille could still be friends with her, but there it was.

'And how is Grainne?'

'She's very happy. As far as I know. Buying up and letting houses in the Leicester area at a furious rate I think. At least that's what she tells me. Playing lots of tennis too. You know!'

'Is she still on her own?'

'I don't think she'll ever live with anybody, Rosie. That's not for Grainne. She's too fierce, she scares them away. She once told me she'd be a lesbian if she had any interest in sex at all. But after her previous work, she says she doesn't. She's interested in making money – providing for her family back home, and for Sean.'

'And Ron? How is Ron?'

'He's coming down by coach this evening and staying till Sunday. I'll have nearly the whole two weeks on my own. Bliss! He sounded alright on the phone. We're going out on Saturday night in Brighton, to the opening night of an exhibition; canvases, canapes and cheap champagne – and then dinner. I'm really looking forward to it.' She laughed, then coloured a little. 'The thing about Ron is: at least he wants me. Which is quite flattering after all this time. Not that I tell *him* that of course, although I should be more grateful, I suppose. But I always wanted a man who would look after me as well, someone I could lean on. Richard did once provide that for me. I wasn't very nice, Rose, not at the time he had his stroke. And I didn't really appreciate what he used to give to me until it was gone. But Ron? No, Ron is only good for one thing, to put it crudely. And I think that like Grainne, I'm not terribly interested in that anymore. Not in itself. But it *is* nice to be wanted.'

Rose nodded her head, but said nothing. She wasn't a prudish woman. But Richard was the last person she herself had had sexual intercourse with. More than twenty five years ago. A quarter of a century. Astonishing! Neither had she missed it. She had had the Boundless Book of Rules and related diversions over the years to make sure of that.

She patted Lucille's hand, said,

'With men generally having a predilection for dying so much earlier than us, I think it's probably quite rare for a woman to find herself still being looked after by a man for very long in the second half of her life. It may be what we sometimes dream of having when we're not so young anymore, but by my age, the reality is that will usually be us looking after them.'

'Uhk-kuh-kuh-illmmmm-eeh-uh!' Richard suddenly interjected, crashing in on their cosy if discomforting chat like a train careering into them off the rails. It wasn't what he said, but the vehement volume with which he said it which startled Rose.

Lucille looked more jaded than shocked. She twiddled her necklace nervously before giving a forlorn, confused shrug.

'That's the *only* thing he has said to me in the last few days,' she said. "Kill me, kill me, kill me.' I can't bear it ,' she added.

'I can well imagine,' Rose replied, in whole-hearted agreement. 'Richard I do think that you might say something else to Lucille before she goes home.'

He didn't say anything, but instead managed to move his left hand up in a benediction or an apology or a peace sign. Something benign anyway. You could tell. Rose looked at Lucille whose face lit up like a lamp.

'You may not *mean* to upset me,' she said to him fondly. 'But you do!'

They talked some more about Richard's diagnosis, current physical state and care needs, and she found she was grateful to him for diverting them from further intimacy. If anyone else had talked to her about him like this, she would have given them short shrift. Very short shrift indeed.

Life was so absurd.

They finished up their tea and Lucille went back out to the Nissan to get Richard's suitcase and unload the hoist. It was a very heavy contraption with its hydraulics and motorised metal arms. And like Richard it needed lowering down mechanically from the back of the car. While Lucille pressed various buttons on her remote control in order to do that, Rose went out to the garden shed for the ramp for her front door so that they wouldn't have to struggle so much to get it inside.

Shortly afterwards having pushed the hoist in together and safely installed it by the bed in the front room, Lucille gave Richard a peck on the side of the head and then hugged Rose goodbye, repeating how grateful she was to her. Rose told her to shut up and turning her around gave her a little pat on the bum.

'Go on, get along with you!' she said. She didn't want it to show. It wouldn't be kind, but she couldn't wait for Lucille to leave, to have Richard all to herself. The fact that he wanted to die meant that she was much closer to him, in terms of being a kindred spirit, than poor little Lucie could ever be.

Lucille picked up her bag from the kitchen table, went out towards her car obviously relieved, stepping lightly, Rose was satisfied to notice, into the immediate prospect of a couple of weeks relief from her burden of duty. Rose smiled to herself as she stood by her open front door, watching her get into her great big car. For a moment they just stared at one another as if from a great distance, then after a mutual final wave, Lucille switched on her engine and drove off down the road.

Rose shut the door and went back into the kitchen where Richard, of course, still sat immobile in his chair staring at her walls.

'Well Richard, she's gone now, your little 'wife' and my little 'daughter'. And, as always, I wonder what it was we both needed from her, you and I; and what we have had in common in sharing her in our different ways?'

He struggled to find words, but she stopped him.

322

'There's always been something terribly malleable about Lucille, hasn't there? Perhaps it is a characteristic of her kind, but we have both in our different ways tried to mould her into what we wanted her to be, don't you think?

Again he was obviously trying to speak, making a repetitive luh-buh-uh sound. Now what was it Lucie had said? R's and W's usually came out as L's. Whereas B's usually remained B's but could sometimes be F's. Ruh-buh? Wuh-buh? Wuh-fuh? What for?

'I'm sorry Richard, its going to take me a day or two to key back myself into your speech. Let me give you some more tea .'

She went over to him and bending, took his great head under the crook of her arm, tilting it up towards her so that she could get some tea down him. She looked at him staring up at her from her breast, his jowls flopping, his now much thinner hair short, fine and wispy. Like a baby's. He seemed to be trying to shake his head.

'Don't you want any more tea?'

He *was* shaking his head. It seemed to be easier for him to do so with her cradling it in her arm. She put his cup back down on the table, but he still seemed to be shaking his head. Again he said 'luh-buh'.

She heard a loud slow dripping sound emanate up from the floor below him.

'Belatedly she reached for his wee bottle which Lucille had left tucked into his chair beside him. "Wuh-buh' meant 'wee bottle' didn't it? Of course it did. I'm sorry, Richard.'

He looked tired and angry. She could almost see the exasperation on his face. Unfortunately it wasn't with himself, it was with her.

'You don't think you said 'Wuh-buh' do you? As far as you are concerned you did actually say, 'Wee bottle'. Well, I wonder how can I put this nicely and in words you can understand, Richard? Let me think. Yes! There is only one word, and it is this: Bollocks. There you are. You didn't say 'wee bottle' at all and you will just have to trust me that you didn't.'

'Lob-bbb-bb-bocks.'

'Oh you can do B's and L's alright and 'Kuh' sounds! But you've got them the wrong way round. The word is 'bollocks', Richard. 'Bollocks'.' She smiled. 'We hardly ever argued when we were married. Now it's the first thing we want to do. We must love it now, we really must.'

Still smiling, she left him sitting in his damp chair while she went back to the kitchen and filled a plastic washing-up bowl with warm water. Careful not to let it spill she took it back to her sitting room, his bedroom now, and placed it on top of a plastic sheet on the floor beside his bed. Then she wheeled him in and proceeded to undress him in his chair.

Having removed his socks and trousers she noticed the back of his enormous sweat shirt had somehow contrived to become damp too. She would have to strip him completely naked.

'In some ways, you know, Richard, and I say this utterly without irony, you *are* a very lucky man.'

She heaved Richard's upper body to his left in his chair and pulled the lurid sweat shirt up and off his right arm. Thank God it was so bulky. Ever practical, Lucille had known precisely what she was doing. Considerate too, leaving him in clothes that were easy to get on and off. Rose went round to the right of him, leaned his large, jowly head towards her and pulled the sweatshirt up and over his left shoulder. Then she pulled it over his head and the whole thing was off. He sat there slumped, but alert, eyes full of knowing, staring like a huge boneless pig out of his flabby, useless, and rather yellowed body. Perhaps he was developing jaundice.

She got a fresh flannel and soap, and getting down onto her knees started washing his feet.

'Lucille hates arguing. She clearly hated having to argue with you about your request, didn't she! But she keeps you wonderfully clean.' She chuckled, 'I'm not sure *I* would actually bother if I had you all to myself.'

She rinsed the soap off his feet with the flannel and then started soaping his knees and calves. Silly woman, she berated herself, you should have started at the top and worked downwards. Never mind.

'I can tell she'll do it for you, though. Eventually. Kill you, I mean. I know her as well as you do; better in some ways. She loves you and because of that she'll do anything for you. She understands what it is like to be desperate enough to want to die. It was the state she was in when I first met her. I never told you that, did I? No! Don't look at me like that! Why should I have? It was none of your business. And here's something else you didn't know: I was feeling the same way myself.'

She started washing his thighs, lifting up first one leg and then the other to clean underneath. She knew he could move the left one up and down very slowly a little way himself, and that he wasn't actually bothering to help her. But why should he? What would be the point? She understood that. She wrung out the flannel, spread his legs apart, and lifting up his testicles mopped up the little pool of water which had gathered between his legs.

'I should have got you onto the bed first. Will I never learn? After all these years! Never mind.'

With a little more gentleness she soaped his genitalia. Immediately his penis stood up.

'Poor love,' she said. 'I know you don't feel anything, but I'll let myself be flattered anyway. Yes, I was feeling the same way. Not sexual – suicidal. And underneath of course I always have, and still do. In my own way I still love you, you know. You *do* know! And I love Lucille. So I cannot let her do it and destroy her own life as well. No,' she stood up feeling almost dizzy with the revelation of what she was about to say.

324

'I think it would be much better if it were me, Richard. Don't you? Me, not her. *I* will do it for you. And I will do it for her. The thought of death has always been a comfort to me, but until now I have really never had a good enough excuse. But you provide me with one. I shall killl two birds with one stone. Yes, that's right. If you want me to, Richard, *I* will kill you. And then I will kill myself. In one fell swoop: two birds with one stone.' She stood up, put her wet hands on her hips feeling marvelous, feeling she had a purpose.

'Well? Do you want me to?'

Chapter 20.

Richard was aware that although he could often make himself understood, at least to Lucille, it did tend to take him a little while to find the right neural pathways between the damaged speech centres in his brain, his vocal chords, mouth and tongue. Having not seen him for three months, and clearly desperate to talk herself, Rose, (as she usually did when he first arrived), wasn't taking enough cognizance of this and was carrying on speaking as if he wasn't going to reply.

Slow down woman, please, he thought. Let me get a word in edgeways.

He closed his eyes and enjoyed the scent of her mingling with that of the soap. He had never had such a good sense of smell as he had since he had been disabled.

'Grief made me mad, Richard. Did it do that to you? I don't suppose it did. You always seemed to take everything in your stride so much better than I did. But when I first met Lucille I was, as it happened, minutes away from killing myself.' She laughed. 'I can see she never told you that, did she?'

As she bent down to rinse her flannel again in the bowl of water he looked at her tightly combed head of grey hair tied behind her head which itself sat like a pink and pale beach ball on top of her plump, friendly body. He felt such love for her that he wasn't surprised his penis had responded. Not that Richard could feel his manhood, he merely observed it from the corner of his eye. His love for Rose was not sexual anymore. But he found himself wanting to cry with love for her nonetheless. She had never told him this before. Poor thing - to feel so bad and not to tell him. But, of course, by the time she must have been contemplating such a dreadful option he had been long gone and married to Mary. It would have been none of his business. Technically. Legally. He regaled the ridiculousness of the human condition. How in real emotional reality could you genuinely have lived with someone and loved them, and it not be your emotional business years later if they are trying to kill themselves?

The way she was talking now reminded him of the woman he once had married: direct, uncompromising, and with a heart big enough for both of them. He had always thought that Luke's long dying had destroyed all that.

To be fair to her, she had herself known she wasn't right in the head, of course, because she was never stupid. She knew she had become an obsessional, anxiety-ridden wreck who was impossible to live with because she wouldn't talk about her feelings. To him there was something oxymoronic about using her grief-ridden craziness to drive the one thing she had been able to be definite about: that their marriage should end. She had insisted upon it, saying that they should part as friends while they still could, and before their despair broke both of them into pieces. There had been no way he could reach past her cold certainty that, without question, it was the right thing to do, so eventually he had acceded to her wishes and left.

And you couldn't argue yourself back into a marriage. Especially if behind your high-status facade you were actually a weak and ineffectual man. Argument would have taken mental energy that the death of his only son had excised from him. That's what he had felt, and tail between his legs he had done what she asked, removed himself from her life as requested.

But now, having just made him her wonderfully kind offer she seemed to have become more authentically herself again, or at least her old self.

For some reason this made him think of Mary, who could access all her emotions with no neuroticism whatsoever, who had offered him everything that Rose had no longer been able to give. He had known he was on the rebound, but it hadn't mattered, so desperate was he by then to be in a relationship with someone who wasn't frightened of what she was feeling. But of course that too had palled soon enough, because after less than a year with her he had begun to realise that good as she was, Mary's self-absorption and her satisfaction in her children, were cloying and boring. Marriage with her could either be cruelly truthful, or false and empty if he lied.

And then there was Lucille. And once again he had been on the rebound. It wasn't sanity he had got from Lucille at all. It was a sense of power, for a while anyway. During the first years of their marriage, Lucille would do anything for him, wait on his every word, always trying to please him in every way she could, which he had found intoxicating. What he saw wasn't just what he got from her. Like Rose, there were more depths to her, depths which he didn't understand, but which made such devotion to him all the more incomprehensible and seductive. Stupid and inauthentic as he was himself, he had known there was something not quite real about her, which he had explained to himself in terms of her disgendered past. The strange fact that she had continued to look after him during these last ten years, despite the rocks upon which their marriage had been foundering at the time of his stroke, had left him now with a combination of gratitude and respect for her. This in turn made him recognise how little he had had before, how much he had patronised her. He regretted how little there was he could do now to try and make amends for that.

Except die.

And he just didn't seem to be showing any sign of doing that.

But nevertheless Rose was right. In many ways he *had* been a lucky man. He still was, under the circumstances. But the ungrateful fact remained that he now no longer had any wish to live at all. It was as simple as that. He'd had enough.

This feeling first began in earnest three or four years ago when he had finally given up fighting the facts of his paralysis. It was ironic that this had coincided with suddenly getting some use back in his left arm. But that, of course, had proved to be a false dawn. When he tried to feed himself he could not always get the food onto his spoon – he had never been a left-hander anyway – and when he did, he still missed his mouth ninety percent of the time. Getting this fragment of mobility had only left him frustrated, wanting more. Despite Lucille's encouragement, he still felt like one of those prize-grabbing machines you used to find in fairgrounds, diving down into the soft toys, pincers wide and ready, and coming back up again with absolutely nothing. Lucille had continued to be delighted about his 'improvement' however, happy to help fill his fork for him, guide it up to his mouth and wipe his face and neck when he spilled food down the side of his cheek. She had fussed busily around him full of misplaced optimism, quite convinced he was making progress. She didn't realise that in doing so she was returning all the patronisation he used to impose upon her before he was he was stricken, and in an equally well-meaning and unknowing way.

So his negative view of himself began to grow in almost inverse proportion to her positivity. The prospect of ceasing to exist, of not slobbering around like this anymore, of not being a constant burden to Lucille, and on these thrice yearly fortnight breaks to Rose, began to consume him. Over the minutes, hours, days, months and years of his life since then, it had grown and grown relentlessly; from being a small soothing worm of warmth in the cold feelingless pit of his stomach, to the all-comforting all-devouring, huge and fiery serpent it was now.

Nothing else interested him anymore. Dying was his sole preoccupation. For a while he had tried refusing food altogether but Lucille's tears had been too much to bear. So, prepared for her sake to go on until the bitter end, the radio programme about evolution had suddenly inspired him: he *must* die both because he wanted to and so that she might live before she become a dried up old maid.

Rose must therefore be stopped right now from twittering on and let him answer her bloody question. He also had to ask her a few himself, but how would he be able to if she didn't give him time to try and reply? He didn't want *her* to kill herself as well.

He wanted to tell her he still felt responsible for Luke. She has been neither able nor willing to share even the smallest morsel of guilt with him. For her own unfathomable reasons she had always had to accrue the blame for what happened to Luke all to herself. She was more than a martyr in so doing. She was so completely fucking selfless it somehow changed it into its opposite as far as he was concerned, making her as greedy, unempathic and egotistical as it was possible to get. So that he came to experience her as selfish for not allowing *him* to take any responsibility for *his* part in what had gone wrong. When, as a doctor, he felt he should have had Rose and himself checked out genetically before they had embarked on bringing a child into the world. The fact that he hadn't, was completely negligent of him. In his own mind and for the rest of his professional life he had struck himself off the register – a con man, not a real doctor. He was a quack, the evidence of whose phoniness was his own son's pathetic trajectory from conception to death.

'And you are not to try and give me any stuff and nonsense about not wanting *me* to go as well. This is the deal Richard: if you want to die I will help you, but I want to go – I *will* go myself as well.'

She placed a towel over him, bent to pick up the bowl of water and took it back into the kitchen. He heard her pouring it into the sink and running some more. Like his sense of smell, his hearing had improved remarkably during the last ten years.

'Did you hear me Richard?' Rose said, sweeping back in again. He followed her with his eyes, his head lolling sideways on his chin and tried to speak. He wanted to tell her how completely selfish his wish was. He wanted to tell her it was so all-consuming that even though there was a part of him that would love her forever, to his eternal shame it was far too small not to succumb to the overpowering enormity of his need to be dead and gone.

He wanted to say all this and it felt as if what few undamaged synapses he had left were stinging with the effort of turning these thoughts into words. He finally opened his mouth to speak. Unfortunately at that very moment Rose took his head in the crook of her arm again and proceeded to take a fresh wet flannel to his face.

When she had finished she clamped a towel over his head and kneaded his features dry. When she pulled it off he said,

'Clag-choolled.'

He didn't realise that was what he said. He realised he may have got the odd pair of syllables back to front. But all in all, he thought he'd made a fairly successful stab at telling her she must not ask him to agree to such a thing. Even though he himself was asking it of her. She must not. Because it wasn't fair – he would inevitably say, 'yes please', and he didn't want to drag her down with him, he really didn't. He still loved and respected her enough to want to say thanks, but no thanks to that.

"Chag-clued?' What do you mean, Richard? What are you saying?'

'Chag-chlood? What in the name of Janus does she mean by saying, 'chag-chlood'? I didn't say 'Chag-bloody-chlood'. Or am I mishearing her?

He wondered for a moment whether she might be sadistically satirising his languaging difficulties. Surely not? She might struggle to

329

understand everything he said, but she wouldn't be derisive. Not Rose. But why, even now, after all this time did everybody – well, both Lucille and Rose – almost wilfully misunderstand him so? Leaving him frustrated beyond measure? The fact that for the last four years he had been able to lift the forefinger of his left hand, once for yes and twice for no, had made no real difference to his levels of frustration. Not when he knew he actually formulated his sentences pretty darn well if they would just take the trouble to slow down and listen. Sl-o-ow dow-ow-n.

'You see the thing is, you consistently refuse to accept that you stopped making sense long ago, Richard. You are always under the illusion, when you make sounds to try and speak, that you are actually constructing proper sentences, speaking perfectly coherently! When actually, of course,' she shook her head, sadly. 'You're not. Not at all. Much as it may annoy you to face it, although I must say I'm surprised that it still does after all this time, you will have to accept that the only way I will even begin to understand what you are trying to say is if you let *me* ask *you* questions. And we'll get there in the end *if* you are patient with me. You're so impatient Richard.'

By concentrating all his energies into his visualisation of a child's swing going backwards and forwards, he managed to get a shake out of his head.

No.

She was wrong. If only she just concentrated on what he said, gave him her attention and listened, she would see that. She must try to understand him. As hard as he himself tried to communicate. Harder.

Because she had to understand that the only thing that would make him feel better was knowing that he would shortly no longer exist. If he was depressed it was of no consequence. Wanting to be dead was a completely considered, rational response to his plight which had been going on for so long. For far, far too long. By the rights of all natural justice it should have been over years ago.

'There is absolutely no point in trying to make any sense beyond a single word. A few single words you can actually do. I do grant you that, Rich. But sentences? No, Richard. Too ambitious. I'm sorry. Whatever you think you are saying, you are actually coming out with – with little blocked glottal stops of nonsense, Richard. Pure nonsense.'

'Collboks,' he said smugly echoing her. He could express himself coherently if he was given sufficient time. It was just a case of stringing words together. He could do that too if she was patient with him. She smiled sadly, said,

'Exactly. Collboks. So I will go back to my first question and you can use your finger in the now time and trusted way, to give me a yes or a no: Do you want me to – to put you out of your misery Richard?'

This question was too important to delay his answer by trying to put it into words. His left fore-finger was immediately and emphatically available to him to lift. So he did. He raised it once.

'Even knowing that I will do away with myself too after I have killed you, you selfish old thing?'

Again he lifted his forefinger once. Then again once more. Grinning. He was sure he was grinning.

'I didn't gather whether that was a yes or a no, Richard?'

He lifted his forefinger once. And then again once more.

'So that's a yes *and* a no, is it?'

He lifted his forefinger a definite once this time, delighting in her recognition of how complex it was for him to convey mixed feelings.

Rose heaved a sigh, her sunken, jowly face beaming like a child's with excitement.

'You need to know, Richard that it will be a great relief to me to be able to go too. I think both us might also feel we will be 'getting one over' on death.' She bustled at him, holding his gaze as if they were sharing a packet of stolen sweets, 'by choosing to go in our own time and in our own manner.'

He agreed with her of course, but his head sank down to his right shoulder and he couldn't find the appropriate facial muscles so he blinked slowly and lifted his forefinger again. Once.

'And how would you actually like to go?' she asked in a pleasingly quiet, matter-of-fact tone, as she opened his suitcase for fresh clothes. So many people had bellowed at him since he'd been an invalid. In contrast, Rose and Lucille both knew how to talk to him appropriately. 'I won't bother putting the rest of your stuff away,' she said. 'There would be no point. I intend the house to burn down afterwards, I've just decided. Make it look like an accident! So I don't suppose it matters how you actually go – the evidence that it wasn't an accident will have been destroyed. But I don't know. What do you think? Just in case? Just to be on the safe side I suppose it might be better if I don't give you an overdose in case it shows up in the inevitable post-mortem examination?' She took his underwear from his neatly packed suitcase and put in a top drawer. The rest of his things followed into their appropriate places.

'Do you have any views about the method of your despatch, Richard? Or is it just as long as you're gone, that's all?'

Again he lifted his left forefinger once, reminded by the number of simultaneous questions she was posing that she had always had an unfortunate tendency towards verbosity. He used to find it charming when they first were lovers. Back before anything.

'Well? Would you prefer to know what I am doing and when I am doing it? Or not?'

His finger twitched, but he didn't feel he could answer this.

'Would you prefer it if you were asleep? I've got an old bottle of Piriton somewhere.'

Reluctantly he allowed his finger to rise once. Then he immediately changed his mind and raised it again.

'That's a yes and no again, isn't it!?'

Rose bent and slipped his underpants on over his feet. She followed this with another pair of track suit bottoms. He had long reconciled himself to the irony of wearing sports clothing when he couldn't move a muscle. With their elastic waistbands and their washing machine-friendly convenience they made Lucille's life much easier than proper trousers. He didn't care.

She put some socks on him and pulled his underpants and trousers up to his thighs. Now would come the indignity of the hoist in order to lift him up sufficiently to get the clothes under his enormous girth. She attached the straps around and under him, said,

'Isn't it awful the way this conversation is both spiritual yet utterly soulless? It's about what we both ultimately want for ourselves, which I feel, at least, can be called spiritual. And yet somehow discussing the nuts and bolts of it is – is like this infernal machine!' She pressed the lifting button two or three times before it deigned to quietly hiss into action. ' Don't you agree, Richard?'

He managed a well-timed grunt and lifted his finger twice as he rose a few inches.

So many of his motor functions had been rendered useless. He wanted to tell her that discussing the practicalities of doing away with him therefore did have a more than merely functional meaning for him. For him their discussion gave a shape to his desire which was perfectly and exclusively in tune with, yes, she was right, his, for want of a better word, spiritual quest to achieve the end of his life.

But even if he did try to say so, she wouldn't be able to understand him.

She pressed the button to lower him back down again and put a fresh sweat-shirt on him.

'There!' she said. 'You look ready for anything.' She rubbed his head. 'I've always loved you, Richard. You know it was because I loved you that we couldn't remain together, don't you? Lucille loves you too. And the fact that you are loved should make you want to live! But it doesn't, does it? Not at all. If anything it is another reason why you want to die. How do I know? Because the same thing is true for me too. We don't feel we deserve it, do we? To be loved, I mean. I speak from the heart because I know Lucille loves me too. And Richard, although our marriage had to end, I don't believe you and I ever really stopped loving each other either. Did we?'

He wanted to hold her, take her in his arms and hug her.

Instead he lifted and lowered his left forefinger again.

'I hope Lucille isn't going to hate us for this. For her sake it must seem like an accident. It will be difficult enough coping with her grief, poor thing. But we have to recognise – to own up – that by doing this together, we are demonstrating she isn't actually important enough to either of us to worry about hurting her. Not that we hate her, of course, she won't think that. Just that we don't – or didn't – care. We are too selfish to care about anyone or anything except our own demise.'

Richard locked his gaze into hers and held it there before again lifting and lowering his forefinger once.

'There we are then! What a pair of hedonists we are, doing what we want to do.' She stroked his brow. 'Are you in a hurry to go? Yes? Well, so am I. No point in hanging around, is there?' She put a hand to her throat, sticking out her tongue, and caricaturing the effect of death by hanging, like some gnomic Hieronymous Bosch figure. He couldn't lift up the corner of his mouth quickly enough for her to see his smile in response. Despite his medical training he had never actually seen a dangler, as they used to call them when he was a student, when making a joke of horror helped stave off the fear that it could happen to you.

His fear now was the horror of carrying on living his life as an animated carcass.

Idly, he wished he didn't feel the way he did, as he watched her empty his suitcase and put his things away in the cupboard after all. 'For authenticity,' she said, sounding pleased with herself. As he became aware of his idle wishing he was also dimly aware of the futility of so doing; that wishing, as Aristotle said, is itself idle. Wish only for the end Aristotle advised. Everything else should be wanted. Well, he wanted the end.

He watched Rose bustling about between his suitcase and the set of drawers inside her cupboard, putting his things away. It had been one of his few pleasures over the last few years, simply absorbing the sense of movement and physical ability that both his sweet carers, Lucille and Rose, took for granted as they got on with what they were doing around him. In some strange kind of osmosis, it was as if he took their mobility into his stillness and himself almost moved with them. And if they moved for him, perhaps complementarily, he had been still for them.

'I think it would be best if I made everything look perfectly normal, don't you? So that not even a hint of our deliberate intent will be evident when we're found,' said Rose, closing the suitcase and sliding it up against the side of the cupboard. She wheeled him back into the kitchen and put on the kettle again.

'I'll make us a nice cup of tea and give you a couple of spoons of Piriton. And then you really should try and sleep Richard. It'll make things easier. For both of us. There really is nothing further to say, is there?'

She was right. Of course she was right. All this concern with trying to get himself understood had just been a smokescreen, a habitual way of denying the fact that actually he didn't want to communicate about anything with anyone ever again. He lifted the first finger of his left hand again. Once.

She filled his spouty mug, tasted it, put in down again saying it was too hot. She pulled open a drawer beside the sink, brought out the bottle of anti-histimine, took a tablespoon from the cutlery drawer and poured two large spoonfuls into his mouth.

'There! That should have you sleeping like a baby in a little while. Oh! While we wait for the tea to cool down, you must let me play you something. I was tidying up, getting ready for your arrival earlier this afternoon, and I came across an old sheet of music. You'll remember it when you hear it.'

Her laugh seemed to contain a hint of residual defiance even though more than quarter of a century had elapsed since he had last heard her play.

Intrigued, he wondered what the piece was. In all the years since they had parted, one thing he had never thought to miss was her appalling piano playing. But now, as she wheeled him into her small back room and sat herself down at the ancient electronic Yamaha they had bought together a quarter of a century ago he found himself feeling emotional.

'It still works perfectly,' she said, smiling. 'And I still can't play it properly! So I must say I am glad you can't say a word!'

The piece was the Andante Spianoto, preceding the Grand Polonaise, opus 22 by Chopin. He felt the faint twitch of a smile trying to surface on the left side of his face. She was right. He had indeed used to struggle – between wanting to praise her for attempting it, and begging her to stop so he didn't have to hear how badly she was mangling it.

Her fingers always, but always, used to get tangled over the keys and her timing become chaotically confused no matter how hard she tried. But she would insist on trying, over and over again to get it right. But Luke had loved it, asking her to play it again and again until, like his son, Richard had come to love it himself for the myriad of mistakes she made.

With a wicked, sadistic grin she pulled at her fingers in mock concert pianist mode and began to play. It sounded even worse than he remembered, but he found he was grinning throughout, could almost feel Luke right there, back in the room with them, frowning, trying to keep his little face serious and solemn, not to laugh at the funny faces he was pulling at him behind her back in reaction to how appalling her playing was.

God, what a monster he'd been.

He brought himself back into the here and now, loving Rose as she bent forward over the keys, sticking her nose into the score because

334

her sight was not what it was. She stopped and started, eventually decided to steamrollered through it, with a huge grin on her tired old face.

His snobbery gone, he delighted in every bum note, was entranced by each one she missed and felt a joy as deep as his need to die in the complete and utter mess she made of it.

When she finished she clapped herself, like Luke had used to do with his little elbows stuck out to keep his chest open and stop himself from coughing.

'What we're going to do will be a joining together of fact and feeling. Lucille felt better when her inner and outer senses of herself were matched, and I know that in our different ways we both will too. There is no question about that, is there Richard?'

He raised his left forefinger twice, again accompanying it with a slow opening and closing of his eyes.

'It is ridiculous to say goodbye to one another,' she said matter-of-factly. 'If there is any such thing as an afterlife we will be going there within minutes of each other – What a thought! Let's hope there isn't. Last chance, Richard. Do you want to change your mind?'

He raised his left forefinger twice.

If he had been able, he might have wanted to tell her that her playing reminded him of the time when Luke had solemnly told him, that if he hadn't been born with Cystic Fibrosis he wouldn't have been himself, that who he was included the illness which was killing him. Similarly, Richard recognised, Rose now wouldn't be *her*self if her piano playing wasn't so bad. 'I wouldn't be me, daddy, without my CF,' Luke had said, earnestly, mustering all the truth that only a little boy of ten who knew he was dying could. At that moment Richard had known his son had come to terms with his life and with himself, in a way which, both then and subsequently, he himself had remained resolutely unable to do. In fact he would die today in his late sixties emotionally far less mature than had his own son.

He would have loved to tell Rose all this, but no matter, she would have memories of her own which would hopefully have brought her to the same conclusion.

*   *   *

Rose wished for a moment that she had some alcohol in the house. Not for Dutch courage, like in the woods all those years ago, but for old time's sake. Then again, she thought, perhaps not. It might anaesthetise her feelings, possibly make her want to change her mind. And that would never do.

Poor Richard. He was so desperate.

She must do the dreadful deed as mercifully and painlessly as she could. It would make it a much easier matter if the Piriton kicked in properly and he had fallen asleep. She would just hold a tea-cloth over his mouth and pinch his nose, gently and carefully. After all, he wouldn't be able to struggle.

But then what?

She looked at the plastic bag with the chocolates and the olive oil lying on the table. She would put some aubergines in a hot frying pan, then spill the olive oil making sure the bottle broke all over the floor. Then she would simply wait for the fire to spread and the flames to consume her. Perhaps by the door. So that when they found her charred body, assuming there were any remains, it would look as if she had been struggling to try and get out. It would give added authenticity to the scenario. Not that she liked the thought of dying painfully. Not at all. But she could see no alternative which wouldn't give away the fact that their deaths hadn't been accidental.

With her obsession for tidiness there would be something quite bizarre about deliberately making a mess. She wrinkled her nose with distaste at the prospect.

She took Richard's head in the crook of her arm again and gave him a few gulps of tea. Lucille had shaved him this morning, the skin on his face was smooth as a baby's bottom, and in his clean clothes he didn't look at all like a man desperate to die. Rose could well understand how hurt Lucille must feel that he still wanted to be dead after all the care and attention she had lavished on him over the last ten years. But perhaps after it was all over – perhaps long after – she would in fact be relieved. It wasn't right having to spend your whole life looking after others.

Rose took the chocolates and olive oil from the Waitrose bag which she scrunched up and put into her little kitchen swing-bin. It was nearly full so she took it out and emptied it into the main dustbin outside her back door. It was one thing to make a mess of the floor with the olive oil, but she didn't feel like changing *all* the habits of a lifetime.

With a slight feeling of déjà vu, she went upstairs to have a quick bath. What with one thing and another today, she needed to freshen up, get focused.

After she was dry, she put on clean underwear and instead of getting back into her usual denims, she looked in her cupboard for something different and a bit smarter for such a special occasion. She struggled into a dress and looked at herself in the mirror, raising a silver eyebrow above her spectacles. Yuck! Never mind, keep your chin up. There's no shame in looking like your mother when you're in your early sixties. There was even a time, back when she was a little girl when she would have been proud to look like her.

Remembering she had a stately pair of ancient heels under her wardrobe which had somehow escaped her purge of all unsuitable, unsensible shoes shortly before she had had her hips done, she pulled them out and blowing the dust off, put them on. She took another look at herself. It could be worse. And it would have to do. She couldn't be bothered to change again now. It must be time to give Richard his next wee. It was certainly more than an hour since he had wet himself.

It *was* a shame, though, that she had nothing alcoholic in the house to drink. It would have helped her feel stronger and more determined to do what had to be done.

Mother had taught her above all else that living in this world was a fight – an endless war against everything other than yourself; that 'Everything Other' included every*one* other. Other people would sting you, or bite you, or otherwise harm you in whatever way they could. You were always at risk from them, always under threat, unless you had taken them under your wing. So Rose had become a professional extender of wings, trying to believe in the capacity of users of her service to be survivors, or even thrivers. Even losers can eventually thrive, Mother used to say. Rose had always tried to pass this hope on to all the desperate families who came to her workplace.

She had also passed on this hope in huge great overdoses to her husband, to her son and to her adopted daughter.

But enough was enough. If heaven was a cessation of all thoughts, feelings and sensations then that's where she wanted to be now, with her son, her father and her mother. Because in the eye of her mother's perpetually defensive storm, there had always been a rosy apple which happened to have looked just like her, Rose, and which Mother used to describe as A Very Splendid Thing when she didn't perceive her as rotten or maggotty. 'Splendid' had been one of her favourite words. So dated now. And when she used it about some trifling childhood achievement of Rose's, which at the time, of course, had seemed enormous, Rose herself had felt splendid.

So it *was* appropriate to look and feel a little bit splendid now. If she were alive, Mother would have understood, Rose had no doubt. Memories of the strange things her mother used to say to her began flooding her mind. For a moment she thought she was going mad, because above and beyond the memories, she could actually hear her mother's voice saying over and over again, 'Suicides aren't sinners, my darling, they're just lost souls. God will find them, even if *we* never see them again.'

She hadn't heard her voice in more than thirty years. It was utterly bizarre to find God and her own sweet mother in the intention to kill. She shook her head, patted her eyes with her paisley sleeves being careful, like a little girl, not to mark the lace cuffs which matched her collar. It

337

wasn't like her to cry at all, and what was more, there was nothing to cry about. It was for remarks like that, that she could be grateful to her mother. If she could actually hear her voice uttering them, it was only because she was feeling at once so frightened and so determined to do away with Richard and herself, that it opened corridors of memory she had long kept shut.

If she had still been alive, Mother would have definitely shown her compassion, even if she hadn't totally agreed with her about what she was about to do. She would have. In fact she might well have scolded her too for being upset, believing that once you've set your mind on something, you should do it and never mind the consequences.

She gave her thinning, steel-grey hair another rub with her towel and then a cursory brush, staring out of the window at the houses opposite, seeing nothing except her feelings and her memories. She put her brush down on the window sill beside the little terracotta basil pot. She had bought it twenty years ago after finding those sad little bundled-up drawings under the floorboards depicting Luke's disastrous French holiday nine months before he died. More than a quarter of a century had now passed since his death, and yet his presence in her heart was still as vital to her sense of self as the rhythm of her own breath. Just like her mother's was. Well, in a little while her breathing would have ceased and she would finally be with them both again.

She really couldn't wait.

She picked off a furled leaf from the current, now very twiggy tenant of the basil pot. Crushing it between her thumb and forefinger, she brought it to her nose. It smelled wonderful. She had always kept some growing in the pot in memory of Lukey, never ever used it in her cooking. For some unknown and completely irrational reason she would have felt like a cannibal if she had.

Instead of going down the stairs, a sudden impulse made her turn and go into Luke and Lucille's old room. She felt possessed, mesmerised, caught up in an intuition she wasn't even aware of, finally driven to complete something she now remembered having deliberately avoided completing when she and Richard had been looking for Luke's treasure map twenty years ago. She had wanted to keep something of what Luke had hidden there all to herself, had been so ashamed of this selfishness that after they had finished looking at Luke's bundle of pictures on the kitchen table and Richard had gone, she had even tried to conceal it from herself by forgetting all about the fact that there had been another little bundle even further along under that floorboard.

She opened the closet. It was empty now, smelled of moths, mustiness and the liveliness of the past. She got down onto her rickety old knees and lifted up the loose floorboard. It came away easily enough. Rose struggled to straighten it up, make it vertical so that she could remove it from the cupboard altogether. Her knees hurt on the floor and her back twinged. She wondered whether she would be able to get up again. She managed to manouevre the board out of the cupboard and dropped it on the floor beside her. Then she lay down on her side and reached in as far as she could, right up to her shoulder, so that she could be absolutely sure she was rummaging and reaching as deeply as possible.

A minute later she was heaving herself up onto her feet again, her head spinning. The lacy cuff on her sleeve was black with dust. She didn't give a two-penny fig, was triumphantly holding a flat little parcel of brown paper covered in curled and crinkled, long-perished sellotape and tied up with string. The string turned to powdery strands between her fingers as she touched it.

With tremors which she felt were rippling like electricity, or influenza, up and down her skin from her head to her toes, she noticed she was shaking. Telling herself to be still, she opened the brown paper-wrapping very carefully. In places it was brittle, in others blue with mould, flaking and soft. Inside was just one small, tightly folded piece of paper. It was a faded and yellow, ruled and margined sheet of A4. She unfurled it as gingerly as she would have a sixteenth century treasure map, knowing that this was itself the treasure she and Richard had been seeking.

In large different coloured capital letters around which he had developed doodles and swirls as embellishment, Luke had written: I WOULDN'T BE ME WITHOUT MY CF.

That was all. Nothing profound. Nothing revelatory. Just that.

But Rose was ecstatic, felt she was floating, exalted. Throughout his ten short years she had despaired of his life because of his Cystic Fibrosis, whereas this was evidence that he himself, in complete and utter contrast, had seen it as an integral part of his very self. If his message was banal, it was nevertheless an affirmation of the lovely little boy who had been her baby, of the boy that he actually was, of his life and of his death.

Just as she and Richard needing to make an ending together now was. We wouldn't be who we are if we lived any longer, she thought.

She went back out onto the landing and made her way downstairs. Very slowly. Dodgy hips and ancient shoes were a dangerous combination at her age, and she very nearly did go tumbling from the very last step when she allowed premature triumph at having almost made it to the bottom go to her head. She was desperate to show Richard what Lukey had written. It was so positive. It *was* a treasure map. She hurried back into the kitchen

Richard was asleep.

Good! Well, anyway, never mind. That was alright. That's what she'd been hoping for before she went upstairs. It would have been nice, but didn't really matter if he didn't see the message from Luke. Not really. She put Lukey's words on the table and wondered what to do next.

Perhaps she should hit Richard over the head with a frying pan first just to make sure he didn't suffer in the flames. Then she would push his chair towards the door and try, if she could, to tip it over with him still in it. If subsequently there was found to be a crack on his skull it would look as if he had sustained it as a result of falling over as they tried to escape from the flames.

She got the pan from the cupboard, and because she didn't want to think about it, closed her eyes, swivelled round on her heels and in one movement hit him with it as hard as she could. She was so cumbersome, old and slow. Nevertheless, something between a clang and a thud reverberated around the room. The blow jarred her all the way up her arm and into to her shoulder. Richard opened his eyes and looked at her, confused at first, his eyes rolling. Then he definitely seemed to smile that lop-sided grin of his as if he understood and approved of what was going on.

'I found Luke's treasure map,' she said, puffing. She picked it up off the table and held it in front of him. His eyes were rolling and he was obviously in a lot of pain so his scalp was clearly unaffected by his stroke. 'It just says he wouldn't have been himself if he hadn't had CF.'

Richard smiled through the effects of the blow on his head. He had clearly heard and understood her.

She hit him again. And then again for good measure.

She looked at him carefully.

She seemed to have knocked him out properly now. His eyes were closed anyway. There was a small cut on the side of his head out of which blood seemed to be welling.

Rather too quickly.

She had better hurry up.

She put the pan on the hob and turned on the heat.

Taking the top off the two litre bottle of oil Lucille had brought her, Rose began dolloping it over her kitchen table, floor and work surfaces in a ring all around her. Plop-plop-plop. Then, again for good measure, she poured half of what little she had left over the front of her dress as well. It dripped down onto the dusty toes of her old shoes, making them glisten and shine. She poured the rest of the oil into the pan, for the sake of authenticity.

Whoops! Authenticity!! She must get the vegetables.

And she better hurry. Without thinking, and forgetting she had been going to break it, she opened the back door and dumped the olive oil bottle in her outside bin. Then she rushed to the larder for the vegetables and almost in slow motion she slipped on the oily floor, landing on her bottom with such a jolt that for a few moments, which seemed like hours, she couldn't move; the pain excruciating her up through her spine and down the back of her legs. She felt faint with it, shaking her head and blinking out the sensation of wanting to sink into oblivion prematurely.

She couldn't black out now. Her scenario wasn't completely set. She had to hurry. Through the stars she was seeing, she could hear her olive oil beginning to crackle over the heat.

But she couldn't move. Even trying to bend her knees sent renewed waves of pain emanating all around her body from her left hip. Oh dear. For someone who was such a perfectionist this was not going to plan at all.

Riding yet another wave of pain as she gave up and laughed at her incompetence, she let herself lie back on the floor and looked up behind her over her left shoulder. A growing pall of dark smoke was beginning to billow up in dark, enthusiastic clouds from the frying pan.

Through the pain in her hips and pelvis she saw the pan become huge, a gaping fiery maw. With an almost contemplative detachment she felt the start of the finest scream of her whole life coming up in the pit of her stomach in response to the flames, so pleased was she to be finally marrying her fortune.

From his chair Richard issued a grunting noise. She turned her head to look at him over her right shoulder. Doing so made the pain in her hip even more intense. Richard's eyes were still closed. Blood continued to pour from the small cut on the top of his head which was already swollen up tight where her blows had landed. He couldn't have remained conscious after the way she had hit him, could he? She'd put all her strength into it.

He could. Richard opened his eyes. It was her life's final mercy that his head was slumped at such an angle that he was looking directly down at her lying on the floor. She smiled back up at him.

Within her, her scream now encompassed every street she had ever walked along the length of her life, every person she had ever known, all the love she had ever given, all the feelings she'd ever had. It became full of joy.

Her scream turned to a laugh.

So she let out a little chuckle.

She felt he looked so happily back at her too, as blood continued to drip from his head into the pool of olive oil on the lino floor beside her. His expression told of being in heaven already. He chuckled back. She reached up to him, and because she was on his left, he was able to reach down and the tips of their fingers met.

Above him her kitchen ceiling was now billowing with thick black smoke curling and curving down around him. The heat was intense. She watched him inhale deeply, smiled up at him, feeling at once sad and glad.

341

There was nothing more she could do.

Chapter 21.

Ronald Symes was enjoying himself. He preferred it when Lucille let him stay at the beginning of one of her holiday fortnights rather than at the end. She was always noticeably happier with the prospect of a whole two weeks ahead of her of being without Richard. It meant she was a bit friskier, more receptive to his advances. And that, after all, was the main reason he came down to see her. He was nearly a decade older than her and she was forty. But still attractive. At least he thought so.

Last night just before setting off for Eastbourne, he'd had a very depressing phone call with Sean whose concrete thinking had, as usual, intensified his own fractures, his own sense of inadequacy and paranoia. He had later arrived at Lulu's flat feeling his old anger with her for having brought Sean up for the first ten years of his life without having a clue about child development generally, let alone considering trying to find him to tell him he had a son.

When she opened her front door his anger evaporated. She greeted him with a warm, welcoming smile in a filmy see-through dark top which invited him to put an impulsive hand up to cup one of her tits and pull her towards him with his other hand for a kiss. In the normal course of events he would have expected her to push him off in the semi-public setting of her open front door. She was very proper, was Lucille, for someone with such a strange background. Instead, she surprised him by welcoming his fondling with a smile and taking his tongue into her mouth when he planted his lips on hers. Seizing the main chance, he immediately moved his other hand down onto her soft, round arse, caressing it fondly and enjoying a good squeeze of each neat little buttock. She hadn't resisted at all, and within a minute he was banging away at her on her bed with her skirt up around her tummy, still fully dressed himself. She'd seemed as desperate for it as he was, judging by the noises she made and the way she had sucked on his neck and wrapped her legs around him as he thrust into her. Afterwards she lay in his arms, holding and stroking his sex till he was up and ready again. He took it more slowly second time round, undressing her properly first and savouring her nakedness, not actually fucking her until his balls were properly bouncing again.

When he was finally spent they had talked into the night and although he became more confused, his anger and paranoia somehow went, as they always did when he was in bed with her. He couldn't in all honesty blame Lucille for Sean, just as he could not really blame her for the fact that over the last few years he had deteriorated mentally again and given up his career in psychological consultancy. He *did* blame her, as he blamed all women, for the longing they induced in him although he recognised this was based on having missed out on essential consistent

343

mothering himself when he was little, on having been put up for adoption. But nowadays, unfortunately, it was far too easy to forget or ignore that insight, and get tangled up in the intensity and confusion of his here and now struggle with desire and blame in relation to the women in his life.

To be fair to Lulu, Grainne was definitely more responsible for his breaking down again than she was, but then there wasn't anything he could do with his anger towards Grainne.

Sometimes the struggle was too much, like it had been five or six years ago when he had had just about enough *nouse* left to understand he was slipping again. starting to believe in the significance of his psychological experience too much, over-inflating its importance. Still sensible enough to recognise the spectre of his psychosis was no longer just abroad again, but was unquestionably right back in his life, he had temporarily given up work and sought treatment. Sadly, none of the medications he was subsequently prescribed at the psychiatric clinic made much difference. Temporary time off work became permanent.

He had been living on the dole ever since, his Ph.D., fading in its frame on his housing association wall.

But life wasn't all bad. As he was dropping off to sleep last night with Lulu in his arms, he was pleased to feel her hand finding its way back down onto his sex again, firming him up and holding on as she drifted off towards sleep. Smiling into the darkness he said he hadn't known her be so relaxed or randy in a long time. Shifting herself beside him and tucking her head more comfortably into his shoulder, she drowsily replied it was true, she did feel happy.

'Why?' he'd asked. 'Has something happened? Have you won the lottery?'

'Better than that. I don't have to kill him anymore.'

'Kill who?'

'Richard, Ronnie. I told you. He was on and on at me to kill him. It was getting so I couldn't bear it any longer. I'm just happy I don't need to kill him now.'

'What do you mean? Is he dead?'

'I'm free,' she murmured, nine tenths asleep.

'Have you killed him then?'

'It's so nice not to have to keep on refusing him all the time,' she replied with contentment, the ridiculousness of the suggestion despite her drowsiness making her sound as righteous as an evangelical. 'I hate not giving people what they want,' she whispered.

She gave him another squeeze, falling asleep relaxed and content. He shook his head, slipped off to sleep himself, feeling happy for her too.

*   *   *

In fact Lucille must have slept with him most of the night because it was now morning and he was still on her bed with nothing on except for his T-shirt. The sun was illuminating the white net curtains of her bedroom. He was lying on his back with his right arm over his eyes to shield them from the brightness. He scratched his balls and hearing the sound of her moving round the room, opened one eye.

Lucille was naked except for a big white towel she was using to dry herself off with. She hadn't noticed he was looking at her so he enjoyed a little voyeuristic pleasure before saying good morning. She peeped quickly at him from beneath her towel, gave him little wave and carried on drying herself off.

His physical pleasure rose up between his legs, grew larger as the friendly smile on her face told him that last night hadn't been in his imagination. Even in the light of the day she was clearly pleased for him to be here. Coming over to the side of the bed she called him her first and last man, and bending to give him a chaste little kiss, passed her hand down his now fully erect penis and gave his bollocks a brief caress. He reached up, put a hand on her damp hair, enjoying the yielding coolness of her lips and the taste of toothpaste on her tongue. He tried to pull her down on to the bed with him. But she evaded him, backing away and continuing to rub her hair.

'No not now, Ron, I've only just had a shower! I have to get dressed. But first I've got to dry my hair, and there's so little time. No,' she shushed him. 'Ask me why in minute. Just let me get on with it now or I'll never be ready. Please!' She insisted.

Still erect, he watched her hurriedly getting into her bra and knickers and sit down in front of her dressing table with her hair drier. Jesus, women could be frustrating. Five minutes later she was making her face up. She caught him looking at her reflection in her mirror and smiled.

'I said I'd be quick, didn't I?' she said, leaning closer towards her make-up mirror, dabbing something on her eyelids. 'The strangest thing, Ron: a policeman, a detective rang earlier while you were still asleep to say he and a colleague, a female officer, want to come round with some kind of information for me, and to ask me a few questions about it. They won't be wearing uniforms, he said, but they will show me I.D.' There was a brittle quality to her laugh as she added, 'Actually, I would prefer it if they did wear their uniforms myself! You feel safer somehow. I wonder what they want. I can't imagine. Can you, Ronnie? Anyway he was perfectly friendly, said he had something to tell me and also just had to make a few enquiries which I might be able to help him with.' She laughed a little uncertainly. 'Isn't that what they say when they've arrested somebody for something? I said that to him actually, and he said not at all, but I'm sure it is. Anyway they'll be here at ten and its half nine now.'

Ron's penis shrivelled.

Police?

Fucking hell. It was him they were after. It must be. What was his crime? There wasn't one, was there? What the fuck were they coming here for then? Had they found him out? For what? He hadn't done anything. Didn't they know he was being treated for schizophrenia again? They should leave mental patients alone. It wasn't fucking fair at all.

Some triggers seemed to catapult him into this kind of persecuted paranoid self-importance quicker than others. He knew that. The very mention of the word 'police' was usually quite enough to send him into an immediate panic. And this was no exception. One part of him – the sane part? – knew it was ridiculous, but whenever it got to him, the sensation of fear began to devour the very foundations of his stability. And sometimes – too often again in recent years – he just couldn't prevent it from getting to him. Fear was like his old cancer of significance used to be. Unstoppable.

He knew he hadn't committed any crime but he *knew* that the innocent are punished. So maybe he *should* commit one. But then again it was too late now. The heel he had been ten years ago, arrogant, clever, womanising, had not been any way likeable, that was true. But he hadn't been a criminal either. Okay, so he had fucked and then left Lucille as planned for a few years, while he went off and tried to educate his son and revive his relationship with the boy's mother. But Grainne had toyed with him in almost the same way that he had toyed with Lulu, initially pretending to be interested in him again, but then once she had recaptured a part of his heart, tearing it out of him and eating it bit by bit as she continually regaled him about his uselessness both as a man, and as a father.

To be fair to her, Grainne also and equally blamed herself for Sean's odd personality. But not herself alone. And not Lucille at all. No. He himself was the other person she blamed. As if he could somehow have magically known he was a father, and as if he could have had something good to give the boy, even though he had never had a father himself. And as if it hadn't been her who had done everything in her power to keep the fact of his paternity away from him.

She was a maddening woman. It was impossible to make any sense of her.

The only one of them who had done Sean any good, she had said, was Lucille. He had tried to dispute that. How can someone who isn't your immediate blood relative truly love you, he'd asked, because it is love that makes you grow. Even if they can, it doesn't help, it just complicates everything. He knew that from personal experience. At least three different women, foster carers and his adoptive mother had all told him at different times that they loved him when he was a little boy. But what good had it done? None whatsoever, he had just become more confused about what the word love actually meant. He had hoped and intended that she might feel his views were supportive of her decision to take Sean back and look after him herself. Children need their parents. Surely she believed that, he had thought, or she would never have reclaimed Sean or had him come to live with her. But she didn't believe it, at least not really. She had had Sean back, she said, not because he needed her, but because *she* needed to repair the damage she had done to him. It was an important distinction as far as she was concerned. Mothering from Lucille could, and had benefited him, but only she, Grainne, could actually repair the damage she had done and she could only do that by having him live with her. She had informed him of this in that old cursory and dismissive manner which she used to use towards him before she left him all those years ago. As ever, it had hurt.

He shook his head to bring himself back to the present.

Obviously in a hurry, Lucille seemed to be stepping into her plain pink frock at almost exactly the same time as she was stepping into her shoes. He admired her grace and the way she managed not to stumble or fall. She looked good enough to eat, but he had lost all his hunger for her now. She asked him to do her up and turned around for him with a grateful smile as he sat himself up on her bed to do it. He fumbled at the catch inexpertly. The eye was so small, the hook too.

'Please hurry, Ronnie. I've got to make the place presentable before they arrive. I don't want them seeing what a slut I can be.'

He couldn't do it. His hands were big, but not usually as incapable as they were just now. He was so fucking anxious he was unable to hold them still. She moved away from him and reaching behind her neck hoisted the dress half way up to her head again and did it herself. 'You better get dressed too unless you're going to hide in here like a criminal,' she said with a grin, smoothing it down again and giving herself a brief nod of approval in the long mirror on her wardrobe door.

'What? What do you mean, 'like a criminal'?'

'Nothing, you silly man! It was just a – a remark that's all.' She laughed lightly, sat down at her dressing table again and reached for a bottle. 'I wasn't serious. You are not very well at the moment, are you?' It must have been perfume. He could smell it from here, as she dabbed it on her neck and wrists.

'I just don't feel comfortable with police around, that's all.'

'Guilty conscience?' she asked with a knowing look, tilting her head as she fixed on her earrings. But he wasn't fetched.

'No,' he almost shouted. 'Not at all.'

'It is probably better if you stay in here then,' she said soberly. 'I'll come and tell you when they've gone. I don't want you to get all upset. Over nothing.'

'No, I'd rather be with you. I want to know what's going on.'

'It's me they're coming to see! Not you.'

'I don't care. I want to be there. Better to know the devil.'

She shrugged. 'Please yourself Ronnie, but perhaps it's private, have you thought of that? Just me they want to see.'

She was a bit huffy, but it was hard to take that seriously when she looked so drop-dead gorgeous. He heard her plumping cushions and tidying her living room next door, then crossing over to the kitchen and flicking on the switch on the kettle.

He wondered what had happened to him, bemused by the facts of his life. He might almost have been surprised except that he believed everybody's life was much the same. Up–down, up–down until the end. But even so, having gone from sick slob to know-it-all and back again, without even noticing when the changes actually happened, it was hard to fathom himself out. Similarly, last night with Lulu it felt like his boat had come in. This morning it had gone out again.

As she showed the police into the sitting room asking them if they would like a cup of tea or coffee, she discreetly pulled the bedroom door to, but didn't actually close it. He lay back on her bed, still wearing nothing but his t-shirt, able to hear everything.

'I'm Detective Inspector Scharff, madam. Jerry Scharff. And this is my colleague, Detective Sergeant Carole Jones. I hope you don't mind, Mrs McElvey, but I will be doing most of the talking and Carole here will mostly be taking notes on her laptop. Unless you object. So as I say, I hope you don't mind. I must emphasise that it's just routine. For our records. Detective Sergeant Jones and myself do it the other way round too,' he said with a pompous and inappropriate bonhomie which had Ron scowling with derision. 'I have full typing and word processing skills. The modern police force is an equal opportunities service, you know. Now you may wonder why the uniformed branch aren't dealing with this, madam, mm? Well they are! But there is some very slight evidence – just a suggestion – that a crime may have been committed. At this stage we are not sure. So it would be most helpful if, with your assistance, we could just iron out a few loose ends. Forgive me for mixing my metaphors, madam.'

Ron heard Lucille repeatedly reply that that was fine and then giggle nervously.

'You look just like a picture I have of my mother when she was your age,' he heard her say. Presumably to the woman. 'Same face, same hair, everything. Except she was never a policeman. I mean policewoman. You could be her double!'

She tried to laugh but she sounded nervous. Rightly so if they were looking for more evidence of a crime. He imagined they were looking serious. Shut up, woman! Ask them what they want.

'We understand you may be a relative of a woman named Rose McElvey?' said the female voice. Carole.

'That's right,' came back Lucille's voice, more evenly. 'Well not exactly a relative, although she has been like a mother to me. She's my husband's first wife actually. Why? Is something wrong?'

Her voice sounded shaky, had risen an octave.

'I'm afraid we've got bad news,' said Scharff. There was silence for a moment as if he was giving Lulu time to gather herself. 'I regret to inform you, madam, that Mrs Rose McElvey's property caught fire yesterday afternoon. It seems to have happened while she was cooking. I'm afraid it's my sad duty to tell you that she and a gentleman in a wheelchair were both er–

He heard Lucie stifle a cracked little scream, like an animal being whipped and crying out at one and the same time.

'Richard! Oh my God! Are they al– ' She choked. 'What happened? They *are* alright, aren't they? Please tell me they're alright!'

'I'm afraid not,' the woman's voice came in with the kind of knowing practised sincerity Ron remembered from his own days as a caring professional. It took one to know one and she clearly didn't give a fuck.

Ronald got up from the bed and on to his feet in one movement.

He had to join in. Protect Lucille. Protect himself. They were bound to suspect him if he was sleeping with Lucille. Bound to. He had to see them, talk to them. Better the devil you know.

He didn't want Lucille turning into a stupid little cow and saying things she shouldn't about him, or even implying them. He couldn't have that. He ignored the small sane part of himself which kept on repeating this was nothing to do with him, stay cool, keep your distance. Instead he hopped with growing irritation around the floor struggling to get his trousers on as he tried to continue to hear what was being said.

'They were both found dead when the emergency services arrived. I'm very sorry. We won't be asking you to identify them as I am afraid that they are virtually unrecognisable, but we will be getting dental records and DNA tests done as part of the routine post mortem procedure. I'm very sorry,' the woman repeated.

'Who is Richard?' asked Scharff. Appropriately sombre, thought Ron. The fuck.

'He's my husband,' Lucille replied.

'My deepest condolences, madam,' said the detective.

Ron did up his flies. One of his shoes seemed to have gone missing. With some urgency and something of a thud, he got down onto the floor and looked under the bed.

'You've got someone staying with you at the moment?' Scharff asked. Ron froze as he heard Lucille not answering. 'That's good. Its important to have friends about at times like this.' She must have nodded then. He would have to join them now, whether she liked it or not. It would invite suspicion not to.

'If you would like to have a few minutes with your friend for, er, comfort..., or if she would like to join us in here, that's quite alright,' said the policeman. We can quite understand that you would need someone to give you comfort and consolation at this time, can't we Carole? Anyone would.'

'That's right, Mrs McElvey. If you like, we can make our own tea and give you a few minutes with your friend on your own. And she is welcome to stay while we continue this discussion. Isn't she, sir? In the meantime, and for what its worth, the fire people said that the first Mrs McElvey's house was built in the sixties at a time when proper fire proofing was not universally built into the walls of houses, so they died quite quickly. Probably of asphyxiation. That won't be known for certain until the pathology reports come back. We'll let you know as soon as we can. There are also bereavement services we can put you in touch with. We really didn't know that one of the victims was likely to be your husband when we arrived here, or I can assure you we would have conducted this differently. In fact we can go right now, if you would prefer.'

What the hell was she going on about, wondered Ron. Lucille didn't need to know about their stupid fucking procedures. This was very suspect indeed. Why would they be offering to go straight away, having just upset her so much? Were they trying to soften her up before getting to him? They must be concealing something, surely, to hide behind all this waffle?

'That's alright. You're very welcome to stay now and ask your questions. In fact I'd prefer it,' he heard Lulu telling them shakily.

Both shoes now on, Ron wanted to know how in hell they had connected a house fire in Balham yesterday with Lucille here in her flat here in Eastbourne. He braced himself then joined them in the sitting room. The policeman was fat and fiftyish, florid-faced with prematurely white hair and little piggy blue eyes. He wore a baggy dark blue suit over a beer belly. The woman was in her thirties with a short boyish haircut and mannish trousers. Dyke probably, he thought averting his eyes as she gazed at him with some surprise on her face.

The Scharff man looked at him with a slightly raised eyebrow.

'Hello, I'm Dr Symes. Ronald Symes,' he said him offering his hand to each of them in turn. 'I'm a friend of Lucille *and* Richard's. I couldn't help hearing what's happened. I'm so sorry, sweetheart.' God, he sounded stilted! He put an arm around her shoulders, felt her tense little frame starting to wrack with suppressed sobs.

Shit. He shouldn't be cuddling her, calling her sweetheart. They'll think he'd been up to something. Guiltily he removed his arm almost as quickly as he had put it there. He shouldn't call her sweetheart either. He never normally called her sweetheart. What the fuck was he being so stupid for?

'Perhaps it would be better if you two did make that cup of tea yourselves,' he said. 'I think Lucille does actually need a few minutes to take it all in.'

'Of course, Dr Symes. Kitchen through here is it?' said Scharff, his expression quizzical and not entirely non-judgemental. He shuffled his girth towards the front of his chair and struggling to his feet, headed for the door. When he got there he turned and pointed at Lucille's adjoining bedroom.

'It's at the end of the corridor,' Lucille said, shaking her head and taking a tissue from the box on the table. She blew her nose. 'Milk is in the fridge.' For a moment she sat looking straight ahead, then suddenly stood up. 'No!' she said more loudly, as the lesbo followed Scharff down the hall. They stopped and turned round looking at her. 'If you wouldn't mind I'd really rather prefer it if I made it for you myself. I just need, you know, to be on my own a minute. And I prefer to be doing something. This is such a shock.'

The detectives stopped in the hallway and returned to the living room. Lucille waited for them to come in again before making to leave for the kitchen.

'I'll come with you,' said Ron. It would be their only opportunity to agree on what line to take with these rozzers and what things to be more circumspect or economical with the truth about.

'I'd rather you didn't, if you don't mind, Ronnie. This is so sudden. I can't believe it.' She left the room, clearly almost tripping over herself in her hurry to get out and away from them all. Ron gestured for the detectives to sit themselves down again.

'Well sir, while you're here, would *you* mind telling me a bit about the deceased? We know very little. Mrs McElvey is the first er, relative as such we've been able to talk to.'

'I don't really know them. I mean, didn't know them. Richard, her husband, goes – went – to stay with Rose three times a year. And I stay with Lucille three times a year too. At the same time. Only for a few days. She can't take any more of me than that at any one time!'

The detectives didn't smile. Ron decided he wouldn't let that phase him. Instead he would take the initiative, ask them questions himself.

'It was an accident, you said?'

'That's right, sir. As far as we know. It looks that way. Of course we wouldn't want to rule out anything at this early stage in the investigation. We wouldn't be providing the tax payer with a service if we did that.'

He sounded so smug and complacent that he must be an empty vessel, thought Ron. But they can be the worst of all, liable to drift anywhere.

'Was Mr McElvey aware that you stay here?' The woman asked him. 'Alone with his wife?'

It was obvious what the bitch was implying but she had no right. Not unless they had some suspicions about him. Fuck. Fuck. Fuck.

'Of course, he was. And he's – I mean he was a medic, a doctor, not a mister.'

'How long had you known him, sir?' She asked, noting it down.

'Ten years or more by now.'

'Can you tell us what he was like? He was found in a wheel chair, so we have assumed he suffered from some kind of disability?'

'Paralysis. He had a series of strokes which left him unable to really move. A long time ago it was now. He could move his legs – one of them anyway – up and down a bit, but he couldn't bend them at the knee without having to have it done for him. By Lucille. And sometimes, as I said, three times a year by Rose, the lady who died with him, his first wife. And of course he couldn't stand up. I understand from what Lucille tells me that he can – sorry – *could* move one of his arms a little. But that was about it. He couldn't talk. Not really.'

Ron began to feel more confident as he carried on speaking. He had had nothing to do with Richard in all these years. Everything he had just said had come from what Lucille had told him.

'It was a hell of a life. If he had been an animal they would have put him down long ago.' He looked at them for some kind of nod of mutual understanding, but the Scharff man just stared right through him as the woman laboriously typed what he'd just said, apparently word for word.

'Would you mind if I asked you, sir,' she said. 'When it was you yourself arrived here? Was it before or after Mrs McElvey took Dr McElvey to er, the first Mrs McElvey's?'

'What has that got to do with this?' Ron said, feeling like he wanted to hit them, but speaking coolly with only the slightest hint of a tremor in his voice. He used to feel like this all the time when he was ill. 'What has that got to do with you at all?'

'No, sir, nothing. You're quite right,' said the fat man.

'As it happens, I came down on a National Express coach,' he said. Better tell the truth as far as possible, give them no reason to be suspicious whatsoever. 'I didn't get here till nine last night. I don't know what time she got in,' he added, nodding up the hallway towards Lucille in the kitchen. 'I still have the return ticket in my pocket. Here, you can see it if you like.' He dug a hand into his threadbare old trousers and fumbled for it, but it wasn't there. Where the fuck was it? It must have fallen out onto the floor when he was looking for his shoes under Lucille's bed.

'That won't be necessary, sir,' Scharff said, 'Not at this point in time. But it might be advisable to hold onto it, if I were you. As a precaution. Just in case.'

'In case of what?' Streams of sweat were suddenly pouring down Ron's brow, embarrassing him, and revealing – what? He hadn't fucking done anything. 'What kind of investigation is this?' he asked, pulling his T-shirt up and wiping his forehead.

'Oh, it isn't, sir. Not any kind of investigation at all. Not really. Not just yet. We're just making routine enquiries at this stage. We were just saying to your friend Mrs McElvey, before you joined us, that we will decide later whether we are investigating a crime. At the moment there is nothing to suggest this wasn't just a tragic accident. As a matter of interest, sir, why do you want to know?'

'Because your partner's question was far too personal.'

'I'm sure you're right sir. I apologise on her behalf. '

The woman nodded her head in apparent humility, properly admonished. They're playing a fucking game with us, thought Ron.

'Known Mrs McElvey long, have you, sir?' Scharff asked, with what had to be mock avuncularity, the patronising bastard.

'Now *you* are doing the same thing. What right or reason have you for asking such personal questions?'

'You're quite right, sir. I was just making friendly conversation, whilst we wait for Mrs McElvey to bring in the tea. I apologise again if I seemed in any way over- familiar. There will be plenty of time later to formally question you should we need to do so.' Scharff beamed, turned round, went to the window and stared out at the grey July day. 'Nice view of the sea from here,' he said, not turning around again. His female sidekick sat on the sofa and stared straight ahead.

Ronald thought the tick of Lucille's clock was phenomenally loud. Where was she? How fucking long does it take to make a cup of tea anyway?

'It would be very helpful if you could give us your name, address and date of birth please sir,' said the woman stonily, avoiding all eye contact now.

'Why? What for?'

'Most people say, 'Yes of course, officer, anything I can do to help,' sir,' said Scharff who still had his back to the room staring out to sea. But the reason why we need your name and address, sir, is that, if for any reason we have to get back to you, or even, as of course at the moment seems unlikely, if we have to start conducting a criminal investigation, we would be able to find you.'

Lucille came back into the room bearing a tray with four cups on it.

'Ah, Mrs McElvey. A nice cup of tea is most welcome at this hour of the morning.'

He asked her for sugar which she immediately went back to the kitchen to get for him with a warm gracious smile, as if she was his little maidservant or something. What the fuck was she doing being so friendly to these fucks? They were only going to lead her on and catch her out so that they could entrap him and pin the deaths of Richard and Rose on him. That was fucking all.

While she was getting the sugar, Ron decided he was getting out of control. He reminded himself that the guilt-free always co-operate comfortably. He would cut his losses, switch tacks and give the woman his name and address. He did so and she wrote it down. Meanwhile Scharff was making a song and dance out of thanking Lucille as she returned, sugar bowl in hand and delicately stirred two spoons of sugar into his tea for him.

'I'm glad I did hear about this from you,' she said to them as she put the bowl down on the tray and sat down. 'It's the most terrible news of my life, but as you are the officers investigating what happened, it's better to have heard it from you directly than from someone who didn't know anything about it. I'm so grateful to you for making the link between Rose and my husband up there in Balham, and me down here. But how did you actually do that? I don't think I packed anything that would have identified him with me, you know?'

She was talking in a breezy, almost academic manner, as if she hadn't got any feelings at all, but it was quite obvious to everyone else except Lucille herself that she was on the verge of tears. Ron knew she could often sound inappropriate, out of sync, but this was ridiculous. What *was* the matter with her? Shock. It was probably because she was in a state of shock.

'We found an empty bottle and a receipt, dated yesterday, for some chocolates and some olive oil amongst the first Mrs McElvey's rubbish bags in the big bin outside her back door, Mrs McElvey. And as the fire seemed to have been started by the olive oil catching fire in the first Mrs McElvey's frying pan we thought it might be helpful to trace the oil's history.' He smiled at the ordinary obviousness of police procedure. 'You paid by credit card. It was a simple matter of getting in touch with the branch of the store where you shopped, asking them to go through their till receipts. We contacted the card issuer for your address. It was all done in a matter of minutes. Easy!'

His professionally concerned, sympathetic demeanour could not quite disguise the self-satisfied smirk which Ron saw and despised him for. Lucille asked Scharff for more details about what had happened. Ron could see she was determined not to cry as she listened to what, on the whole, were evasive non-answers. She was obviously trying so hard not to cry that she wasn't concentrating properly on the replies she was getting, and ran out of questions. Scharff asked them a bit more about Richard and Rose's physical and mental health. Lucie told them about the reality of Richard's care needs and Rose's double hip replacement a few years ago. Finally Scharff informed them that the bodies couldn't be released for burial or cremation until the post-mortem had been carried out. She would be informed when that was, he added with a professional smile, as soon as they knew.

He also asked her, in an easy, straight-forward yet somehow also surreptitious way, how she had met Richard, how long she had been married and what the state of her finances were. He was such an oily old smoothie that any lonely housewife and carer would have been seduced into answering, and sure enough, much to Ron's now well covered-up annoyance, Lucille told Scharff everything he wanted to know, not realising that all his fucking questions were designed to find out what her motivation might be for wanting Richard dead. It was so obvious a child would have seen it, thought Ron. But then, he had to remind himself, she was in a state of complete shock. If she had had her wits about her a bit more she would have realised she should always be much more circumspect with Plod. So he mustn't be angry with her.

The way Scharff couched everything he said to Lucille in such a solicitous mannner was also designed to put her at her ease, lull her into a false sense of security, and make his bad news as palatable as possible. Well, at least that wasn't working. She looked as white as a sheet now, had lost all her usual vivacity. Stupid cow, she should at least pretend to be all right, like she was doing a few minutes ago, not draw suspicion upon herself by acting guiltily.

'I didn't,' she said, ten minutes later, after she had shown the police to the door and he immediately confronted her about this. 'I'm not guilty of anything. I was upset, Ronnie. That's all. Richard and Rose were the two people I was closest to in all the world and now they're gone.' She blew her nose, and with a bright smile very similar to the impersonal one she had given the police when she said goodbye to them, exclaimed, 'I don't know what I'm going to do now. I've got nothing to do anymore.' Ron realised, it was finally beginning to dawn on her just what he was concerned about. She left him in her living room saying, 'You're the one who acted guiltily,' and went out the door and into her bedroom.

A few minutes later he followed her and found her crying silently on her bed. He sat down beside her and put a hand on her hip. She curled herself up like a baby, shutting him out.

'You're right,' he said. 'I'm sorry about Richard and Rose.'

She ignored him, covering her face with her hands. He looked at her lying there in her pink dress, her body shaking now and again, until it dawned upon him that she didn't want to share her distress with him at all.

Nevertheless he continued sitting there, staring down at her until eventually the reality of what she was suffering somehow softened the edges of his paranoia. He shifted closer towards her on the edge of her bed, moved his hand up to her shoulder.

'Leave me alone, please, Ron,' she said in an almost inaudible voice.

He nodded, got up, went over and sat down on the stool by her dressing table. He avoided his own reflection, fiddled instead with her earrings which adorned a little tree-like stand, like flowers or fruit. He hadn't really noticed it before. It turned round on itself. He started flicking it around; faster and faster until an earring flew off and dropped onto the floor. He retrieved it and found his bus ticket at the same time. Eventually Lucille sighed, reached for a tissue on her bedside cabinet and blowing her nose got up. He reached for her, but she brushed past him saying she was going to make them both another cup of tea, and could he *please* stay out of her bedroom.

A few minutes later she joined him in the living room with a couple of mugs of tea, but she didn't even try to drink hers. She went back to her room leaving the door open, lay still on her bed with her head in hands for the rest of the day. Ron didn't want to intrude on her grief, occasionally going in and stroking her head and then leaving again because she just lay there, not responding at all, as if she was dead herself.

In the evening he switched the television on and tried to coax her to join him saying he would make them some scrambled egg.

She ignored him.

Five minutes later he heard her get up and go to the bathroom. When she came out she said, 'I don't like scrambled eggs', went back into her room shutting the door and locking it firmly.

He went to sleep on the sofa in his clothes. He didn't wake up till the sea gulls were flocking overhead the next morning, complaining about the weather. He heard the sound of Lucie washing up his egg pan from yesterday in the kitchen sink and went to help her. She looked terrible in her big white dressing gown, empty and dehydrated, eyes and cheeks hollow. He didn't fancy her at all. She managed a smile for him although he could see she was forcing it, and asked him if he would like any breakfast. Her normal bubbly contralto had lost all its liveliness. She no longer sounded unhappy, just somehow automated, almost disembodied like she was a loud speaker at an airport or a fucking bus station announcer or something.

He would help her get a grip.

All morning he tried to engage her in conversation, alternating between wanting to cheer her up any way he could, and trying to stop himself talking about his fear that they were going to be suspects in a murder investigation. It was inevitable. She responded only once, ignoring all his subsequent attempts to continue the discussion. 'We haven't done

356

anything wrong, Ronnie. At least I haven't. Have you? So please, for my sake, stop being paranoid. Anyway the truth is, Richard wanted to die. He'd been going on and on about it. I was telling my friend Paula about it earlier this week. And Rosie, well Rosie would have been pleased to go too, if she had to. They made some kind of pact between them. That's what I think.'

She put on her trainers and went out to the shops for some more milk at midday and didn't return till three, saying she had been up to Beachy Head. Occasionally wondering where the fuck she had got to, Ron found his alarm about the visit of the police yesterday continually preoccupying him while she was out. He tried to watch the television, but although his eyes and ears were focused on it, the pictures and sounds all went past him.

If the deaths were not yet suspicious, it was clear that they did not appear completely accidental either. Otherwise, why would the police have dissembled about whether they were conducting an investigation? They were working on the theory that the fire had been caused by the cooking oil which they had proof Lucille had purchased. They were much more likely to think she had killed them than that it was an accident or a suicide pact, of course they were. And if they suspected her, then they were bound to suspect him too. He was sleeping with the dead man's wife, for fuck's sake. He hadn't been able to produce his bus ticket for them yesterday. They would be fitted up. How could they not be? It was the police's job to 'make a case' and make a case they surely would. It was inevitable. He felt it with a strength as significant as anything he had ever felt since the dark dim days of his 'cancer' twenty years ago. The irresistible feeling that he would have to do something drastic became overwhelming.

He tried to say as much to Lucille when she got in, but she neither replied nor appeared to be listening as she unpacked her shopping and put things away.

'Do you still want to go out with me to the opening of Neil's exhibition?' she asked when she had finished.

'Who the fuck is Neil?'

'Ronnie! Don't talk to me like that, please. I told you the night before last. A friend of Paula's. I've only met him once, at a New Year party a couple of years ago. But Paula says he's very good.' She gave him a bleak smile. 'Life must go on. They'd both say that, Richard and Rose. Paula told me he does big colourful pictures. They might cheer us up.'

How could she possibly be talking about such trivialities at a time like this? Of course he didn't want to go to a fucking exhibition. Anyway at least she was speaking to him again. So he would make an effort not to let his angry anxiety show. The trouble was it tended to slip out anyway.

'I want to talk about what we are going to say to the police if they come back. And they *surely* will come back,' he said. Then, seeing the set of her face, he added, 'I don't mind going out with you, that would be great, but we need to talk about this okay?'

'Okay. I'm going to have a bath, try to relax a bit, Ronnie. There's nothing we can do now, is there?' She must have been talking to herself really because she started nodding her head as if in agreement with her own advice, but when he moved towards her soothingly, she flinched and pulled away, shaking her head and saying, 'I can't believe it. I can't believe any of it.'

'What are you talking about? What can't you believe?' Then he twigged. 'Believe it! They're capable of anything, the police.'

'I am *not* talking about the police,' she said, icily and it dawned on him that had she been the type she might have liked to have hit him then.

'Oh, yeah. Yeah, it's terrible,' he said.

He knew he sounded lame. It was only understandable if her ice became fire. He thought she would bawl and shout, but she simply shrugged and went into her bedroom to get undressed. He followed her, but she asked him to leave. When she went into the bathroom she locked the door.

Three hours later, during which he had been unable to stop himself worrying and ruminating about how everything would lead to him, and railing about the existential unfairness of that, Lucille emerged from her bedroom in an off-the shoulder wine-red velvet dress, with her hair all fluffed up and her face all made up, looking like a porcelain doll. He immediately felt like fucking her, and realised she was right. They did need to let life go on.

As she drove them over the Downs to Brighton in her big Nissan, he found himself feeling angry with her for not wanting to talk with him about his fears. After all they too were a real part of life-going-on, but she just ignored it whenever he tried to bring up the subject. 'I told you this morning what I think, Ronnie. I'm not going to tell you again.'

At the exhibition she put in a fine performance, sipping white wine, holding onto his arm making admirous remarks both to him and to other people about the paintings. He thought they were childish crap himself, all fluorescent dots and indeterminate swirls. Irritatingly bad. She insisted she wanted to stay till nine thirty in case Paula showed up. Through the milling, expensively dressed little crowd of people she pointed out the 'artist' himself, Neil, a soft-looking man in rimless spectacles with what Lucille said she felt were sad, kind eyes. Ron just thought he looked a bit shifty, himself. He had an effeminate mouth and sweaty palms when he shook hands. Gay probably.

By quarter to ten when together with two or three other people, they were the only ones left in the gallery, he pressed her and she thankfully agreed to go. They said goodbye and good luck to Neil, and left. Paula hadn't made it.

They went on to an Indian restaurant. It was decorated in swirls of dark blue Hessian and each candlelit table was bathed in its own little pool of blue light. Perhaps that was how they justified their prices. He could hardly see the menu, let alone the food that eventually came to them. He could however see enough to notice that Lucille was only picking at hers sporadically, leaving most of it and saying very little. He finished his own meal quickly, devouring it in the same way that his angry anxiety was devouring him. When he had finished he reached over with his fork to spear at her vegetable Biriani, which she had hardly touched and which she'd stopped eating altogether now. His fork-full spilt on the table as he tried to bring it back to his mouth.

Now and again he tried to persuade her that they had to have a convincing and mutually supportive story for when the police came back. 'I only mention it,' he said, trying not to make an issue out of it.

But she was consistently not interested.

At the end she peeled the paper off her courtesy mint chocolate and looked him straight in the face.

'Look, Ronnie, I really don't *care*! I don't care whether the police want to ask us more questions. If they do, I will tell them anything they want to hear, because I don't care. Now, can we change the subject?'

'Fine. If you don't care, then why not do what I'm telling you,' he said. 'Give them answers which put them off any idea that you had anything to do with Richard and Rose's deaths, okay?'

'Alright, Ron,' she said, looking at him oddly. He felt like a specimen of something nasty picked up with tweezers from under a stone. He didn't trust her look, or her tone at all. She patted his hand, gave him another of her bland, bimbo smiles, and looked away across the other tables. She fucking knew he didn't trust her. It must have been written all across his face.

He could see her face clearly lit in the lift as they went back up to her flat on the second floor. She looked older. The vacated expression in her eyes told him she had changed. She wasn't the woman he knew. There was now a look in her eyes which suddenly repelled him, reminding him of the strange wild creature, the kid with the shaven head, who had helped Grainne in the park nearly a quarter of a century ago. No gamine adolescent now, of course, and not androgynous anymore either, but unmistakeable nevertheless. The feral look of permanently startled and permanently wary vulnerability was identical. He didn't like it, and he didn't like her for not hiding it from him.

Nevertheless when they were back inside the flat he found he wanted sex, despite his anger with her. She shrugged, rather than actively demurring and when he came on to her she stroked his cheek once, then turned for her bedroom where she raised her arms passively into the air for him to take her clothes off.

He could do what he liked then.

He pulled her towards him and reaching down over her behind he pulled the velvet skirt of her dress up, putting his other hand down under her knickers and squeezing her rump. It was full and soft in his hands so he turned her round, asked her to take the knickers off and kneel down on her bed on all fours. She shrugged, but straight away did so. Her skirt had fallen down over her bum again. He flipped it back up, admiring the roundness of her rear again as he unzipped his fly. Then he humped her from behind, like an animal. She pushed back against him, whimpering as he entered her, and he came quickly.

When he had finished he looked down and noticed her head was down between her hands and she was crying.

But what could he do?

He pulled out of her. She remained motionless as if she would never move again. Well, she could stay like that as far as he was concerned, if she wanted to. He might even come back for more if she did. He put his trousers back on and realised he had forgotten his underpants. He picked them up off the floor, and seeing her bum was still up in the air and semen was now seeping from her fanny, he wiped her with them. As a kindness. Then he pulled her dress back down, patted her behind one last time for good measure and left the room.

He went to her living room, and lay on his back on her cream-coloured sofa staring at her old wedding photograph in the corner above her small collection of china shepherdesses. What did she call them? Her Little Bo Peeps. She'd recited the rhyme to him once. He looked at her Little Bo Peeps, and he knew that he could never just leave things alone and let them come home bringing their tails behind them. He was the kind of person who had to do something about situations he had no control over.

So he decided on a plan.

On Monday morning he would ring Detective Inspector Scharff and inform him that Lulu had told him that last Thursday night, the night before they had died, Richard had asked her to kill him. He would mention that she had also told him she'd spoken with her friend Paula about it a few days before.

So his story would check out.

He would let Scharff know all this as part of his civic duty.

He didn't really know why exactly he suddenly needed to become a good citizen. He was paranoid, he knew that, and telling Scharff everything he knew would help to ease that a bit. So he would tell him everything, answer every question. He might even tell him about Lucille's common law legal status as Richard's 'wife'. There was definitely still a part of him that wanted proper revenge on her after all these years, give her something to really chew on. She had, after all, fucked up his relationship with Grainne when they had first been living together and then, by not not bothering to look for him, find him and connect him with Sean, had destroyed any possibility of his having a proper relationship with his son as well. To add insult to injury she had always taken his goodwill and his sexual desire for granted.

And anyway, who knew? Maybe she *was* guilty. Maybe she had killed Richard and Rose, or, at the very least, got them to kill one another.

It would be better if he never saw her again.

He slipped out quietly at six a.m., walked down the steep, zigzagging pathways through the shrubs and bright flowery borders below the promenade, on to the shingle; from there across the stones to the sand and the sea.

The early morning tide was out and he was alone on the beach. He stepped across worm casts and sea weed. The odd tiny scuttling crab and hoards of nervy, garrulous sea birds hurried out of his way. He walked on to the edge of the water and watched it calmly continuing to recede, willing it to stop and come back in.

Three hours later the tide had completely turned and he was sitting in his seat on the coach back to London, a small satisfied smile on his face.

Chapter 22.

'Grainne? Grainne?'

Lucille's voice almost shrieked down the phone. Grainne moved it away from her ear. She was so loud and hysterical-sounding, that at first Grainne didn't recognise who it was talking to her.

'Hi, Luce,' she said, once she realised. She sat down at the kitchen table, immediately sensing disaster. 'It's great to hear your voice. But what's up? You sound like you've seen a ghost.'

'It's Richard and Rose. They're – they're dead, Grainne. They're just dead.'

There was complete silence for a whole minute, except for the disembodied sound of their breathing. Grainne watched the second hand of her kitchen clock doing one complete revolution around the dial, so she knew it was a whole minute before she whispered, 'You poor thing. You poor, poor thing. I'm so sorry.'

'They died in a fire.'

'How?'

'I don't know. I don't *know*! That's what the police asked me. As if I'd know! I mean, I don't know, Grainne. I don't know anything.'

'What happened? Tell me everything.'

'I don't *know*,' Lucille repeated, almost wailing. 'All I know is they died in a fire and the police are probably – no, not probably – definitely going to formally interview me after they've decided what questions are still unanswered about how it happened. They told Ron that when he rang them. They interview everybody, they said, as many times as necessary. It's routine. So they might even interview you. I don't know.'

'Do you want me to come down? No, Lucie, don't answer that. I'll come to stay with you for a few days. Is that alright? I need a break. I'll be there tomorrow morning before twelve.'

'It's not nec– I mean, you don't have to Grainne.' Everything about her tone of voice spoke of relief, of thank goodness, of please-please-do-come-quickly-I-need-you desperately.

Grainne found it a bit much, said,

'I know I don't *have* to. I want to, and I'm going to. But I'll have to put Ron off. He rang me a couple of hours ago saying he was coming over to see me and wanted to stay the night. He had something long and difficult to explain, he said. Well, I've heard his long and difficult explanations before. I'll ring him and put him off, that's all. I'm not having him here getting in the way in the morning when I'm trying to leave.'

'No, Grainne, don't! I mean I think you *should* see him before you come. He was with me when the police came round. It was so frightening. He was on at me all the time to tell them lies. Why, Grainne? I don't know.

I've never done him any harm at all. Not that I know of. So why? I don't understand it. I don't want to lie ever again.'

'Uh-huh. I thought he sounded kind of flustered when he called. No wonder.'

'He's changed beyond recognition, all paranoid again,' said Lucille. She sounded terrified. 'And so angry! I don't understand why he is so angry. Yesterday when he saw I was angry with him – and I was, I really was – he didn't care at all about Rosie and Richard, just his own skin, you know? It was horrible – but when he saw I despised him for that he, I don't know, he turned. He turned into someone else. Some *thing* else, almost. Something I don't understand. All I really want to do is cry. I'm scared. I just said to you I didn't want to ever lie again, but I'd tell them anything, Grainne, I really would. Anything! The police, I mean. Even though I haven't done anything. But I *feel* like I have. And it was my olive oil.'

'What was your olive oil, Luce?'

'It probably caused the fire. The police told me. They found the receipt for it in Rosie's bin. I don't care – I mean I don't want to care – about that, but I do because Ron's got me all frightened. I should be all upset – I *am* all upset about Richard and Rosie, but I'm all confused too. I don't know what I feel anymore.'

'Listen to me, Lucille, Ron can just fuck right off. Come on! He's crazy. He's always been crazy.'

'He contacted the police again. Rang them up. Before he rang you, he rang me to say he had been on the phone to them and told them Richard had asked me to kill him. Told them about – about my past.'

There was a resounding silence.

'Why Grainne?' she wailed. 'Why did he do that? And what's your past got to do with *them*? Why did he have to tell them that? I don't understand. He rang me straight after speaking to them, said he had to be fair, he had to tell me what he had told them. I didn't mind at first. I thought it was all true what he was saying, but then when he said he'd told them about my awful history too, I started shaking. I couldn't stop. I mean that's so personal, and so irrelevant, and I know I *shouldn't* be ashamed, but I am. He knows I am, and I think that was why he told the police, just to make me ashamed. You know? I asked him what had that got to do with Richard and Rose dying. I can't remember what he said, but then it dawned on my tiny bird brain that he was trying to get me into trouble, as though their deaths weren't an accident, they were murder, and he wanted me to be the prime suspect. I was so shocked it made me dizzy. I had to sit down. I still feel giddy now. I don't understand why he would tell them personal things they don't need to know about me and blame me for something I did not do. It's so scary.'

'Lucille, he's a fuckwit. You know he is. I don't mean to be horrible and I know he means far more to you than he does to me, but face it, he's a complete narcissist.'

'I won't be happy till you're down here with me, Grainne.

Ron is mindlessly egotistical. You know, don't-care selfish. Everything has to revolve around him. Remember him once telling you he'd killed Milly? Selfish. Completely fucking selfish.'

'Oh, yes. Sure, that's so true, but I'd kind of come to love him, you know. And now I'm so hurt I don't know what I feel.' Grainne heard her voice choking and then breaking into small discreet sniffs. 'I can't wait for you to get here, Grainne, help me see sense. Ron said I would need an advocate. Will you be my advocate? '

'It's a solicitor you need for that, not a friend. I'll help you find one tomorrow. *If* you need one.'

'Paula, my friend Paula knows solicitors round here.'

'Ring her then, get a name and a number just in case. Give me her number too while you're at it. Now you're not to worry. Luce! Ron has gone a bit rabid that's all.' Lucille's laugh at this statement sounded like a strangled scream. Grainne felt guilty. 'He's not credible, Lucie. The police will be sensible enough to recognise that, I'm sure. He knows he's not credible, and that's another reason why he thinks it's okay to act crazily and do horrible things to the very people who care for him. I think you should try to sleep now. Face the mess that idiot might have made, tomorrow. And it is only 'might have made', don't forget. I think you should put all this nonsense to one side, if you possibly can. I'll see you in the morning. Promise. So, DON'T panic! There's no crime and there's no evidence of one. Don't you see that because you're unhappy – bereaved – you're bound to be distressed and frightened and vulnerable at the moment! Vulnerable to being infected psychologically by the rantings of a– well, never mind what he is. Don't be diverted from what you are really feeling. Let your dam burst, Lu. Have a good cry. I'll see you tomorrow.'

'I don't think I can cry. I feel angry. I haven't felt so angry since my dad– well, since my dad. And I loved *him* too. In my own way. I never feel angry.' She made a little screeching sound followed by an incongruous trilling. 'I hate feeling angry and I hate feeling hate.'

'Get some sleep, freshen up. Then, when we talk about how to deal with this together tomorrow, your anger can drive you on again.'

'I don't want it.'

She put the phone down and felt sad. She'd always liked Rose, and whatever she had thought about Richard before his stroke, he had been suffering so long since, poor man, that she couldn't help feeling sad. How awful to take ten years to die. Then she felt angry, fiercely angry with Ron. What was that weak, stupid *eedjit* playing at? Ringing the police and trying to fit up Lucille with something that wasn't even a crime, for heavens sake? Just a tragedy, an everyday little tragedy, but a tragedy all the same. A terrible tragedy for Lucille. Well she would ask him herself, directly, when he arrived. Get it from the horse's mouth. He had always been *such* a tosser, that man. She'd met so many fantasists like him back in the bad old days before Sean's arrival had put paid to her previous profession. Even during his successful years there was something unhinged about him, the way his only interest was in the workings of his own mind and his monstrous assumption that everyone was just like he was. What was all that rubbish he had told her about once believing he suffered from a cancer of significance? What was that all about? And all that ridiculous PET stuff he worked his Ph.D. around, what was that about really, if it wasn't an attempt to regulate the bizarre workings of his own stupid, *stupid* mind, Ron's interest in Ron ?

But what on earth had he got against Lucille? It was so hateful if it was true what he had done. Lucille certainly hadn't sounded like she'd been lying. Why should she? As she said, she still loved him really, stupid idiot that she was. Why else would she let him come and stay with her three times a year? No. Grassing someone to the police by trying to fit them up with circumstantial rubbish was something only someone full of hate could do. Grainne had never seen Ron's hate before. Whatever had Lucille done that he should be directing his hate at her so viciously? He had certainly never mentioned anything about it to her, so whatever it was, it must have been fairly recent. Years ago he had once or twice made it clear he still carried a little bit of ancient resentment about her role in the break up of their own relationship many years before that. But really, that was ages ago. And he had also sometimes grumbled, but only very mildly, that Lucille should have told him she was fostering his son. But if these things were what his gripe was about, they could both be equally said about her too. So what else might Lucille have done? There had to be something else, something more driving his cruelty towards her now.

Or maybe less. Maybe he was just so egotistical and so self-important that it wasn't as if she or Lucille had ever even really existed for him at all. Not really. And because of that, it wasn't actually possible for them to *do* anything to really get his goat, even if they'd wanted to. You can't do anything if you don't exist. She herself had certainly tried to annoy him over the years. Many times and it hadn't made a blind bit of difference. He had treated her exactly the same as if she had been trying to please him, with a complete lack of any kind of close involvement or care at all. Yes, the more she thought about it, the more she was sure that she and Lucille were just there to be used or abused as necessary in order to meet his own needs. That had to be it: he was just so self-absorbed that he didn't care what happened to Lucille, she just didn't figure. And if he was becoming more deluded and persecuted again, he definitely wouldn't mind what damage he did to others – whoever they were – as long as he himself was out of the woods.

The bastard wouldn't give a toss. That was it in a nutshell. It was his lack of consideration for others which was driving this disregard for Lucille. Simple as that.

It had always been the thing that Grainne herself had felt was most annoying about the man from the very first time she met him. It meant his betrayal of Lucille was probably a barmy act of self-preservation, rather than an active act of thought-out hatred for her. He wouldn't have even considered imagining what the effect of what he had done would have had on her. The stupid, selfish git.

But not so stupid that he couldn't be made to understand what he had done once he got here. She had his measure. She would read him the riot act, get him to phone the police again and recant. If he wanted to be a psychopath he could go and be one somewhere else. A hospital preferably. But not in her life and not in Lucille's.

She began packing a bag. She would get in the car first thing and drive down to the south coast for a few days.

Linda! She must ring Linda, her office manager, at home. Tell her she was going away for a little while. A holiday. Ask her to keep things ticking over till she got back. She only had one major deal to close and all the paperwork bar the final signature was done, but compared with this crisis it didn't rate. It could wait a couple of days, or a couple of weeks, till she got back; and if it couldn't, well, she had wasted time and money worse than that during the course of her life. If she lost it, she lost it. Too bad.

After coming off the phone with Linda, Grainne found herself glowing with the thought of Eastbourne. They'd have a nice time and it would be great to get away from her business for a little while. It was a good time to go and it would be lovely to see Lucille again. Her own residual resentment towards her was long gone. Prehistoric. The more she had become reacquainted with Ron and his insistence on being the great idealised father, the more she had felt that Lucille could keep him. For all the smooth presentational skills he had developed when he was earning money off gullible fools interested in his ridiculous little psychology seminars, he had still actually been the same old Ron. She'd realised that almost as soon as she'd met him again that night at Rose and Richard's, when they had both been introduced to their son for the first time. Well, his first time, and her first time for more than eight and a half of his ten little years at that time. All Ron had been interested in was what he wanted to do for Sean, not in Sean himself at all. And he had continued like that ever since, completely out of touch with the person who was his son, foisting reams and reams of crackpot advice and spurious scientific papers upon him. Despite all this and despite all the terrible things she had herself done to him during her pregnancy and his early years, Sean was fine, thank goodness.

She smiled. He'd been gone nearly a year now. Into adulthood, looked after by no-one but himself anymore. He'd just completed his first year at Durham and for the last couple of weeks had been picking up casual work at tourist resorts when he wasn't windsurfing. He had rung her the day before yesterday to say he wanted to come home for a few days to see her, would be travelling by night bus and arriving early tomorrow morning. Shit. She would have to ring him and explain what the crisis was. He would understand. He was such a nice boy nowadays. His successful transition to an easy, socially skilled young adulthood had probably not had much to do with her and certainly nothing to do with his father bamboozling him with ever more obscure developmental theories and waving endless research study outcomes at him whenever he saw him. The fatherless little Asbergery boy Sean used to be may have lapped up everything Ron gave him for the first two or three years of knowing him, but little by little, he came to terms with the fact that nothing Ron gave him was actually even the slightest bit helpful and he'd definitely had his father's measure by his early teens.

Nevertheless, in a curious way contact with his father had done him some kind of good. At least he had learned that he wasn't the only oddball in the world. The difference was that his father was mad, whereas it was debatable whether Sean even suffered from a syndrome. Whatever, he had successfully adapted himself around it. He had learned to navigate the world of emotions, feelings and relationships – The Waterworld, they used to call it when he was little, Lucille told her, because it could often lead to tears – and had eventually learned to function in it as if he was a normal human being. And what makes you a normal human being if not functioning like one? Ron had never been able to achieve a similar consistency.

Her doorbell chimed. Face set hard, she went to her front door.

'Grainne, I've done a terrible thing,' said a dishevelled-looking Ron, barging in past her without a bye your leave.

'I know you have,' she replied. 'Come in, do,' she added with heavy sarcasm. She could not be bothered to hide her irritation with him. Closing the door, she added, 'But you're not staying! I'm off down to stay with Lucille shortly.'

He pulled up smartly, head and shoulders visibly shaking like he was having a fit, or as if she had just stunned him with a shot of electro-convulsive therapy, which if it made him see sense was just what he needed, was her sour observation. Well, she hadn't intended to be subtle.

'Whatever are you trying to do to her, Ron? Fitting her up like that? For goodness sake! I know you've been in touch with the police! Deliberately tried to get her into trouble. She told me.'

'Yes, it was a bit cruel and everything, but–

'A bit cruel! Ron, you are a prize get! A prize fucking get.'

'I was frightened, Grainne. You know what it's like. You were often frightened when you were a little girl. You told me.'

'*You* are not a child, Ron. And what have you got against Lucille? Why did you do that to *her*? She's always been good to you. Always. She still is. What's the matter with you?' She tapped the side of her head with her forefinger, waved it around in the air and rolled her eyes. 'Going dulally again, are we?'

'She took me for granted,' he replied flatly. 'She always took me for granted.' He made for the kitchen and put the kettle on, making himself at home with her, taking *her* for granted. 'Can I make myself a coffee?'

She ignored him, shaking her head as he ignored her too, poured half her Cafe Direct straight from the jar into a mug.

'Did you just want to make sure no finger of suspicion pointed in your direction, you poor, pathetic coward of a man? Is that it?' She could hear the anger and disdain in her voice reverberating around the room. Even as she spoke she could tell by the stolid way in which he hunched his shoulders, like some television penguin waiting out an ice storm, that it was true. He didn't look too bothered about it though. He was used to her contempt, of course, but he really should have been more ashamed about it. It made her so angry she felt like killing him.

'Something like that and,' he trailed off, his concentration caught up in levelling his teaspoon of sugar. The stupid man liked it absolutely flat. He shook some sugar off the spoon. She could see he was vaguely aiming for the bowl, but most of it seemed to fall on to her expensive marble work top. He did the same thing twice more while Grainne remembered that he'd given up sugar in tea and coffee years ago. She closed her mouth, her heart skipping a couple of beats. He always used to have three spoonfuls of sugar in his tea back in the bad old days twenty years ago when he first started becoming ill. She was right, she must be: he was going bonkers again.

She breathed deeply. It meant he had got to be handled. As carefully as a sick punter.

'And what, Ron?' she said, trying to sound gentle, a haven of refuge, a port in a storm.

It didn't come easy and it didn't come over. She knew it didn't. She was almost crackling with anger for him.

'Dunno. I just thought: she can do anything, Lulu can! She'll be able to deal with it. The police, I mean. But I wouldn't. I mean, I knew I wouldn't.'

Grainne felt herself explode. She didn't try to resist it. She *couldn't* treat him like a punter. He was too fucking annoying.

'You are always and forever one great big booby, you bastard. You wouldn't have had to deal with anything at all,' she said, not bothering to keep the screech out of her voice. 'If you had just kept your stupid mouth shut! It was never even a crime, just an accident. An accident, Ron. *Now*, if this nonsense does lead to the police trying to build up some kind of criminal case against her, you – YOU, Ron – will have to deal with courts, lawyers, cross-examinations, the whole caboodle, won't you? Let alone the problem of perjury afterwards once they've found out you were framing her. You are a complete nutter. I've never really been surprised about that, but what does never cease to amaze me is what an eedjit you really are too. Completely fucking stupid. How you ever achieved a Ph.D., I'll never know. Did you buy it from some notional university in the American mid-west or something?'

'It was easy,' he replied, ignoring her question, not phased or upset in the slightest. 'You just had to put your mind to it and work, not stop till you got to the end.'

'Well, put your mind to this, we – No! *I* have got to think of a way to get Lucille off the hook and since you are here and since you put her on it, you can help me how.'

'I really did just concentrate,' he went on, still talking about his academic career. 'Took my medication and applied my mind. My thesis–

'I'm not interested Ron. I'm not interested in *you*. All I want to know is what possessed you to complicate things like this and how can we simplify them again? Return to the truth. It was already a tragedy for Lucille, losing her husband *and* her friend and mentor, and now you have turned her tragedy into a personal hell. Why, Ron? You're trying to get Lucille into trouble. You're trying to get her locked up. Why?'

'I just told you. She took me for granted too much.'

Grainne could tell by the affected gravitas he adopted as he spoke that he really believed this was a good enough reason. Self-important bastard. His accompanying smile as he turned round and took a sip of coffee was cunning and smug. 'Anyway, I knew she could deal with the police.'

'But why tell them about her medical history?'

'I thought it was relevant. It would make them more interested in her.'

'Relevant to what, precisely?'

'Well, um, to er, making them interested in her, making them think she might have, you know, done it.'

'Why would it, Ron? And why would *you* want them to think that?' She felt herself bridling. 'What about your medical history? Perhaps you're psychotic again. What have *you* done?'

'Nothing! I just told you: I put them onto her so they wouldn't think it was me. I'm frightened of going to prison.'

The great oaf spoke in a horribly rational, calm tone of voice, like a diagnostician, a medic. Not a patient. He looked complacent, unbothered, not trying to appeal to her sympathy or understanding at all, just stating his position, imperious and matter of fact. Like a psycopath rather than a raving loony.'

'You're already in prison, Ron, and you always will be. But are you really telling me you are so pathetic that fear of being banged up yourself, in a real cell with real bars, was a good enough reason to try and get someone else – someone innocent – banged up instead? You are a nasty piece of work, Ron, that's all I can say.' She felt so mad with him she wanted to rant. Instead she felt her own cunning come creeping out of the cupboard Uncle Frank sometimes used to sometimes lock her in if she didn't promise to be very, very good.

'Perhaps it was *you*,' she said, her voice cold, equally matter of fact. 'Perhaps it was you that killed them. Perhaps *I* should ring the police and tell them that. What do you think?'

Again he shuddered, at last looked frightened.

Good.

Then he marched past her into her living room and removed the telephone handset from its cradle on the little side table by the wall. He put it in his pocket, smug self-importance replacing the grim anxiety on his face.

Jesus, Mary and all the stupid saints! She had never seen him deranged in this way before. In all kinds of other ways, sure! But never with this fascistic, bullying certainty. He'd always been too frightened to ever do anything to challenge her. But now he looked and sounded so certain of his own importance and rightness that she knew she ought to feel terrified of him, but actually she just felt angry.

'Ron! What are you *on*? How dare you?'

'I'm not on anything.'

'So what do you think you are doing?'

'I feel scared, Grainne. I feel as scared as I did when you told Sean I suffered from schizophrenia that Christmas Eve when I came round with a new computer for him. Remember? He asked you what schizophrenia was. And you? You made sure you told him in a way guaranteed to undermine all my credibility as a father.'

'Don't make me laugh, you stupid, stupid man. You'd already lost that with all your silly books and articles about Asperger's. He knew they didn't make a jot of difference to how he felt at all. If anything – if you want the truth – which of course you don't, but I'll give it to you anyway – it made him feel less lonely and have more respect for you to know *you* weren't normal either.' She looked at him, narrowed her eyes, when again she saw priggish self-satisfaction wrinkle his vertical lines with little horizontal puckerings around his mouth and eyes.

'As, I see, you well know. You'd succeeded academically despite how fucked up you really were. I actually think he admired you a bit more after he learned about that. Anyway, this is irrelevant, Ron! We had all this out at the time. I wasn't prepared for him to live with a lie between himself and his parents. That blighted my childhood. It wasn't going to blight his. And, happily, it hasn't.'

'It didn't help him to learn you had been a whore.'

'It *did* actually. It wasn't as if I ever brought my work home. And besides, you know perfectly well I stopped all that after he came by the leisure centre after school and could have caught me with a punter. I didn't hide it, but I didn't impose the truth on him either, shove it in his face all the time, like you did with your antics. I just told him about it.'

'Once it was over! Once you'd stopped. Which was fine. For you. Very convenient. But I was different. I couldn't just give up being myself, like it was a job. My, my schizo-fucking-phrenia was – is – a part of who I am.'

'It's such a shame, Ron. It truly is. My heart bleeds for you. But we get what we get, don't we. Anyway, like I just said, I'm sure he admired you more after he learned about it, so this whole discussion is spurious, phoney crap. So, now, do please be nice, and plug my telephone back in. If you're not silly, I promise I won't be either. But I would like to know why you shopped Lucille? Before you *go*.'

'I told you,' he said, wrapping the cord around the phone and continuing to hold it.

'No, you didn't,' she replied, feeling less frightened of him again now, equilibrium restoring itself as she realised what a performer he was, even if he himself didn't realise it. It shouldn't be too hard helping him see that he was following a script, but he would have to feel understood first. 'Not everything. Did she wind you up the wrong way or something?'

'I wanted revenge. I looked at the sea this morning, all calm and flat, and cool and misty – and I thought to myself I'm the opposite of this. I'm boiling with rage cos I've been let down by women all my life. My mother. All my mothers. You! Yes, and Lucille. All taken me for granted. It just felt fair, if I had to pick on anybody, to pick on Lu. Cos she shouldn't have been the same, shouldn't have been like all the rest, you know? She should have been a bit different. With *her* history. But she wasn't. So I decided just then that I wouldn't care. I am sorry now, but that doesn't mean I feel any guilt about what I did at all. Anyway, if she didn't kill those two old farts, then she will be able to convince the police of that, won't she?'

Grainne shook her head. Sorrow without guilt? The man was positively evil, as well as mad and stupid. He must have once been clever, or clever enough anyway, to have achieved what he had, but he had since become so stupid. Because if the police did get convinced of Lucille's innocence then they would inevitably have to turn their time and attention to wondering why he had wasted their time by trying to make them believe she wasn't. What he had done was almost guaranteed to achieve the opposite of what he had intended. It would make them want to investigate

371

him, once they had established Lucille's innocence and ascertained that he had shopped her.

'I'm not as stupid as you have always taken me for granted as being, Grainne. I do actually know the difference between facts and feelings. But I've been thinking about it a lot recently and I came to the conclusion that sometimes it's a mistake to discriminate between the two. I was fed up being relied upon to behave predictably all the time. I wanted to be unpredictable. So I thought about it and decided I would merge facts and feelings, like you women do so much. Just occasionally I would be right fucking on, let myself go, ignore the facts and follow my feelings. And yesterday morning it *felt* like she did it to me deliberately. You know – deliberately arranged things on purpose so that the police would come round just then when I was there. I *knew* she hadn't, not in fact, but that's what I felt. So I decided, fair do's, under the circumstances a little revenge was okay. If that was what I felt. Not just against her, you understand. Against all women. And not just for that. Of course not. For everything. She was just a good person to have revenge upon. I mean she *chose* to be a woman, didn't she? Anyway, it can't do any real harm. It's not the end of the world. Not if she's innocent.'

'Of course she's innocent, you stupid man. And you are *completely* wrong: she didn't choose to be who she is at all. That's really why you fitted her up, isn't it? Because, all your life *you* have felt like a fitted up innocent who never had any choice. Well, welcome to the human race, Ron.' You prat, she managed to think silently to herself. You arbitrary, psychopathic prat.

He raised a questioning eyebrow, looked both triumphant and apologetic and took too big a sip of coffee, scalding his lips. He grunted, licked them and blew, panting air out on them a few times to cool them down. Like a dog.

Perhaps he wasn't human. Grainne could recognise barking when she saw it.

'I don't want revenge anymore,' he continued, 'I'm over that now and I recognise I did do a bad thing fitting her up. I told you that when I came in. But I did what I felt. And I'm going to carry on doing what I feel. I feel now that I am not going to let you out of this flat until I know that *you* are not going to go to the police. I don't want them getting me for perjury, like you said.'

'Ron, you are utterly revolting, you know.'

'Yes. It's true.'

Moving very fast he went over to her front door, bolted the latch and turned to face her with his coffee steaming in his hand.

Oh shit. Oh shit. What with the phone, and now the door, there was no mistaking it, he was threatening her in her own home.

She felt her pulse quicken and her consciousness detach itself and find the safe place within to which she had always gone whenever she could not escape from something; her safe place within where she had the strength and memory of an elephant, and where she always went when she felt her oldest, most terrible sadness, which only got switched on by fear. The place she'd found inside herself when she was eight years old and hid in her mother's wardrobe trying to get away from Uncle Jack who was baby-sitting while Ma took her sister's into town for their immunisation jabs. She'd locked it from the inside and he told her that if she didn't come out and let him do what he wanted he would have to break Ma's little dressing table statuette of Our Lady Queen of Heaven. Grandma had bought it for Ma from Lourdes one summer. It was more precious than anything to her. So she did come out then, but he smashed the statue on the floor afterwards anyway. It had meant so much to Ma, that ornament. She had cried on her bed for hours after hitting Grainne repeatedly around the head for breaking it. Sobbed and sobbed. And Grainne had felt her skin become thick like an elephant's, and her memory longer. Her safe place within had been like a savannah, Ma's blows like the sun.

She felt herself wandering across her savannah again now as she wondered what to do.

She wasn't going to scream for the neighbours. She turned round, went to the kitchen and poured herself a glass of water. She went back out into her hallway and leaned against the wall, slurping, almost sucking the water from the glass as if she had a trunk.

'Ron! If you don't let me go you will be in serious trouble, you know, because *I* will go to the police afterwards when you're finally done with this bullying. I will definitely go and tell them myself what you've done.' She laughed too loudly. 'If that's what you want.'

'You won't.'

'Oh? Why not, pray?' Although she felt this pathetic attempt at her old, all-powerful insouciance rang hollow, Ron looked just a little disconcerted for a moment, which gratified her.

'I just told you,' he said. 'Because I won't let you. Not till I know you're not going to. You're going to have to convince me.' He smiled. 'I don't know how you'll do it.' He spoke in a slow, sing-song manner as he repeated this statement to her, patronising her, teasing her as if he was talking to a simpleton. 'I don't know how you'll do it.'

Despite her fear, she felt herself colouring with astonishment and rage. In all the time she had known him, he had never been like this with her before. Never. She could well understand the hysteria she had heard in Lucille's voice earlier over the phone.

'Are you threatening me, Ron?' she whispered. The feeling of being trapped, of helplessness and of not being in control made her voice sound like a little girl's. Be here now, she told herself. Deal with this like a grown up. She cleared her throat, straightened her shoulders.

'I'm just telling you,' he said, as she glared at him.

'You better let me out, Ron, or I don't know what I'll do.'

She did though. She knew she would have to be prepared to kill him if necessary, sacrifice the self-confessed scapegoater on the altar of her blighted life if that's what he insisted on making her do.

'It's good to see you looking how I used to feel,' he said with a maddening, friendly cheeriness.

'What do you mean? You cannot possibly know what I am feeling.'

'I can though. I really can. But I'm afraid it means I'm going to have to stay by this door all night and all day if necessary. And all the next day too. As long as it takes.' He gave her a flat smile which she didn't return. 'As long as it takes for you to convince me you are not going to speak to the police. I can't have you threatening me, Grainne. I'm sorry.'

'You haven't got a clue what sorry means. And you're the one who's threatening me.' He was crazy. Stark, raving bonkers. She would have to use every grain of ingenuity she had to extricate herself from this.

He shrugged with a sad little smile, and leaning his back against the door, slowly slid down it onto her inside front door mat, setting his coffee mug on the floor beside him.

Then they talked for hours about anything and everything, but mostly about him. Fueled by the terror she felt at being trapped, her perception was heightened. Her ears grew enormous – like an elephant's – so that she could hear everything. She could hear the anxiety in his voice and knew that what he was actually staring at so fearfully from her front door, what he actually wanted to get away from at all costs, was not prison. Not really. It was the rest of his life in mental health hostels, psychologically broken. Grainne could hear and make sense of the frightened discussions going on in the back of his mind better than he could himself. She could understand what was driving him. And her understanding gave her a plan.

She would lull him into a sense of security, make him feel there was no problem which could not be solved, ease all his anxieties, smooth his ruffled brow till he believed there was nothing he could not laugh off as trifling and insignificant. She would humour him, flatter him, have sex with him if he wanted, talk with him till she had sprung his trap and entrapped him back; by which time he would either have got up and left her flat, temporarily convinced and fearless that things could only get better, or he would have fallen asleep. At which point she would roll him over away from the door and leave. If he woke and tried to physically stop her, she might even have to kill him, perish the thought.

But try as she might to get him to relax his guard and chill out, she couldn't help arguing with him about certain things as the night wore on. It just wasn't true that she had treated him like a plaything when he had tried to woo his way back into her affections while they both became acquainted with their son ten years ago. After he had followed her up to the Midlands, taken a studio flat in Mansfield, she used to let him come round and stay every other weekend for a while, sometimes let him take Sean out on a weekday evening as well. She had actually been trying to be nice to him, but for Sean's sake and for his sake only. If Ron wanted to view that as toying with him, well, that was his problem. At no time had she ever led him to expect that he might get inside her knickers again.

She heard her overly-defensive tone of voice as she said this to him, realised she was getting caught up in his shit and changed the subject, returning as stealthily as she could to the task of trying to lull him to sleep, calm him down, get him to be less tense, to trust her, and move far, far away from all his paranoid ideas. Secretly she kept on reassuring herself she was strong as an elephant. But perhaps just because she did feel trapped, and just because she felt as helpless as she had when she was a child, it seemed to take hours and hours. The trouble was that although her childhood experiences with Uncle Jack had left her feeling that being forced to do anything was anathema, nevertheless the traumatically ingrained familiarity of being trapped by a man had a disgusting, compulsive quality to it which also had to be resisted.

So she wasn't very convincing at all.

She was a bad actress at the best of times and this most definitely wasn't one of those. She wheedled, she pleaded, she cajoled and she begged. 'I won't say anything about you to the police, I swear it,' choked out in almost-tears – she could never really cry – was no more or less effective, than coldly trying to appeal to his logical faculties. He was impervious to everything.

At one a.m., according to the digital display on his watch, he started yawning, but by two he seemed almost wired with wakefulness again, his eyes flashing, the veins on the back of his hands pumping, absolutely alert. Nothing daunted, Grainne kept up her gabbling. Half an hour later he was yawning again, and she got up to make them both a cup of tea. He asked her to put three sugars in it. She wished she had some odourless, tasteless poison to put into it too, but she didn't even have any paracetomol. She brought the tea to him with a biscuit. She bent, placed them beside him, picked up his old coffee mug and standing up again, discreetly altered the setting on the dimmer switch so that her hall was almost, but not quite dark. From the floor below on which he was now reclining, he greeted this action warmly, saying he needed to sleep soon and couldn't she just tell him, like she meant it, that she wouldn't contact the police.

She did continue to try. In as many different ways as she could call upon. But nothing she said, nor any way in which she said it made the slightest bit of difference to his ridiculous and bullying determination to stay planted exactly where he was.

Nevertheless Grainne could be patient. She had had a lifetime of disrupted nights one way or another, and she knew he would eventually drop off to sleep before her. But it was a shame she would be late getting to Lucille. What a pity she had left the mobile phone in the car yesterday or she'd have called her up now and explained what was going on.

Grainne had plenty of time to ruminate as they talked. She allowed *her*self to go mad for a while too, let *her*self feel that her overriding desire was to be selfish and amoral. Extraordinary situations called for extraordinary measures so she let herself feel she would just love to be a psychopath like him, do precisely what she wanted too, take revenge on all men, on Uncle Jack, on all her punters by scapegoating this one man, Ron. Just as he had done on the mother he never knew and on all women by fitting up poor Lucille.

There had always been something too alike about Ron and herself which she would have preferred to deny because it undoubtedly made her feel uncomfortable. She too could be inconsiderate about getting what she wanted. Unlike Ron however, she wasn't afraid of prison. She had always known, as he had not, that she had been in one all her life. It would make no difference to her whatsoever whether the walls and bars around her were made of bricks and steel.

At three a.m., his eyelids looked leaden, began to quiver as finally he began to struggle to stay awake. Grainne smiled. She was in control of this. She would be in Eastbourne well before midday, no question. She could even chide him about it.

'You're falling asleep, Ron! You don't want to do that, remember?'

'I don't care. I'm doing what I have to do. You can't do anymore than that, can you?' Then his tone changed. 'But I really don't care,' he mumbled, sounding less driven. 'This isn't really me. I'm possessed, that's all, by fear. I'm not really like this. You know that don't you, Grainne? I'm not really frightening.' He spoke slowly and fitfully, nine tenths asleep now and probably telling the truth, as he saw it anyway. She wasn't worried now. She could say what she liked, he would definitely be out like a light in a little while.

'No, I don't actually! I know you well enough to know you really are not very nice at all. Shopping Lucille, and now confining me here. It's seriously nasty. What's the point, Ron, except to be horrible? You actually want to be horrible. Well, people get what they want in life eventually and so, quelle surprise, yes, you actually *are* now horrible, Ron. Well done! Really horrible. Congratulations. What an achievement! But what I cannot understand is why you would want to be? You claim you once loved me. And Lucille loves *you*. You know she does. She always has. So why, Ron? Why are you doing all this?'

He didn't hear her. He was snoring. Wake up, you bastard.

'Why are you doing all this?' She said again, very loudly. He gave a little start, settled himself more comfortably across her doorway.

'I don't know. I just told you. I'm possessed. I think. I meant well. At first, anyway. I know what the police are like. I wanted to protect Lucille from getting herself into trouble by saying the wrong thing. You know? I didn't want her to incriminate herself. And then I found I also wanted to take revenge on her. And, well, you've got to do what you feel.'

'You can't have it both ways, Ron. You can't have your cake and eat it too.'

'I can though. That's what I have found out. I can.'

Grainne said nothing, watched his chest rise and fall rhythmically. He was away with the fairies. Sound asleep. She stepped quietly over to him and reached down into his side pocket and retrieved her phone. She padded silently back to her sitting room and shut the door without a sound. She dialled Sean's mobile. He replied on the first ring.

'Hi, Mum.'

'Sean! I have to whisper. It's your father. He's gone mad. He's lying across the front door on the door mat and he won't let me out. I have to go to Auntie Lucille. Her husband, Richard, and her friend Rose have both died. Yes, I'm sorry, darling. I know you were fond of him. In a fire. Your father told the police that Auntie Lucille started it, deliberately. He has as good as fingered her for their murder. Now he won't let me go to her. Goodness knows what else he might have done to her, but he has just fallen asleep, so I am hopeful of finding some way of getting past him and down to the car. He may be here when you arrive, but I'm afraid I won't be.'

'I'm still an hour away, Mum. This coach doesn't get into Leicester until six a.m. What do you want me to do?'

Good boy. A nice practical question.

377

Chapter 23.

It was ten thirty a.m., Grainne would be here soon, thought Lucille. Everything would become much easier, simpler, clearer. Grainne was so good at being easy and simple and clear. She would tell her what to do. They would talk together – and laugh! – about how to deal with police when they arrived, cover every angle so that the truth could be preserved and everything would be alright. And then they would laugh about it all again, and she would be free to cry at last about Richard and Rose.

Lucille had déjà vu as she prepared Richard's room for her. Earlier she had been rung by a policeman from the coroner's office who told her the most horrible things in the kindest of voices. She resisted the urge to weep as he said that the post-mortem had been completed and the bodies could now be released. He told her there would be an inquest later, the coroner's office would let her know when. He explained she would have to find an undertaker to deal with the bodies, advise about funeral arrangements and so on. When she said she didn't have a clue where to begin, he suggested she look in yellow pages, advised her to ring around and not be afraid to haggle about prices. There was no question as far as he was concerned that she wasn't responsible for what he delicately called the respectful disposal of both bodies. So she hadn't questioned it either.

Rose didn't have any relatives as far as she knew. Richard had a cousin in Canada. She would also ring Mary. It wouldn't be fair not to. She would have them cremated. It seemed easier. Invite his old friends and colleagues to the funeral service once she had arranged a date with a crematorium. They hadn't seen any of them in years, but one or two would certainly want to be there. Ever practical and sensible, Paula had suggested on the phone this morning that she get it all done here in Eastbourne – one straight after the other. It would make it easier. Lucille just had to hope that Rose's little address book with the pictures of medieval gargoyles on its covers had survived the fire. She could only think of one or two friends of Rosie's herself to contact about the funeral, and they would take some finding. The police had said all three ground floor rooms as well as the downstairs hall and the stairwell were gutted, but with a little luck her address book might have survived the inferno. She used to keep it upstairs beside her bed. She always liked to be in bed when she did her phone calls.

Remembering that made Lucille want to start crying. Instead she shuddered, needed to sit down for a moment to gather herself. She didn't want to be thinking about these things. She felt tears rising again and again, but each time suppressed them because they were only for herself. She was sure Richard and Rose were alright.

She got up, went to the mirror and checked her face, shook her head then went out on to the balcony overlooking the sea to water her geraniums. She looked out at the hot close sky. Over the Channel she saw flashes of lightening shrouded in the blanket of cloud that merged almost perfectly with the horizon. It felt positively tropical. Beads of perspiration formed on her brow and on the back of her neck beneath her hair. She looked up along King Edward's Parade watching for Grainne's distinctive black Toyata. No sign.

She was dressed for the funeral already. Loose black silk top, black skirt, black court shoes. She hadn't even bothered with her hair, just put a dark purple hair band in it to keep it out of her face. No jewellery of course. Just her wedding ring. She didn't know what else she was supposed to do. Were you only supposed to wear black for the funeral? Whatever, it felt right. She was in mourning, or would be if there wasn't so much to have to deal with.

Again, tears threatened to come. Again, she suppressed them.

Gone. Richard and Rose were gone. It felt like her spine had gone too, turned to jelly, all soft and wobbly, but full of pain. She didn't have the strength to let herself actually feel the loss of either one of them for more than a moment at a time. It was as if her grief had taken physical possession of her backbone, trapping her between spinelessness and self-pity when she allowed herself to feel it. But if she did, it felt too much and she just wanted to crumple.

It made her so ashamed she couldn't cope with her feelings, that a large part of her just wanted to walk out into the sea and join Richard and Rose.

Not an option, though. She had to see that their remains were properly attended to first. It was the least she could do. And she *could* do that. If the poisonous anxiety and fear that Ron had injected into her would have been impossible to deal with without Grainne's support, she could at least make sure that the final arrangements for Richard and Rose were properly and respectfully carried out.

As long as her back held out. She had never had back problems in her life before. The pain seemed to come and go, was at its worst when she concentrated on it. Whenever her thoughts and feelings turned instead to how truly depressing and horrible the loss of Rose and Richard was, which was actually the only thing she could really think about now, it seemed to take her mind off her spine. But it was all so physical. She could feel their absence in her very body. But she didn't want to cry. Crying was so physical too.

She straightened her shoulders, put a hand to the small of her back and tried to massage it. It didn't help. She went back inside and through to the hallway, opened the utility cupboard just inside the front door. She reached for the desk fan which she kept on the top shelf, brought it into her living room, plugged it in and switched it on. It was a bit yellowed, more than ten years old and it hummed too loudly, but at least it worked. She had bought it for Mum when she was in the nursing home. She turned it down a setting.

The feeling now was exactly the same as when Mum died, except then she had been expecting it. This was so sudden. This feeling now which made her want to burst was of Richard and Rose being absolutely present inside her heart and her head whilst at the same time being absolutely absent in fact. How could they be both here and not here at the same time? But that was how she felt and that was just how she had felt when Mum passed on too, together with this same horrible feeling of nothing else really mattering, the same sensation of being completely abandoned. And the same feeling of neither knowing nor caring who she was anymore, now they weren't here to confirm it for her anymore.

She felt the same sense of dissociation she'd had with Ron on Saturday when he taken her from behind. As if she was anybody. Hardly even a person. And she had felt so much love for him the night before. How could things change so dramatically? It left her feeling like she didn't exist; or if she did, that it certainly didn't matter who she was anymore.

Memories of Richard and Rose and Mum loving her anyway, despite her contradictions, even loving her for them, came flooding in. She tried to hold them back, but they wouldn't be stopped.

She tried not to cry, but the more she tried, the more impossible it became. So she was quietly weeping when the doorbell rang.

Grainne! Thank goodness.

She took a tissue from the box on the coffee table and blew her nose, then gave a cursory dab to the corner of each eye as she hurried to the door and opened it. If she was still a bit smudged, it didn't matter. She didn't have to look like the perfect widow for Grainny.

'Good morning, er, madam,' said the Detective Inspector with a huge empty leer. Oh no. This was the last person she wanted to see just now. Oh god! She had forgotten his name. And why was he addressing her in that snide tone of voice? Oh, yes, of course. Ron. Ron had been so cruel. She couldn't really care less about herself at the moment, so the facts of what he had betrayed didn't hurt as much as the betrayal itself, the terrible timing of it, and what it meant about his relationship with her. That was what was so *un*loving. In her own strange way she had always loved him. For almost as long as she could remember. She really would have let him do anything he wanted to do to her. But had he really had to do this? Oh God. She shook her head. She must concentrate, tell the police the truth and trust that they'd believe her.

The scary, overweight detective was again accompanied by the woman sergeant, Carole something-or-other who had come with him last time. The phone started ringing. She would let the ansaphone deal with it, ring the person back.

'H-hello. Come in officer – Officer...? I'm so sorry, what with one thing and another I have forgotten your name.'

'Scharff,' he paused before exaggerating and emphasising her title. 'Mrs, er, McElvey. Thank you. Just a few more questions to clear a few things up. If you don't mind. Thank you.'

'I was expecting somebody else.'

In the background she could hear dear Sean's rasping young baritone on the ansaphone, saying he had heard she could be in trouble and was following his mum down to see her in a mate's car. He left her his mobile phone number in case she didn't have it, ended with a cheery 'Bye Mum'. She smiled. She hadn't heard from him for at least six months, if not more, but it was cheering to know she wasn't completely alone at this time.

'Oh yes? Who exactly, if you don't mind my asking?'

She sighed, focused on the policeman and with a humble smile replied in as bright a voice as she could muster, 'A friend of mine, actually.'

'Well perhaps he or she'll be along presently,' he said stepping past her into her hallway. 'Shall I make my way through to your lounge? Funny word, 'presently'. It has two conflicting meanings. It's not like the same word with different spellings and two different meanings like, for example, the word 'wear', meaning to be clothed in one sentence, and a geographical question in another. Or 'tart' which has a number of different meanings although it is always spelt the same. No, 'presently', is an impossible word in my opinion, because it actually has contradictory meanings. It means both 'now' and one of its opposites, 'later'. Isn't that strange?'

'Very odd,' chipped in Carole. 'Now if it meant two completely different things that would be understandable wouldn't it, madam? And yet there it is. Plain as plain. We were just talking about it on the way here, weren't we, sir? Words with opposite and contradictory meanings. We tried to think of other words like that. 'Imflammable' was one we came up with. Did you know it means both combustible and not combustible? I didn't. Detective Inspector Scharff just told me that in the car. Yes madam, on the way over here. I never knew. You would think it was impossible. Like being both a man and a woman. Impossible.'

'Yes, you're right, you would think so, wouldn't you?' said Lucille feeling strangely unafraid, although her heart was all aflutter with anxiety and trepidation. This was so obvious. She wasn't completely stupid.

They all sat down at the same time. The detectives in an armchair each, with Lucille alone on her sofa between them. She certainly felt intimidated, but curiously ready for anything they had to throw at her too.

In real life it was quite possible to have contradictory feelings. More than possible, it was fact.

'Has there been a crime?' she asked them, attempting a bland smile. 'Am I a suspect? Are you formally arresting me? And if not, could you tell me please why you are here again? Because I don't really understand and it's making me feel a bit, you know, anxious. Dr Symes told me he informed you that I had gender reassignment surgery twenty two years ago. He also said he told you what Richard had repeatedly been asking me to do in the days before he died. Well, that's alright. I don't mind the truth coming out. In fact I want it to. Of course I do. Both things *are* actually true. Richard did ask me to kill him, but I told him I wouldn't, and that I never would. And before you come out and ask me directly: No, I didn't change my mind.' She must not let herself feel guilty when she wasn't. They would sniff it and turn on her, like dogs.

'As to my gender,' she looked at the woman with wordless appeal, hoping she might be moved into restraining Scharff from actually behaving like a dog because he was staring at her like a big albino Rotweiler, sighing as if panting, and looking her over with no discretion at all. It was so horrible it stopped her in mid-sentence, his smile making her feel like some plastic bone he wanted to chew. She glanced down at herself, then angrily drew herself up again. There was nothing undone, no embarrassing stains. He was just trying to make her feel uncomfortable, that was all. 'I don't think that that's any of your business really, is it?' she said coolly.

'Absolutely not, madam, absolutely not,' said Scharff. 'Unless, that is, you were living under false pretences, or unless it was a material fact relevant to the commission of a crime. Then of, course, we would have to investigate, because in that case it would be our business too.' The phone started ringing again.

'I would rather you didn't answer that, if you don't mind. Now what was I saying? Yes. In this country you are entitled to call yourself anything you like,' Scharff continued, staring her down with his flat professional smile. It seemed to be permanently fixed onto his fat face like a sick moon. 'Of course you are. So long as you are not committing a crime. Criminal deception, for example, is an arrestable offence. So, no, we have not come to arrest you. Not at all.'

In the background she could hear Grainne's pretty Irish voice on her ansaphone asking if she was there and telling her to come to the phone if she was. Then she heard her say something to someone else, before apologising for not being down already, but Ron had given her a few problems. She promised to be with her in two or three hours and said goodbye.

'We just need to ask you a few more questions, that's all,' Scharff continued over Grainne's voice. 'If you would prefer to accompany us to the station to help us with our inquiries, and we may have to ask you to do just that, I'm afraid, you are more than welcome to call a solicitor or an advisor or a friend to represent you at any time. More than welcome. But at the moment, as I say, all we are doing is asking a few more routine questions. In fact if you want a solicitor to be present right now, you do have the right to have one. I wouldn't want to discourage you in the slightest, even though we do in fact only want to ask you a few more questions.'

He was really very scary and Lucille found herself wanting to hate him, but maybe because it was so hot and maybe because she had been so shocked these last few days, she actually began to find that underneath her fear of them she still didn't really care.

Scharff was ogling her. There was no doubt about that. But was he just trying to make her feel uncomfortable? She crossed her legs, arranged her skirt. Let him. She didn't care. Mum used to say if a man makes you feel uncomfortable, imagine him just as he is in front of you without any clothes on, then you'll laugh instead.

'I have got nothing to hide,' she said, speaking to the woman because Mum was wrong, the thought of this man naked wasn't funny at all. Carole. That's right, her name was Carole Jones. 'You can ask me what you like. I will answer every question as honestly and truthfully as I can, Detective Jones.'

The woman looked up at Scharff who had rather laboriously got up again out of his chair and moved to stand by the open balcony door. Something about him reminded her of her father. One thought led to another and for a moment she couldn't help vaguely wondering what he would be like in bed. She shuddered, shook her head, disgusted with herself. He took his jacket off, folded it in two and laid it over his left arm. She was pleased not to invite him to hang it up or place it over the back of a chair. She noted the ghastly sweat stains under his arms and felt even more shaky inside. She didn't want his smelly jacket hanging on one of her hooks, thank you very much. She felt herself relax, breathe a hidden sigh of relief when he turned around and looked out at the sea, like he had last time he was here.

'Detective *Sergeant* Jones, madam. But you can call me Carole.'

'Lucille,' she returned with a small clipped smile, instantly angry with herself. Why had she allowed herself to be inveigled into letting the woman call her by her first name?

'I should tell you that I will write down what you say and whatever you say could be used in evidence later. Is that alright? I'll read you the full formal caution which advises you that what you don't say, and if it is relevant the fact that you didn't say it, can also be used in evidence, for your information. But as D.I. Scharff just said, we just want to clear up one or two loose ends and at the moment. We are not, erm, not *presently* conducting a criminal investigation. Just making routine preliminary enquiries.'

Lucille wasn't born yesterday. When she had finished reading out the full caution, Carole's smile was about as genuine as the glittering watch on her wrist was gold.

'That's fine. Ask me what you like, Carole. I'll answer everything.'

Scharff turned round and draped his jacket over the chair in front of him. It reeked of sweat and Sure for Men. Just like her father used to wear. Perhaps that was the connection because he otherwise bore no resemblance at all to Dad, except for being over-weight. Lucille bit her tongue as the man put a hand up to stop the Jones woman speaking and instead himself asked,

'Would you mind me asking you one thing then?'

'Not at all. I think I just said that to your colleague,' Lucille replied. Sighing, she got up, took his jacket and put it on a hook in the hall after all. She didn't want her armchair to reek of her father once they had gone. That *would* be too much.

'Did you know that in her will Mrs McElvey left her property and all its contents to you?'

'Oh my god, no! Oh Rosie!' She staggered back to her chair feeling emotion she couldn't control flooding into her face. 'No, I didn't know that,' she said, unable to stop herself starting to cry again. She pulled a couple of tissues from the box on the coffee table in front of her, blew her nose and gathered herself. 'No, I didn't know that at all.' She didn't want her house or its contents. She wanted Rosie back. And Richard.

'So you also wouldn't know she redrafted her will to that effect just last week?'

Lucille shook her head staring into her loss so deeply that for a few moments she forgot the police were even in the room with her. Then out of the corner of her eye she noticed Carole glance meaningfully at Scharff before switching on her compassionate considerate look again..

'We also need to inform you,' said Carole, 'that initial forensic and scenes-of-crime examinations of Mrs McElvey's kitchen reveal that your olive oil was probably deliberately poured over her kitchen surfaces including chairs and table which means, I'm afraid, the fire was probably not an accident. But as I said we are still at the preliminary stages of this enquiry. If Mrs McElvey did murder Dr McElvey and then had a tragic accident herself, as looks more than likely, then we are not at the moment looking for anybody else. If you follow my drift, Lucille.'

Oh no. Poor Rosie. Poor Richard. Could she have done such a thing? She could. She could do anything, Rosie could; take in waifs and strays, wander the streets, kill. Yes, she could have.

Lucille felt numb. She felt she couldn't talk anymore, even if she had wanted to.

'First I need your full name,' said Carole.

'Lucille. Lucille Emily,' she said through her sorrow. 'McElvey,'

So she could still talk after all. It was a shame really. She could guess the next question. She should have joined the police herself. 'Nee Farouk.'

'And your date of birth, and the name on your birth certificate, please?'

Lucille rattled them off mechanically. Thanks to the change in the law her birth certificate had been altered, but she was nevertheless transported, despite her grief, to her pre-operational shame. The question was designed to humiliate her. It could have no other purpose.

Where was Grainne? Something must have happened to her.

'You call yourself Mrs McElvey but, excuse me, we understand that, um, you are a transsexual female.' Did Carole actually sound a tiny bit apologetic as though she might be able to understand how humiliating this was?

Why ? What possible relevance did her gender or her marriage have?

'I am half French and I was married in France. In a little village just outside Toulouse. Women like me were legally recognised in France long before we were allowed to marry in this country. They've always been more enlightened over there.' She sat up straight and with her most fragrantly false smile said, 'If you cannot bring yourself to call me Mrs, then Madame McElvey would be perfectly in order.' She stuck out her chin, daring them to challenge her. 'I have a French marriage certificate.'

She remembered her wonderful wedding outfit and Richard, with whom 'in love' would have been an insulting understatement of what she felt for him at the time, carrying her across the threshold of their honeymoon gite set in an olive grove on the side of a hill overlooking the town. He had even recruited the then still tiny Sean to stand on a chair and throw confetti over them as he carried her in.

Lovely, precious memories. They were too much for her just now. She must deal with these horrible police people in the here and now first. What could have possessed her to let them in? She should have waited.

'It won't be necessary for us to see that, Mrs McElvey. Not for the moment anyway,' Scharff said, wiping his brow with the back of his shirt sleeve. He was disgusting.

'Could you tell us why the first Mrs McElvey would have left her house to someone who might be seen as, ahem, a rival?' he asked.

'I could tell you, yes. I imagine so anyway. I mean I can guess. She didn't tell *me* though. I had no *idea*.' She heard the potential screech in her voice as she spoke, told herself to get a grip. She must not let them see her cry.

'That does happen, of course, in wills. Even dying within a week of making a will often happens, but I think, yes, it would help us greatly to know why *you* think she was so generous to you.'

He spoke in such an obviously sarcastic manner that she found herself feeling angrier still. All these feelings she was going through. It was too much. She looked up at him and saw a sad, fat, motherless man behind his belligerent complacency. Even so, she wanted to stick her tongue out, or spit at him. Thankfully, just then, the woman said with more emollience,

'You must have been on remarkably good terms with her, Lucille.'

Being understood could be dangerous, but it was so *nice* it made her tears want to return immediately.

'She was like a mother to me! She loved me. She was always generous to me, right from the moment we first met.'

'I see. Could you explain why exactly?'

'Because, because…I don't know why,' she wailed. 'And I don't know what *that* has got to do with this.'

'Probably nothing, but it would help us understand,' Carole said with such a soothing, sisterly voice that for one mad moment Lucille just wanted to sink into her not insubstantial arms for a hug. Watch out, she told herself. Beware. Don't slump.

So she straightened herself up again. Her back immediately felt better. Chest out, small of the back in. Like her father had once tried to drill her into doing when she was a child. Be my little soldier boy, he had said, and one day you will join the Foreign Legion. But then he got exasperated by the girlish way she marched up and down for him, so as soon as he gave up on her she went and hid inside Mum's wardrobe for the rest of the afternoon and played with her shoes instead.

Feeling a bit bemused by this memory of her father intruding at such a time, she found herself wanting to imagine instead that Mum was sitting beside her right now on the sofa. Immediately a mental image of her became so vivid that it was like sitting next to her ghost. Lucille could have gone dizzy with shock because it was if Mum was right there smiling at her, and what made her more real than anything was that fact that she could *smell* her right next to her too, that lovely mother fragrance that was like no one else in the world. It was ten years since she had last breathed it in. So she inhaled slowly and deeply through her nose, smiling secretly to herself. It was so wonderful to have her there beside her that all her fear melted away.

Hi Mum.

Hello, hen.

She would let herself fall into *her* arms and these two would never know it. There. That felt better.

She picked a short grey hair off the front of her skirt. It could only have belonged to Scharff, she realised, wanting to flick it back at him and immediately wash her hands. She glanced at him with a shudder of distaste and deposited it in the bin beside her. *Black can be so difficult,* she heard Mum saying beside her, *everything shows up on it.*

It felt so nice having Mum there, that she wanted Rose to join them too. Sit on her other side. She'd really be alright then, sitting between them and it wouldn't matter then that Grainne hadn't actually arrived.

She pictured her mother at her most glamorous in the yellow Taffeta dress and the little matching Spanish hat she wore to the school Water Sports Day one summer. She was much the most beautiful lady present, all her friends told her later. Sitting here now she felt so proud that nothing could daunt her.

In contrast, she pictured Rose in the old clothes she had first seen her in when they met again in Holland Park having had neither sight nor sound of each other for seven or eight years. The clothes were clean now and the gash in the hip of her skirt where her bread knife had cut it when Ronnie knocked her over had been mended as if it never been there.

Hi Rose.

They are menials, my darling, don't let them get to you.

Lucille imagined the two of them both sitting there happily, one on each side of her and felt serene. She actually felt so safe surrounded by ghosts she could hardly believe it. She wanted to laugh out loud. Instead she looked at Carole and said,

'Understanding, and more, was what she gave me.' She was ready to answer their questions now. 'She gave me everything my mother gave me. She gave me my self, and I would *never* have killed her if that's what you two are wondering.' Her smile at Scharff and Jones was almost kind. Not having known Rosie or Mum they also couldn't know what she meant, even if she took all day to explain. So in the kind of sing-song voice she used to affect all the time when she was nervous, she smiled at each in turn and hardly feeling nervous at all asked them, 'What else would you like to know?'

'What kind of understanding?'

'The understanding kind, of course! The kind that doesn't assault you or arrest you or make you feel small. The kind that holds you and cares for you and sings to you and makes sure you're alright. Do you know what I mean?'

Scharff harrumphed, not interested.

'I think Carole meant: how did she show it? What form did er, er—

'Rose. Her name was Rose, as you know perfectly well.'

'Yes, thank you. A momentary lapse. My sincere apologies. What form did Rose's understanding actually take?'

387

'She looked after me when I had no future. She gave me my life.'

'And then you took her husband,' Scharff said, nodding his head.

Her instinct was to become defensive, to tell him the truth, to say, no, he was remarried and on the verge of divorcing his second wife when I first met him, but Rose frowned at her and shook her head, intimating that telling him the truth in this way would gratify him too much as it would be just the kind of response he was looking for. So she said nothing and glared at him, agreeing with Rose and telling herself she wouldn't let him get to her no matter how hard he tried. She would *not* let herself be pushed around and she would *not* be bullied. She would not.

'No offence intended,' he said, 'of course, but that's what it boiled down to, isn't it?'

Lucille tilted her head, smiled her sweetest smile at him and without warning found herself flashbacked into childhood. Almost blinded by its intensity she was transported back to a long forgotten memory of Water Sports Day at school when she was ten years old and could remember every detail so well that for the first instant it was like it was happening all over again:

She had had a natural talent she hadn't had a clue about until the kind Miss Holmes who had a beak instead of a nose, poor thing, but who would otherwise have been as beautiful as her mother, encouraged her with a few simple instructions. The school had a small outdoor pool built in more optimistic times some years before. With Miss Holmes's support the little boy she was then had been performing precise splashless arcs from the spring board, and back-flipping perfectly from the high board all week in the run-up to the final on that flaming Friday afternoon. Everybody had been telling her that she would win, and she had wanted to believe it, to try and ignore the fact that it was a complete fluke that she could dive at all considering she hadn't been taught for more than a few weeks and could hardly even swim. She'd never been good at anything before except maybe drama and domestic science and then only when she wasn't in a daydream. Her pride about being good at something compensated for the shame of having to expose her upper body in boy's swimming trunks. They were bright scarlet, baggy and long so she could feel they were nearly like a skirt around her small body. She caught sight of Mum waving to her among the spectators as she climbed the last few steps onto the high board and waved back. She had turned flamboyantly at the top, like a Spanish dancer, to fix her toes on the edge of the board. Then, just as she was readying herself and all the school and all the parents, what few there were, had hushed, Barry White, (for obvious reasons, his name was still unforgettable), who was by an open window with his mates in one of the upstairs classrooms which faced out towards the pool, had said something stupid about girlie-boys. The people below beside the pool probably didn't hear him, but up there on the board *she* did. She also heard his cronies' sycophantic laughing. She tossed her head ignoring them, then pushed her unfashionably long hair behind each ear as she prepared to take her dive. In so doing she inadvertently looked up into the sun. Temporarily blinded, she waited for what felt like forever for her vision to come back and lost all her focus as throats cleared below and the sound of whisperings started to mount. Again she heard what she was sure was Barry's voice whisper loudly about chickens. Several silly squawking noises followed. So she hurried, half slipped as she went up onto her toes, tried to make the dive anyway. But it was really a fall and she belly-flopped, landing with a loud, painful smack on the water with less grace than a pancake on a kitchen floor and a great deal more of a splash. Under the surface she swam to the steps wanting to cry, but managing not to. It wasn't the first time she had ever been humiliated. Skin smarting, she got out of the pool pretending her pride was still intact and wrapping herself in her towel went round to meet Mum. She heard a few sniggers from Barry and the boys about the way she now had her towel done up high over her nipples and under her armpits like a girl. Teachers and parents muttered, and the lovely Miss Holmes pointedly led the clapping. Turning failure into success Luke Farouk, who knew she was Lucille really, had waved, proud of what she could have done if things had been different, took happy little steps, almost skipping her way back to Mum, deliberately mincing, like she was on the catwalk in a fashion show, basking in all the attention she was getting. She hadn't failed. She'd been put off by a bully. That was all. There was no shame in that. She held her head up high as Mum embraced her, sat her on her lap and rubbed her down warmly. From the comfort of Mum's breast with her thumb in her mouth she just stared at Barry and his little gang emerging from the school block. If she was crying, she didn't care. She really didn't. When the final relay event was over and she got off Mum's lap there was a big dark damp patch right across the front of her lovely yellow skirt, but Mum hadn't cared about that, not minded it at all. She had been proud too.

Lucille pushed this memory away, shaking her head and returning to the here and now sitting, as she still imagined, between Rose and Mum, with Scharff and Jones opposite her like dogs so excited by her scent they didn't care they were swimming in a sewer. If they were going to bully her, she would dive in with them and bully them back. That's what she would do. She certainly wouldn't let herself mind about their unpleasantness, or the scary sense of doom identical to what she had felt on that day on the diving board. She knew that if she descended to their level, whatever she did in this sewer of theirs, she would, like them, sadly come out of it smelling of shit. There was not other word for it.

And they gave her no choice, so she might as well get on with it.

Amazingly her back felt alright now. She had a spine again, she felt empowered. She would execute a perfect jack-knife and twist.

She readied herself, heard Mum saying *go on you can do it*, and made her sweetest smile at the police even more dazzling. She nodded her head and steadied herself, Rose massaging her back one last time and giving her a final reminder that – *quite right* – she was *not* going to let these two make a victim of her because she, Rose, wasn't going to let her. Lucille took a deep breath and then she went, with a perfect arc into her dive, saying,

'And I find the manner in which you asked that question extremely rude, Detective Inspector. I would like to complain to your superiors. Is that possible, Carole? I don't think he can just walk into people's homes and insult them like this. Do you?'

Heart beating over-time, she shook her head, camping up the tuts and sighs and blinking and shaking her head, then looking at Carole for confirmation that what she was saying must surely be true. Discomforted, Carole's face changed colour and she looked at Scharff.

'Alright. That's it!' He said, glaring at his colleague with fixed angry smile.

He spoke so loudly that if Lucille didn't jump out of her seat, Rosie and Mum certainly must have done so, because with his shout they were both gone again as if they had never been there. Straightaway Lucille felt scared and alone once more, frightened of this brute of a man. To assert herself she had had to dive into the doo-doo. The dive was over and she was as deep in shit as she had ever been in her life, but she felt proud of herself all the same for taking him on. He strode over to her hallway and returned with his jacket

'Detective Sergeant Jones, we're going back down to the station. I like to do everything above board and by the book, *Madame* McElvey, and if you wish to make a complaint you have every right to do so. We will continue this interview on video down at the station so that we can have a full, accurate and visible record of our interview and you can have a legal or para-legal representative with you. I will furnish you with details as to how to make your complaint when we are down there. In the meantime it is my duty to inform you that I am now arresting you in order that you may help us with our enquiries. Would you kindly read this person the caution again, Detective Sergeant Jones, whether she or he wants you to or not, and then we will all make our way back together. Thank you.'

*   *   *

Four hours later she still hadn't been properly interviewed. Scharff and Jones left her with a uniformed WPC who went through her belongings in the presence of slim young Asian man in his early thirties who said he was the Station Sergeant and got her to sign a document she didn't look at, after her bag was taken away from her. They wanted her shoes as well, but just then Scharff came out of the gents loo and shook his head. 'It's okay. Leave them, they haven't got laces.'

The WPC took her by the elbow showed her to a cell and locked her in.

She immediately sat on the bench and stared at the oppressive proximity of the whited brick walls. They were thick with paint as if they had to be redone every few weeks. White had always been her favourite colour, she reminded herself, trying to stay positive now the arc of her dive was over and she was swimming in a cesspool.

It was shocking, absolutely shocking and she found herself shaking like a leaf.

She thought about Grainne. She had given up any hope of seeing her now, but wondered what *she* would do if she was in this situation and this was happening to her. Grainne would certainly be telling her off for being willing to talk earlier – not that she had – and she would be advising her to say nothing more now until she did actually have someone with her. She had wanted Carole to ring Paula to come, but apparently that wasn't an option either, as she was a possible witness in the event of a prosecution, so she had to have someone one else. Lucille couldn't think of anyone so the Jones woman said she'd arrange for the duty solicitor to come and see her. Then they would want to interview her.

Lucille tried not to panic, to stay calm, think normal thoughts. This cell wouldn't be too bad, she thought, if they just put a bunch of flowers on the window sill and maybe brought in a little coffee table or a bookshelf and some magazines so that people had something to do while they waited for the due process of the law to take its course. She would tell them that as a kindness when her solicitor arrived and they came to get her.

These last few days had changed her. It would never again be so easy to hide behind a show of simpering grace or serene politeness, because somehow with their dying Richard and Rose had left a part of themselves behind with her. Neither of them had ever possessed such dubious qualities themselves and they'd never personally been interested in them in her either. But she couldn't help thinking that if only she had used one or the other with Scharff earlier she might not now be sitting here sadly realising stupidity and injustice were not just other people's problems.

She wanted to cry, instead she steeled herself. She would be strong. She would use a combination of Richard's skill at social manipulation, driven by Rose's wilfulness to play these people at their own game. Her days of cloying acquiescence were over. They had to be. The thought of prison was just too scary. She would be sent to Holloway probably. They surely couldn't remand her in a men's prison, could they? Perhaps they could. She felt so frightened she wanted to scream, like she was a child having a nightmare whose mother would come running as soon as she heard her.

She turned angrily on herself, demanding that such feelings went away. This was not time for feelings and she wasn't going to behave like a child. She was determined they weren't going to remand her at all. She would fight for her freedom, with teeth and claws if necessary.

She *was* innocent, after all.

But what could she do?

It had been really helpful imagining Mum and Rose being with her in her imagination before they brought her here. She would do the same thing with Richard while she sat and waited for her solicitor and her food to come, see what effect his presence might have on her. Imagine what he might say. When he had been able to talk she had long stopped listening to him. It would be good to listen to him now.

She couldn't remember ever having such an active imagination in her life before. The effect of fear on her was like she had taken drugs or something.

She sat back against the hard wall and closing her eyes envisaged Richard in his prime when she was still madly in love with him and before he started treating her in private as he had always done in public, as his trophy wife. She imagined him in the blue pinstripe suit she thought he looked best in at the time – without a tie – in the kind of thoughtful reflective state he came home with in the evenings after work, his eyes lighting up at the sight of her in that way that later would annoy her so, but which now prompted a wistful smile. She found herself recalling him speaking to her about the difficulties involved in trying to tell at least five or six people each week that they were dying. It had been his main preoccupation for a while to find a personal blueprint, a standard script he could feel comfortable with for telling people the worst. But as he had said, quoting her mother, it takes all sorts to make a world, and in the end he had reached the conclusion that the only formula he could follow was that you have to be guided by what people needed from you.

She closed her eyes and in her mind leaned against the man that he was then, letting him hold her and telling him what she needed from him. What shall I do, Richard? Tell me how to get out of this mess, please. She wondered what he would say, and immediately it came to her. As someone who seemed to love his own power, Scharff was likely to be afraid of someone who pushed powerfully back.

She felt like wailing that that was what Rose had suggested and look where it had got her.

So she was sceptical. What can I *do*, Richard? He was silent and she slumped and felt her back pain again. She wasn't powerful at all.

She straightened back up. She must *not* be weak and wobbly. The worst thing about the police perception of her as a criminal was that it was just so wrong. And so un*real*. She was not the person they were trying to fit her up as at all. It made her so mad that they could be doing this to an innocent person.

She heard Richard and Rose's voice ringing with that sentiment too, encouraging her to be furious with Scharff and Jones for completely and wilfully misperceiving her like this. They should be objectively looking for the truth, not building a case against her. It was horrible.

There was the sound of footsteps outside in the corridor, then the automated whirr of deadbolts being electronically withdrawn. A uniformed woman came in with Scharff. She had natural, orangey red hair tied in a pony and was bearing a tray. Without giving Lucille even half a glance she put the tray down on the bench beside her, announced that the plastic cutlery should be treated carefully because it easily broke. Lucille smiled at her anyway, thanked her and watched her leave again. Her hair colour reminded her of Grainne's.

She was alone with the professional shit swimmer.

'I just came back to inform you Detective Sergeant Jones and I spoke to your friend, Mrs

Paula Stone earlier this morning. She confirmed that last week you told her that Dr McElvey had repeatedly made it clear that he wanted to be killed. She also said that you had refused to even consider it.'

Lovely, lovely Paula.

She smiled sweetly up at the revolting man who was standing far too close for comfort. She recoiled away without him noticing, drew her knees closer together and raised her eyebrows. How dare he stand so close! Did what he had just said mean she was going to be released then?

Her heart leapt into her throat, her eyes felt like popping.

'However, she also said that you had admitted to '*feeling like killing him sometimes.*' She said it was understandable, anybody would in your situation, but I told her I didn't join the CID, more than fifteen years ago now, to let murderers get away with their crimes – that not everybody would actually carry out such a dreadful deed, so everybody at whom the finger of suspicion even briefly points has to be investigated, if only to eliminate them from the enquiry. You have not yet been formally interviewed and I so am not at this point, I'm afraid, able to consider letting you go.'

What did he mean he was 'afraid'? It was her who was afraid. The monster was such a liar. But was he trying to be friendly again? He had been so rude in her flat. And why was he talking so much? It wasn't as if she needed to know the finer points of police procedural thinking. But, Paulie, how could you have told him that? Probably because it was evidence as far as she was concerned that she would never have actually done it. But, of course, a policeman wouldn't see it that way at all.

'In fact, in court,' Scharff continued, his revolting gaze fixed on her breasts rather than her face. 'Her testimony on its own would be enough to convict some people. Together with the receipt, the deliberately spilled splashes of cooking oil, and the will, and some further reports from the pathologist suggesting that both of the deceased sustained some physical injuries before the fire actually started, I think there is little doubt that we have sufficient corroborating evidence to ensure that you will be successfully tried for double murder, and are likely to have to remain in custody for a very long time indeed.' He leered triumphantly. 'As I think Detective Sergeant Jones explained, in view of the fact that Mrs Stone may be required to submit a statement or be subpoenaed as a prosecution witness, I fear I cannot let her be your personal advisor at this time. The duty solicitor will be along, shortly and then we'll begin your interview,' he said. 'Madame.'

He made to go, adjusting his trousers at the same time. Her eyes were briefly drawn down to what looked odiously like arousal. She didn't feel so overwhelmed by what he had just said that she couldn't look at his fat face with disgust. She glared at him with all the disdain she could muster, hating him.

Then she felt stupid.

Suppressing all hint of her own embarrassment about what she was doing and even though it required a complete perversion of what she actually felt, she tried to turn her look of hate into one of longing for him.

And failed. It felt ridiculous, and he grinned unpleasantly, seeing right through her to someone she wasn't, a murderess, and now an old whore. Flushing, she shook her head, and resisted sticking her tongue out or throwing her food tray at him. She stared instead at the shit-white wall and he left, his triumph rampant. She heard the deadbolts clunking into place behind him.

It was his power over her that had turned him on, not her.

So she had humiliated herself. Again.

Oh well! There were worse things to have done.

What now?

Grainne! Where was she? Why hadn't she come? Although she wasn't dead – at least – oh God! – she hoped she wasn't – Lucille wanted to do the same imagining exercise with her that she had done with

394

Richard, Rose and Mum, imagine she was here now in the cell with her, advising her. But she wasn't able to imagine anymore. Not here. Not now

Then her imaginative faculty returned.

Simple, she imagined Grainne saying with an evil grin, *beat yourself up before your solicitor arrives and say it was him. They'll throw the case out before it's started! You've just been alone with that fat bastard in your cell. You won't get a better opportunity.* But that would mean a split lip or horrible black eyes, and hurting! I don't like pain. I can't *bear* it, and why should I have to?

Do you want to forever be known as 'Transsexual Wife who Slayed her Disabled Husband'?

Lucille shook her head. Why in her imagination did everyone close to her take the same line?

She took the plastic lid off the food on the tray, looked at the fluorescent pink ham, soggy lettuce and celery inside. Yuck. She couldn't eat a thing. But that didn't mean she felt like beating herself up. She felt shaky, uncertain, and so lonely. Being reduced to imagining her loved ones were here and recommending resistance by harming herself was so desperate. And wrong.

A little money spider, brown against the black of her top and too small to be scary, was making its way purposefully down her front from her shoulder. She put a finger below it and after a little hesitation it climbed on. She moved the tray of food on to the floor, climbed up onto the bench and tried to place it on the window sill. It didn't want to leave her. She didn't want to hurt it, so she let it start climbing hurriedly back up her sleeve.

For some reason it reminded of her Ronnie. She could forgive him now for what he had done. He had been scared. She could well understand that now, she really could. Being scared makes you want to do things you shouldn't. If she ever got out of this mess she would tell him that. Being scared made you prepared to do anything. She could understand that now and she could forgive him for it.

She got down off the bench, as she did so accidentally placing the pointy toe of her shoe too near the edge of her food tray causing it to tip the tray up a tiny bit and spilling water and vegetables onto the floor beside. Sighing, she sat down and used the very small tissue on the tray to mop up some of the water from the floor. It was fully soaked before she had made any inroads on it at all. She dropped the wet tissue on the tray and glared at her own incompetence. It was so vexing, she could have really done with a little drink of water but now it wasn't possible. She could be so contrary sometimes. She bunged the bits of salad back on the tray and slumped back against the wall.

She tried to justify giving herself bruises. She would definitely have had some sympathy for someone else doing that if they were in this position because it was as if Scharff was beating her up anyway by fitting her up like this. Leaving marks on herself would just go to show it. It would be him doing it really. Not her. She would never have dreamed of behaving in such a way herself. Never.

With an only half-ironic shrug of thanks to her imaginary Grainne for her ever-so-not-very helpful suggestion, she gritted her teeth and closed her eyes. Deliberately hitting yourself was such an evil thing to do. She knew it was, but she couldn't see any alternative. She had to do it to give herself a chance of being freed. Two wrongs don't make a right, but in this case the wrong she was about to do would have to make an exception. She gritted her teeth, felt as if she was back on that high diving board at school determined to do her best however bad it was.

She readied herself; raised her arms up wondering if it would hurt her hands as well as her face to slap herself and tried to look at them as if they were someone else's; steadied herself by taking a deep breath and holding it; told herself that when she let her breath out again it would be time to go, to just get on with it.

She exhaled.

But she couldn't. She just couldn't.

It simply wasn't possible, not for her.

Agitation about this prompted her to get up, pace around the cell. Without concentrating on what she was doing she stood up too fast and too carelessly, slipped on the spilt water beneath her feet and went flying, banging the side of her head against the brickwork of the wall and knocking herself out cold. In the instant of losing consciousness she found herself drifting in a dreamlike state of enhanced imagining and emotional disconnection. The last thing she knew, a multitude of judges with angels' wings were all giving her a perfect ten for her dive off Beachy Head as she floated serenely upon the surface of the dark brown sea, staring up at the sun.

Twenty minutes later Detective Sergeant Carole Jones came to escort her up to the interview room to meet her solicitor and take a formal statement from her. Though she was still lying face down on the floor, Lucille was conscious again. She could remember nothing of her fall or the blow to her head, but realised what must have happened from the dampness of her skirt and the hardness of the floor beneath her. The sensation of pain in her head felt a bit like waking up after facial plastic surgery had twenty years before. She felt strangely safe, as if nothing they could do to her emotionally would really perturb her at all now her head was hurting. For a brief, panicky moment she wondered whether she had attacked herself after all. She could certainly now understand Grainne in a way that she never had before. The skin on her forehead and around her right eye felt terribly tight, it was certainly bruised and swollen and might have split in places. She could not feel any enjoyment in it, hoped there would be no scarring. She could taste blood. She must look frightful. If only they had allowed her to keep her bag she could have looked in her mirror.

Through her unhurt eye she could see Carole kneeling down on one knee on the ground beside her looking at her worriedly. Good.

'Hi, sweetie,' said Lucille.

'What happened?'

'I'm so sorry. I'm ready to see my solicitor now.'

'I'll have to call the duty PS first to have a look at you, see what he says about your fitness to see the solicitor. You may have to go to hospital. How did this happen? No. I'm sorry. Not now. Don't try and tell me, Lucille. You need medical attention first.'

'P S?'

'Police Surgeon – doctor. We have one on twenty four hour call. I've only got first aid training. You've hurt your head. You mustn't be moved. Or try to move'

Lucille attempted a grateful, graceful smile. She was wet and she wanted to get up. She heaved herself up onto one side, then lay back down again on her back

Life was so strange. All she had ever wanted was to be normal and it seemed as if normality was the one thing she had never had. So in a curious detached way what was happening now seemed as if it was something she was accustomed to. All she had ever known for certain in her life was who she was, but now even that was gone. The illusion of respectable married womanhood with a disabled husband and a part time lover was history. She was a sorry slab of meat on the floor of a police cell.

Two or three minutes later the Jones woman was back with a large hairy man of about Lucille's own age with a swarthy olive Mediterannean appearance. His white shirt sleeves were rolled up and he carried a medical case. He immediately got down on his knees, started feeling for her pulse. Then he held her face gently in his hands and studied her bruises by sight and by feel with his fingers. She liked the sensation and squinted at him through the slit which was all that her left eyelid would allow. He looked vaguely familiar, certainly she felt she had never seen such hairy arms before except on – on who? Oh yes, on David, the first boy she had had sex with after her operation. This couldn't be him, could it? He wouldn't be too pleased to see her, if it was. She had unceremoniously dumped him after he became embarrassing with his declarations of undying love twenty years ago. He had raped her hadn't he, sort of anyhow, didn't stop when she had asked him to anyway. And hurt her. If it was him, he had put on a lot of weight and lost most of the hair on his head. She might normally have been intrigued to meet him again, but not under these circumstances. She closed her eyes.

He probably wouldn't recognise her anyway under all this swelling, she thought, as he asked her to try to open her eyes and follow his finger with them. She couldn't open her left eye but she opened her right which was fine and watched his forefinger move from left to right and up and down. When she returned her gaze to him as he wrote something down on a pad of paper beside him, she was sure he didn't realise he had once known her, if it *was* him. Thank goodness her name was McElvey now, not Farouk. And what a small world it was. Or did this kind of thing only happen to her?

He took a little torch which seemed to also double up as some kind of microscope or something, lifted her eyelids and got down right up close to look, he said, for any damage to the retina. Gentle as he was, it still hurt more than the actual fall had and she combined a long wince and a sigh with all the silent grace of a screen goddess. That's what *she* thought anyway. He asked her if she had lost consciousness at all. She didn't reply.

'How did this happen?' Carole asked from beside him. 'How did you do this to yourself?'

'I don't think she did,' said the doctor who looked like David. 'I'm not a pathologist but I would say this injury is consistent with having been attacked – hit – by someone else, I'm afraid. She is not a big woman. She hasn't got the weight and she wouldn't have the strength to do this to herself even if she had wanted to.' He picked up her be-ringed left hand. 'It was a breach of procedure not to take her jewellery from her when you arrested her, wasn't it? One really wonders what goes on at this station sometimes. How long has she been held here?'

'Only about three quarters of an hour,' Carole Jones replied in a sombre voice.

'I would say that this has certainly been done within that time,' he said.

'Schar–

'No! That's just not possible.' Jones interrupted her before she could go any further. 'But she was absolutely fine when I brought her down here.'

'Who's been in since?'

'Only my boss and the WPC who brought the food tray in.'

'Scharff did it,' Lucille whispered with as much pathos as she could. It was a good performance and both the doctor and Jones looked shocked. She found this curiously upsetting. She would have started shaking her head if it had not hurt so much. Instead she just winced. It was no good. She couldn't lie either. 'No, he didn't,' she said. 'I was joking.'

Neither of them smiled.

'He didn't,' said Carole. 'He couldn't have.'

'I'm anyway going to have to report this to the Station Officer and write it up for the Commander who can decide what to do about it.'

He pointed to Lucille's right hand which was now lying palm down on her tummy. 'Look, there would be swelling on her knuckles as well if she had been punching herself. The swelling on the side of her head is extensive, it's even under her hair. It may be just tissue damage – she has sensitive skin, but as a precaution she needs to be taken to hospital right now for an EEG, MRI, the works.'

'MRI?'

'Brain scan. She might have had a cranial haemorrhage, possibly a stroke. With all this damage she needs her head examined.'

Well that had always been necessary, thought Lucille.

'I want to plead guilty,' she said exercising her prerogative to change her mind. 'Scharff didn't do it. I did. I'm a slapper,' she said. 'And I want to confess to murder.' She smiled through her pain. 'Although I warn you, I might always change my mind.'

Chapter 24.

'Talk to me, Ron, please, or I'll fall asleep at the wheel.'

The traffic on the M1 was heavy as they got closer to London.

'You are the only one I ever really loved, Grainne. I mean, I love Lulu too, but it's not the same. I would have married you.'

'Oh, would you! I think I would have had some say in that, thank you, and believe me, it would *never* have happened. Anyway, after what you've done I don't actually believe you,' she said, concentrating on the road, occasionally nipping into the middle lane to overtake the slower trucks and coaches on the inside, so-called slow lane. She liked the slow lane, it could be so much faster.

'Well, you should believe me, Grainne. I wasn't myself yesterday, or last night. I was all paranoid, but I'm better now.'

'If you can change so suddenly you can also change back. So I don't trust you one little bit. What's actually made you stop being so paranoid all of a sudden? I think you are just manipulating me, Ronald, because you have got no choice.'

He shook his head in denial.

'Don't argue with me, Ron. If I hadn't woken you at six o clock this morning, waved the phone in your face and told you Sean knew everything and would be on his way to the police himself if he didn't get a call from Lucille by midday to say everything's alright, you would not now be coming with me to Eastbourne to repair the damage you've done, would you? Not at all! You would still be keeping me under house arrest; a jailor at my own front door, my own fucking front door!'

She hated him. He was only accompanying her on this journey down to Eastbourne because she had insisted on it. He had got to repair the damage he had done. When all this was over, she would never have anything directly to do with him ever again.

'I don't know. Maybe you're right, but that's not what I feel,' he replied without a trace of shame. 'What I feel is you.' She was aware of him looking at her, idealising her like the big baby he was. It made her feel so uncomfortable that had things been different she would have simply stopped the car and told him to get out.

'Change the subject, Ron. You're record is stuck'

'*You've* stopped me,' he blathered on. 'What you say may be true; I mean it is true, but it is all incidental. I don't deny I want our son not to be ashamed of me. That is true. And I don't want Lulu for go down for something she didn't do, not any more, but it is *you* who's stopped me. I shouldn't have done what I did. I know that now.'

Grainne shook her head from side to side, trying to control her anger with him and concentrate on her driving. A large truck was tailgating her. She felt like suddenly braking, teaching the truck driver a lesson, giving Ron whiplash and getting a new car from the insurance all in one go. Instead, as law-abiding, courteous road user she put her foot down on the accelerator.

'You can *not* just suddenly change, just like that, overnight.' she said, between gritted teeth once there was a safe enough distance between herself and the lorry.

'It wasn't sudden. Listening to you talking last night made me realise that what I'd really been feeling all along underneath was, well, it was what you were saying last night, that I was being selfish, unthinking, not really following my feelings at all, just trying to tell myself that I was. I was anxious and frightened and I thought that was a feeling. But you weren't frightened of me last night and I realised fear isn't a feeling, it's an angry short-sighted sensation banging away inside your skull, like a wasp or a hornet or something, buzzing against a window pane.' He looked at her again. 'You helped me let it out. Feelings exist in relationships.'

'Jesus Christ, Ron!' she almost screamed. 'I cannot believe how, inspite of everything, inspite of the fact that you are a mad as a hatter, you are also a complete phoney! About as genuine as,' she couldn't think. 'I don't know.' Seeing her thumbs on the steering wheel, she nodded. 'As the colour on my finger nails.' Her anger did not dissipate.

She was aware of him staring at her as she spoke.

'Stop looking at me like that, Ron. It is irritating and it's putting me off my driving. If you do mean what you say, then prove it. Prove you are not just talking. Prove you care. Prove Sean and Lucille are actually real to you and that you've got real relationships with them by doing the right thing.'

'I want to,' he said uncertainly, 'I will. But then what?' He shrugged. 'What will I have achieved?'

'Does telling the truth have to achieve anything?' She asked with withering scorn. Can't you just show your love for what it is? No, of course you can't. Everything for you always has to be about something else, doesn't it? You are such an arsehole, Ron. You truly, truly are.'

'I suppose so,' he said. 'But really, why do I need to prove I mean what I say? Who needs to know? I know I'm telling the truth.'

'*You* are such a fucking narcissist, Ron. You'll never get it, will you? Never! I'll try to put it to you straight, one last time, in words of one syllable.' Her voice rose an octave. 'Who needs to know you mean it when you say you care? Well, *you* do, you selfish eedjit, and actions speak louder than words, don't they?! Lucille does too. She *really* does. She is in trouble because of you. I do too. And Sean does! When I told him what you'd done on the phone a few hours ago, he said he was going to kill you. He did not sound as if he was simply expressing his feelings, Ron.'

She was actually worried about Sean. When they had spoken on the phone a few hours ago he had simply said his father was a bastard and he would kill him. Don't do that, she'd replied, all reason and common sense, Ron and I will be gone in a few minutes. Let yourself into the flat when you arrive and if Auntie Lucille or myself haven't rung you by midday, just get in touch with the police and tell them what I've told you. She didn't want her lovely son getting himself into trouble as well, doing something stupid. But then he had telephoned her from his mobile saying he'd borrowed a car and was going to follow them down. Ron was ranting at the time and she had felt it politic not to say too much to Sean in case Ron lost it again. Their differences over Sean had invariably been the main bone of contention between them these last few years.

'How?' Ron asked, with more certainty and determination in his voice.

'How what?' she replied, distracted. She must try ringing Sean again when she stopped and could get out of the car and speak to him out of Ron's hearing.

'How do I make everything right again and get Lucille off the hook?' Ron asked.

'I don't know. I don't care *how* you do it. Just tell the police the truth.'

This morning after phoning Sean, Grainne had kicked the great lug awake, showed him she'd got her phone back, told him she had used it and insisted he was coming with her down to Eastbourne to tell the police he had concocted a lie to frame Lucille with. He grumbled and groaned, but got up off the floor, docile and compliant, having been woken from his sleep into an apparently more honest, less barking state of mind. They had a quick cup of coffee which she made with two heaped teaspoons to help them stay awake and then went down to the car and set off for the south coast. Ever since then, he had been going round in circles castigating himself for shopping Lucille, repeatedly regretting he'd followed his feelings, as he put it. They weren't to be trusted.

God, he was moronic

It was ten past eleven in the morning now. Sod's law had decreed that there should be an accident amongst the road works on the M1 and the journey down to the M25 which should have taken an hour or an hour and a half had taken four. Half an hour ago as they slowly filtered through more motorway road works she had been rung by Lucille's friend Paula who had been distraught. She had told the truth and now regretted it terribly, she said, to a man and a woman who had identified themselves as plain clothes CID officers when they came round to see her in her office at 9:30 am. She had found their purposefulness menacing. They said they'd had come to 'chat' with her about Lucille's relationship with Richard of all things, and then informed her in no uncertain terms that they would 'almost undoubtedly' be interviewing her again more formally at a later stage. She had felt very frightened as they assured her she was not herself being investigated in connection with any crime, and were confident she did not need telling that she should not interfere with police business by alerting Lucille to the fact that they'd been asking questions about her, because that would be an offence for which she could be charged and if found guilty, imprisoned. Before they went they told her about Richard and Rose's deaths. It put all their earlier questions and the way they looked at each other when they heard her answers into shocking context. It had made Paula feel sure they intended to obtain a warrant for Lucille's arrest straight away. She'd felt shaken, tricked into compromising her friend. For a while afterwards she'd felt paralysed, till it occurred to her to call directory enquiries for the number of O'Riordan Real Estates, knowing Grainne was Lucille's oldest friend. Once she'd explained to Linda at the office that she needed to contact Grainne urgently on a personal matter, Linda had given her her mobile number. What had they asked her about? Richard wanting to die and Lucille's response to it. They had been very interested, far too interested she felt, when she told them Lucille had last week admitted to her she did sometimes *feel* like killing him, weren't interested at all in the fact that she'd been adamant that *actually* she wouldn't.

That call had made Grainne feel even mores anxious on Lucille's behalf than she had before. She'd tried ringing Lucille again just now, but got no reply, had to leave a message. She was probably 'helping police with their enquiries' at this very moment, poor thing. What with the circumstantial evidence of the receipts, they probably felt they had enough to keep her in custody, for a while anyway. It was a mess. Ron must tell the police the whole truth.

'That would prove you care and that you are not a liar anymore, and it will get her out of jail. Because that's where I think she is right now, thanks to you.'

'Yes, but *how*?' he repeated. 'I don't know how. If I tell them I was lying yesterday about Lulu they might arrest me.' Grainne was aware of him shaking his head and gave him a quick glance. He did look very torn, both frightened and determined not to be, which was a good sign. He was going to need to be determined when they finally got to the police station in Eastbourne. 'It was my stupid fear of arrest that started me off in the first place and I've fucked Lulu over because of it.'

'At least you're trying to understand it and make amends now,' she replied in a more soothing voice. He needed support or he would chicken out.

He over-reacted, became embarrassingly effusive.

'I do love you. I still love you, Grainne,' he said. 'I haven't changed at all. Not in how I feel about you.'

'You don't *know* me, Ron. Not anymore, and you never did. Not really. Who you love is your own fantasy, that's all. Not me at all. I don't know about Lucille. Maybe that's a bit more real if only because you've been having sex together, but it showed no care of her whatsoever getting her into trouble so you could avoid it yourself.'

'I love you,' he insisted. Then he narrowed his eyes. 'But I don't want to be arrested.'

'You don't know how to love. What you did to Lucille yesterday wasn't loving at all. It was completely despicable. To be loving you have got to think about how you are you going to get her out of the mess you've got her in, and then you have to do it.'

'I don't know.'

'Think about it, Ron, please, between now and Eastbourne. Lucille is my friend and your girlfriend andd we are going to be loyal to her whatever it takes. Either you think of something or your son will go to the police about you. And I promise you I will not stop him.'

'You don't have to threaten me, Grainne. I'm going to do the right thing. I just don't know what it is yet.'

She bit her lip. He was right she should not threaten him. Her own life had been ruined right at the outset by bullying and threats. It was just that she was so fed up with lies and the effects of lies. She'd hadn't really known either of them very well, but she felt some admiration for Richard and Rose. If their deaths weren't an accident then the only credible alternative was that they must have entered into some kind of suicide pact together. She had, at least in part, to admire that, although there was an element of unkindness in the fact that they had not considered that Lucille would be heartbroken. That was selfish. But nobody's perfect and by killing themselves they had presumably managed to be loyal to the truth of what they felt inside.

Well, she wanted to be loyal to her friend. All her life, really, she had been loyal to Uncle Frank by finding ways of depersonalising herself, treating herself like someone without feelings. Prostitution and Estate Agency had both been about that. Now she wanted to be loyal to something better by being loyal to her friend and by not abusing Ron. He couldn't help it that he was such a stupid prick sometimes.

'You're right,' she said. 'That was a bit uncalled for. I am sorry. But, Ron, you – we – have got to think of way of getting her safely out from under the noses of the police. We need a strategy and a plan.'

They drove on in silence for a few miles, joined the M25 and headed east.

'Mad,' he said. 'I'll have to be mad. That way my lies will be seen for what they were, the paranoid ravings of a psychotic loser. If they still feel they have to arrest me they'll have to take me to hospital as a nutter rather than to jail as a criminal. Hospital I could cope with.'

'Brilliant. You're a genius,' she said, reaching over and patting his hand. She noticed her mobile sitting in its stand on her dashboard was off and felt angry with herself for leaving the car charging lead indoors. Her phone battery had run out.

*   *   *

At 2:00 pm that same day, roasting inside his lion suit, which the woman with damaged teeth in the fancy dress party hire shop had said was last used in an amateur dramatic company production for the part of the Cowardly Lion in The Wizard of Oz, Ron went into the police station in Eastbourne and demanded to see Detective Inspector Shaft. He had left Grainne in the nearby pub where he had changed into the costume. Thankful for small mercies, he was glad that at least it only had a hood with ears, not a complete face mask as well. The heat of that would really have been too much. You're supposed to use face paints with it, the woman in the shop had explained, showing them a full set of colours at a ridiculous price. They had declined her offer and just took the suit. Their plan was that he would retract everything he'd said to the police about Lucille and at the same time undermine all his credibility as a sane and respectable member of the human race. Grainne had wished him luck and didn't think he would find it too hard.

'Shaft was a black man,' Ron tried to say with righteous indignation when the smiling desk sergeant took the trouble to personally get Scharff from the main CID office to meet with him, presumably to watch his reaction. Covering up his own nervous grin by shifting his weight from foot to foot, Ron went on, 'A question has been bugging me ever since I first met you and it is, 'Why?'. Why have you hijacked the name of a fictional cinematic character, Officer Shaft? How can I tell who you really are, and how can I trust you with the information – the important information I have to impart – if I have to deal with a policeman who is clearly more than just institutionally racist, he is also pretentious enough to have appropriated the name of a famous African American detective from the seventies? It is extremely hard to take you seriously, under the circumstances, Detective Shaft. Extremely hard.'

'Scharff. My name is Scharff. My father was German. What is it you want to see me about so urgently, Dr Symes?'

'Ah! So?' Ron raised his eyebrows, which Grainne had made more leonine in the car with an eyebrow pencil, into a stereotyped nazi leer. 'But surely you cannot have a racist ancestry?' he said, bending his head back, flaring his nostrils, looking all around him then staring down his nose at Scharff. 'No, seeing all the politically correct posters around us here, I know I can be confident you would not have become a policeman if your father had been a racist or if you didn't care for all the colours, creeds, ethnicities, genders and such like which together make up the society you have committed yourself to serving and protecting so well. Completely confident.'

Ron solemnly nodded his head. Scharff's expression went satisfyingly near apoplectic, his face puce. Ron was pleased, almost triumphant to note he was having such an effect. It was so very strange that he, of all people, should be pretending to be mad. Despite his undoubted expertise, he wasn't sure he was actually putting on a very good performance though, and he really needed to. Scharff wasn't stupid. He would be able to see right through his pretence if his performance wasn't perfect. He was thankful he did have a certified mental health history to help him feel more confident in the role. If he provoked the man too much, or if he did manage to see through it for the charade it was, it would make him so unkindly disposed towards him that he might lock him up straight away. Nevertheless, Ron couldn't resist a further little dig. 'On the other hand, if your father wanted to come to this benighted country and he *was* a racist, he would have felt completely at home with its imperialist history and its oppression of minorities. So I really don't know. Have you been vetted by MI5 or the immigration authorities? Or did you perhaps come into the country under a lorry as an asylum seeker?'

'Make no mistake, Dr Symes, you will be arrested and charged if you continue with this insulting behaviour. Sergeant Harris said you wanted to see me about something? If you haven't come in to sign or to add to the statement you made over the phone yesterday which was automatically transcribed and is ready for you to sign should wish to do so, then kindly state your business. Or leave right now.'

It was time to get a bit loopier. Pick up on anything said to you and distort it, Grainne had suggested earlier. That's what you've always done when you're at your most deranged, so it should all come very easily and naturally. Combine grandeur and paranoia. You know how good you are at that.

'How can I shine anything out here?' Ron replied to Scharff in the best tone of dense moral outrage he could muster. 'I'm not going to polish my private business out here where people can observe me!'

'Polish?' Scharff echoed, cold intelligence finding him out for a phoney. Ron winced beneath the dim perplexity he was trying to put on his face.

Fuck it, it's too late to stop now.

'What if I was? What would that have got to do with anything?' Ron asked in the grand manner, before kindly condescending. 'But as it happens, no, I am not Polish. I'm as English as the next man. Well, not you, Shaft, but, you know what I mean.'

'I am not sure I followed you, sir, when you said you are not going to polish your private business?'

'Well, we're all square then because I didn't really understand what you meant by shining it. I can't believe you might be suggesting I change my statement? Are 'polishing' and 'shining' police euphemisms for altering it?'

'I said nothing about shining anything, Dr Symes.'

'What do you take me for, Commander? Just another member of the public? Well, I'll have you know I have some extremely important information which – make no mistake yourself, Shaft! – you will regret not hearing if you do not allow me to share it with you. In private. In one of your interview rooms please, not out here. You never know who else might be listening.' He leant forward and in a stage whisper, added, 'I do not trust your colleagues.'

Scharff looked at him with calculating jowls, making it clear he knew he was being set up, but for now was prepared to play along because he was intrigued as to why and, after all, this was his turf and he had the power. Despite the air-conditioning, Ron felt the heat turning up. He became even more sweaty inside his cowardly lion costume. His courage wobbled and his anxiety grew as Scharff let him through the door into the station proper and asked as did so,

'Why not? Do you wish to lay a complaint against an officer this station? You can do so in complete confidence.'

'Why do you think I am dressed like this?'

'Oh, I do like a guessing game!' said Scharff, rubbing his pudgy, pink hands together as if he had found him out and wanted to play along. 'Are you going to a party?' He asked with a disturbing jollity, clearly not phased at all by these antics. Beneath his costume Ron reminded himself he was doing this for Lucille and Grainne and Sean, but he felt his courage slipping further down as the detective continued in the same vein. 'Although that's unlikely at two o' clock on a Tuesday afternoon.' He pantomime-scratched the back of his head. 'Are you raising money for charity, perhaps? I don't know. You tell me.' He opened a door. 'In here.'

Scharff showed him into a room with a white plastic table which seemed to be bolted to the floor and on top of which was what looked like a small computer. Presumably it was used to record interviews. It was housed in a transparent box bolted to the table. Light-weight plastic chairs were arranged around the table and above it a one-way screen made it possible for people to look in on the room without being seen. On the other side of the room light from the afternoon sun streamed down through the closed windows onto the sills. There were no papers, no pictures or notices on the walls, nothing of any kind except the table, chairs and computer. The noticeable chill of the temperature in the room and the whirr of air conditioning coming down from the vents in the ceiling, told of the closed, artificial, yet functional environment he had so stupidly insisted on being seen in. He braced himself.

'I am doing it for you, Commander. I am wearing this costume in order that someone like you with a name like yours might take me more seriously than you would otherwise do.'

He felt a sneeze coming on. He made sure to express it as loudly as he could and then blew his nose with the end of his tail. He hoped he wasn't developing a summer cold. He sneezed again. He had once or twice suffered from hay fever over the years. Maybe that's what it was.

Scharff grinned, his face becoming as round, red and white as a poisonous toadstool.

'I wasn't born yesterday, Dr Symes. It may help you to know that I will not be riled by your attitude in any way, although I would like to understand it, if you wouldn't mind putting an end to this little charade. Nor, for your information, will the different titles you are giving me cause me any concern whatsoever. However, unless you get to the point I will have to have you taken to a holding cell until such time as you *are* ready so to do. Am I making myself clear?'

'Yes, thank you very much.'

'Well?'

'Well what?'

'What are you doing here, or have you simply come to undermine your credibility as a witness?'

It was Ron's turn to do apoplectic, but it wasn't an act. Fucking hell, the fat policeman had rumbled him before he had even sat down.

He sat down, thinking hard. Then he stood up again to sweep aside his tail which had nearly buggered him. If you can't beat them join them, he thought. But stay mad.

'We lions should stick together,' he said.

'Have you come to withdraw your statement? For your information I can tell you that finger prints on the olive oil bottle which was used to pour oil all over the kitchen in the first Mrs McElvey's house up in Balham and which was found in her rubbish bin outside her backdoor, matched those taken from her ten years before when, I believe, she was living on the streets of London and was more than once taken into temporary custody by my colleagues in the Metropolitan police. They are now of the opinion that that she herself started the fire. There is certainly insufficient evidence to charge anybody else at this time.'

Ron's elation was boundless. He was the king of beasts. He wanted to roar.

'So unless you have got anything else to say to me, I'm going to the holding cells now to tell er, the second Mrs McElvey that she can go. We no longer require her help with our enquiries.'

Ron reminded himself to admit nothing, avoid being charged for perjury or wasting police time.

Keep your feet on the ground till you've got out of here, he told himself, getting up out of his chair and resisting the temptation to whoop or get down on all fours on the floor and rub his head against the policeman's legs.

'I'd like to go now,' he said, pawing at the door and growling. A caged lion, but a coward no more.

'That's fine, sir. Please do. Mrs McElvey had a fall while in our custody but has refused to be taken to hospital, which our surgeon did advise her was necessary to rule out neurological complications. She may therefore be a little unsteady on her feet and need your help. But if you would like to wait, we will have processed her discharge within five or ten minutes.'

*   *   *

Three hours later Grainne and Ron came out of Accident and Emergency. Between them Lucille put on a pair of dark glasses and a white, wide-brimmed hat given to her by a plump, bespectacled middle-aged woman in pink and black. Sean thought she looked much better than she had before she went in. The bruise on her head was now discreetly screened and she was hanging onto their arms, apparently exclaiming how glad she was she had not cracked her skull or something. Sean couldn't really tell because from where he was he could not hear their conversation and could only surmise what they were saying. She no longer looked so pale or so shocked. He watched them saying goodbye to the plump woman and then piling into his mother's Toyota. Mum pulled out into the road with her customary speed and élan. She was a good driver.

Following two cars behind, Sean broiled in his friend Mick's ancient Micra which he had borrowed as soon as he got home early this morning. He hadn't seen him since Christmas, but Mick had handed over the keys without demur, told him the electrically operated windows wouldn't open but it was otherwise just about roadworthy and to bring it back with a full tank of petrol. As the sweat poured down him now, nearly nine hours later, Sean glowered, trying to make sense of what he'd seen so far. Mum stopped outside a fancy dress hire shop. He braked too and pulled over inconspicuously some distance behind her. She got out of the car and hurried into the shop with a bag. Presumably it contained the costume his father had been wearing, but why wasn't *he* taking it back? He'd been the one wearing it and she was the driver. It didn't make sense and he didn't feel reassured at all. A minute or two later his mother was back in the car and heading out towards Seaford.

It was mid-afternoon and the heat of the day was at its most intense, but she still hadn't rung him. It was worrying,

He had called her himself as soon as he was on the road this morning, but she'd answered his questions in worrying monosyllables, agreeing yes, it was difficult to talk freely at the moment; yes, his father was in the car beside her; no, she would prefer it if he didn't know that he was following them down to Eastbourne; so yes, she would ring him herself again later. But she hadn't. The only thing she said this morning was that they would be going to the police station. So he had followed them there and waited discreetly nearby, slumped low in his car seat so he wouldn't be caught sight of.

When he'd seen Auntie Lucille coming out of the police station earlier, he had hardly recognised her. She was dressed in black and looked terrible. The side of her head was bruised and swollen, her right eye puffy. Next to her, his congenitally ridiculous father was dressed in a mangy, extremely sleazy-looking pantomime cat suit, the tufted tail of which was dragging on the ground behind him. When they got into his mother's sleek black saloon car he observed that she was delighted to see Auntie Lucille, and that neither woman seemed obviously angry with Dad despite what he had done. Unable to fathom what was really going on he decided to continue to stay out of their sight watching and waiting until he had some sort of clue, or unless he heard from Mum. He followed them at a discreet distance as they turned into the hospital, watched them park and then get out of the car and go into A and E. He got out of his oven of a car and placed himself in shade far enough away that he would not be seen from the entrance unless they were looking for him. Mum should be keeping an eye out for him, although she had not seemed to have done so outside the police station. He reckoned she should get the chance now to go to the Ladies toilet or somewhere away from Dad where she could safely ring him and let him know what was going on. If she didn't he would have to just continue observing them from afar.

As he followed her now, driving up over the Downs, he felt disappointed with himself for not having found some way of contacting her whilst they had been at the hospital. He was stupid. He should have left a note for her on her windscreen or something. But then again his mad dad might have seen it and asked her awkward questions, so that would have been stupid as well. Two feelings had a hold of him: he was disappointed with himself and he felt angry with his father. How could Dad have done that to Auntie Lucille? It was unbelievable. Wasn't he supposed to be her lover? It made him feel ashamed to be his son, with a slow anger like lava, hot and heavy. It felt as if he himself was generating the heat in this noisy little car.

In fact he was always angry with his father whenever he thought about him. His anger with him weighed so much because he had been carrying it around for so long. At first when he was a still a little boy it may have been an irrational response to having had no real father at that time to model himself on. Richard had been nice enough but relatively remote. Later, on and ever since, his anger had been about being a disappointment to his father. Dad had been disappointed in him for almost as long as he had known him. It had probably begun when he had insisted on clinging to the surname on his birth certificate. Auntie Lucille, who had effectively been his mum when he was little had always insisted that he should be proud he was an O'Riordan just like his mother not a McElvey, which in those days he had wanted to be because she and Richard were. So shortly after he went to live with his mother in Leicester and his father arrived on the scene, his sense of identity became confused. He had insisted he was Sean O'Riordan when his father with an equal insistence had said he was really a Symes. They had ended up shouting at one another in Macdonalds. Mum had been sympathetic when he got back home. At first he wouldn't speak to her so she had asked Dad what was the matter with him and then they had had a row. His fucking father thereafter always looked at him with a gloomy expression on his face as if was too Aspergered to understand. That had prompted him to understand one thing at least, he didn't want to fit his father's view of him. So shortly afterwards, as a young adolescent, when Dad started bombarding him with geeky papers and endless psychologising he came to the conclusion that the papers and the psychologising said more about Dad than they did about him. He made a deliberate decision not to behave in any kind of way which would fit his father's view of him, became geeky about not being a geek. By the time he was fourteen he had come to loathe the contact with him that Dad had applied for legally through the courts and refused to hide from him the fact that he could see through his bluster even if Dad himself couldn't see through it to him. Shortly afterwards Dad moved down south again which curiously had also annoyed him, as if Dad couldn't even give him a good fight.

No, what he could do was pick on women and children. He was just a fucking bully that was all. As the Micra laboured up the next hill, Sean felt he shouldn't be angry about being a disappointment to a bully. But he was, he was still mad as hell.

At the bottom of the next Down, his mother suddenly turned right under the trees into a car park. There was another car park on this side of the road so he turned left into that, found a space and parked there. He got out quickly and looked at the information board, the sweat dripping down him front and back. He had to hurry or his mothers and father might see him. Apparently he was in the Seven Sisters Country Park and this was the Cuckmere valley, an ancient glacier-formed river estuary and now also the start of a walk called the Seven Sisters Way which ended at Beachy Head. They could hardly be wanting to go all that way, could they? And not now. They weren't dressed for it for one thing. Perhaps they just wanted to take a stroll down to the sea. What the fuck was going on?

He considered confronting them, but even as he did so found himself instead following day trippers, dog walkers and backpackers in their dribs and drabs on the long path towards the sea. He would get well ahead of his family and spy on them until he could either catch his mother's attention or he could understand what the situation was now so that he could know what to do.

The seashore was deceptively far away. He could not see it or hear it as he followed the wide valley path towards the expanding horizon between the Downs which must lead to the sea. The old river snaking serenely beside him with a timelessness which took his mind off his rage was almost completely still, the whole place a haven of peace and tranquillity. Sheep chomped at the grass and above, the sky was a cloudless blue with the occasional seagull gliding lazily on the hot afternoon thermals.

He hurried on, occasionally breaking into short bursts of running till he felt sufficiently far ahead of anybody walking at a normal pace to be able to look around at them. He couldn't see his family and for a moment he panicked thinking they might have just stopped for an ice cream or something and weren't going to be walking this way at all. He was almost at the point of turning back when he saw three people coming towards him in the distance beyond the old man with a fat black Labrador who he had just passed a minute ago. He peered intently at them until he could make out it was a man and two women. They were too far away to be sure but one of the women was certainly wearing black with a white hat and the other one was in trousers. The man beside them was obviously much taller than they were. It had to be them. It was them. He turned back towards the sea which was still at least half a kilometer distant and went into a quandary. The path forked in two directions. One branch went straight on presumably to the sea, while the other on the left sloped up the hill towards the cliff tops of the Seven Sisters. He knew this because there was a sign post. Which should he take? He chose to go up. It would provide him with a view either way.

Continuing to trudge as fast as he could, he was high up the side of the hill within minutes. There was a definite little breeze up here, although he wasn't sure where it was coming from, and he could see the sweep of the sea stretching to the horizon and across to the other side of the bay that the Cuckmere opened into. It looked very calm. His family were still far away, obviously just strolling. That would probably mean they weren't coming up here, but then again, the relaxed way they were walking together suggested that perhaps things were less fraught between them than they had been. He lay back in a chalky hollow and rested, the sun burning his face.

Five minutes later he sat up again and looked back down the way he had come. Mum, Auntie Lucille and Dad were standing at the fork in the path down below, two hundred metres away below. They couldn't see him, but even if he had stood up he was still too far away to be recognised unless they were looking for him. He watched them choosing to come up the hill. He scrambled up out of his hollow and moved fast, well away from the worn path through the grass which was heading in the direction of the cliff tops. He sat himself down amongst rabbit dropping and thistles in another small hollow and waited. A little while later he watched the three of them come trooping up in a line along the path he just left. None of them so much as even glanced in his direction. They were too busy talking and climbing and occasionally looking out at the sea and horizon below. Mum was in the front setting the pace, Auntie Lucille was behind her, walking bare foot, hat and shoes in hand, with Dad at the back looking grim. Just the sight of his stupid face was enough to cause a surge of anger in Sean's breast.

Gradually, as they got higher the soft warm wind carried more and more fragments of their conversation through the air towards him.

'... that's all I need to know, Ronnie,' his auntie was saying. 'I mean, did you lie about me to the police because, you know, it's alright to lie about a liar? Please tell me. I need to know.

'Tell her the truth, Ron,' his mother said. As always her voice was loud and clear.

'I lied because you scared me,' Sean heard his father eventually grunt. The breeze and the fact that they were now passing him and moving away from him towards the top of the cliff made the rest of what Dad was saying less audible and blew some of it away altogether. '...I'm going to scare you...more than that...don't care...' and '...die,' was all he heard his father saying before they were out of earshot.

Sean grimaced. If it came to a fight he was probably stronger than his father. He was younger, fitter and just as tall, if less burly. There was no doubt that despite the way they were walking and the open way they were talking with him, his mum and Auntie Lucille were placing themselves at huge risk from Dad. Had they thought there was safety in numbers or something? That he wouldn't do either of them any harm with both of them there together? If so they were quite wrong. Dad wouldn't be constrained by the fact that they were out in a public setting. It had never constrained him in the past in the bad old days when he used to lecture and adjure him.

If he was more violent and dangerous now, which he clearly was, they should never be trusting him like this. But perhaps they weren't. Perhaps, despite their apparent nonchalance and freedom to move and speak, the women had been coerced into coming up here. That would explain the fact that his mother hadn't rung him. Dad must have taken her

413

phone from her again. And if he knew his former foster mother at all he knew she would surely have changed her shoes first if she had wanted to go for a walk. She had always been such a stickler for doing things properly when it came to venturing into the outside world.

He would have to follow them, make sure they were safe, but it would be much more difficult to keep himself from being seen. The women were always turning round to speak to each other or to Dad as they filed further on up towards the cliff top. They were bound to notice him when they did so. Would that be a good thing? Yes, it might help to reassure them that they weren't alone with his father the madman. And if they did call out to him, that would be fine too. It would show either that there actually was safety in numbers, or that despite the overwhelming evidence to the contrary, he had got it wrong and there was no need to worry anymore

Some hope! He rejoined the path and followed them, not bothering to hide himself at all. They walked on for a full five minutes and never once turned round. The path had widened and straightened out now they were at the crest of what must be the first of the Seven Sisters. All three of them walked next to each other again. Together they stopped to look over the very edge of the cliff down to the sea and stones below. Silently Sean came up close behind them. Auntie Lucille sounded sad above the gently rising crash and boom of waves washing the bottom of the cliffs below.

'I blame myself. I should never have taken Richard to stay with Rose. It wasn't fair on either of them,' Sean heard her say. 'I was selfish, that's all. I did it for myself, for the break.'

'I think that's right,' said his father with his usual combination of commitment to truth and insensitivity to the feelings of others. His mother shook her head, turning away in disgust. So she was the only one to see Sean coming and he saw her grinning with delight the very moment he put his head down and charged.

When his son connected Ron was saying not to worry, everyone's the same, we can't really help it; selfishness can't be condoned, but we can all understand it.